Lecture Notes in Computer Science   1933
Edited by G. Goos, J. Hartmanis and J. van Leeuwen

W0231942

Springer
Berlin
Heidelberg
New York
Barcelona
Hong Kong
London
Milan
Paris
Singapore
Tokyo

Rüdiger W. Brause   Ernst Hanisch   (Eds.)

Medical
Data Analysis

First International Symposium, ISMDA 2000
Frankfurt, Germany, September 29-30, 2000
Proceedings

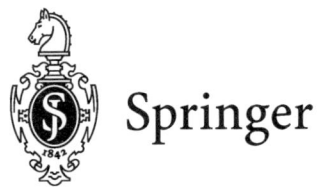 Springer

Series Editors

Gerhard Goos, Karlsruhe University, Germany
Juris Hartmanis, Cornell University, NY, USA
Jan van Leeuwen, Utrecht University, The Netherlands

Volume Editors

Rüdiger W. Brause
Johann Wolfgang Goethe-Universität
Fachbereich Biologie und Informatik
AG Adaptive Systemarchitektur
Robert-Mayer-Str. 11-15, 60054 Frankfurt a.M., Germany
E-mail: brause@informatik.uni-frankfurt.de

Ernst Hanisch
Johann Wolfgang Goethe-Universität
Klinik für Allgemein- und Gefässchirurgie
Theodor-Stern-Kai 7, 60590 Frankfurt a.M., Germany
E-mail: E.Hanisch@kkDortmund.de

Cataloging-in-Publication Data applied for

Die Deutsche Bibliothek - CIP-Einheitsaufnahme

Medical data analysis : first international symposium ; proceedings /
ISMDA 2000, Frankfurt, Germany, September 29 - 30, 2000. Rüdiger W.
Brause ; Ernst Hanisch (ed.). - Berlin ; Heidelberg ; New York ;
Barcelona ; Hong Kong ; London ; Milan ; Paris ; Singapore ; Tokyo :
Springer, 2000
  (Lecture notes in computer science ; 1933)
  ISBN 3-540-41089-9

CR Subject Classification (1998): I.2, H.3, G.3, I.5.1, I.4, J.3, F.1

ISSN 0302-9743
ISBN 3-540-41089-9 Springer-Verlag Berlin Heidelberg New York

Springer-Verlag Berlin Heidelberg New York
a member of BertelsmannSpringer Science+Business Media GmbH
© Springer-Verlag Berlin Heidelberg 2000
Printed in Germany

Typesetting: Camera-ready by author
Printed on acid-free paper   SPIN: 10781200   06/3142   5 4 3 2 1 0

Preface

It is a pleasure for us to present the contributions of the First International Symposium on Medical Data Analysis. Traditionally, the field of medical data analysis can be devided into classical topics such as medical statistics, survival analysis, biometrics and medical informatics. Recently, however, time series analysis by physicists, machine learning and data mining with methods such as neural networks, Bayes networks or fuzzy computing by computer scientists have contributed important ideas to the filed of medical data analysis.

Although all these groups have similar intentions, there was nearly no exchange or discussion between them. With the growing possibilities for storing and analyzing patient data, even in smaller health care institutions, the need for a rational treatment of all these data emerged as well. Therefore, the need for data exchange and presentation systems grew also.

The goal of the symposium is to collect all these relevant aspects together. It provides an international forum for the sharing and exchange of original research results, ideas and practical experiences among researchers and application developers from different areas related to medical applications dealing with the analysis of medical data.

After a thorough reviewing process, 33 high quality papers were selected from the 45 international submissions. These contributions provided the different aspects of the field in order to represent us with an exciting program.

We would like to thank all people and institutions who contributed to this symposium: the authors, the members of the program committee and the additional reviewers, the keynote speakers and all those involved in the local organization.

September 2000

Rüdiger Brause
Ernst Hanisch

General Chairs

Rüdiger Brause, Frankfurt am Main, Germany
Ernst Hanisch, Frankfurt am Main, Germany

Program Commitee

S.K. Andersen	Denmark
A. Babic	Sweden
R. Bellazzi	Italy
L. Brobowski	Poland
S. de Campos	Spain
L.M. Chillemi	Italy
G. Dorffner	Austria
N. Ezquerra	USA
U. Gather	Germany
L. Gierl	Germany
A. Giuliani	Italy
O.K. Hejlesen	Denmark
R. Hovorka	England
E. Keravnou	Cyprus
J. Kurths	Germany
M. Kurzynski	Poland
P. Larrañaga	Spain
N. Lavrac	Slovenia
R. Lefering	Germany
J.A. Lozano	Spain
A. Macerata	Italy
V. Maojo	Spain
S. Miksch	Austria
A. Neiß	Germany
E. Neugebauer	Germany
C. Ohmann	Germany
L. Pecen	Czech Republic
N. Pliskin	Israel
B. Sierra	Spain
J. Šíma	Czech Republic
H. Sitter	Germany
D. Sleeman	Scotland
M. Stefanelli	Italy
J.-M. Vesin	Switzerland
B. Zupan	Slovenia

Table of Contents

Keynote Lectures

Time Series Analysis

Bayes Networks

Neural Nets

Machine Learning

Architectures for Data Aquisition and Data Analysis

Medical Informatics and Modeling

Genetic and Fuzzy Algorithms

Medical Data Mining

Medical Decision Support Systems

T. Wetter

University of Heidelberg, Germany
thomas_wetter@med.uni-heidelberg.de
http://www.med.uni-heidelberg.de/mi/home.htm

Historically medical decision support systems (DSS) emerged from medical biometry and medical informatics. Both disciplines haved pursued different approaches over decades, with only minor exchange or mutual fertilization. Therefore, it is timely to work towards exchange of concepts and possible integration of methods between these and other newly delevoping disciplines such as Artificial Neural Networks (ANN). It is the purpose of this abstract to identify underlying assumptions of different approaches and how they relate to present developments in health care. Among these developments the intension to base decisions on as much information as possible and to improve quality of care are most closely related to the targets of DSS.

Major directions of DSS are known as knowledge based systems (KBS), cased based reasoning systems (CBR), machine learning systems (ML), artificial neural networks (ANN) and data mining systems (DMS). I would like to categorize these as to

- their relation to data
- they way they convey knowledge
- their relation to requirements on and practice of medical decisions.

In the first place, all methods except KBS directly rely on or incorporate data. Roughly speaking, data lead to sets of rules (ML), coefficients (ANN), or factors (DMS), or they are the decision supporting asset themselves (CBR). KBS, on the other hand, classically start out from experts' experience made available in interviews, think aloud protocols and other methods from the social sciences.

Therefore, in data based methods we have to ask ourselves how good the data are and how to justify the transformations of data into decision supporting entities. Both questions are not trivial. Knowing what is a good case requires that it is fully documented in a standardized way and that the outcome can be validly observed. Knowing e.g. that the impact of high blood pressure treatment (in terms lower risk of cardiac infarction or stroke etc) or of cancer treatment manifests itself after decades and that very few studies manage an

R.W. Brause and E. Hanisch (Eds.): ISMDA 2000, LNCS 1933, pp. 1–3, 2000.

unbiased follow up for such a long period demonstrates one of the problems. Transformations, on the other hand, tend to be mathematically well justified, while domain knowledge plays a less prominent role.

In KBS methods we have to ask ourselves whether we get access to the true knowledge of the expert and to what extent this knowledge truly reflects the domain or rather a personal view of an individual. These questions are not trivial either, but we will come to an alternative below.

Knowledge as the second category to distinguish DSS could be worked out in textbook of almost arbitrary length. I will take a rather pratical stance here, namely knowledge to be such information that suits the objective context of a problem and the subjective contexts of a person which allows the person to conduct purposeful action. Medical knowledge must relate to observable symptoms, suggest available procedures and the physician must understand the suggestion of the system. I will concentrate on the latter requirement here, because it is here where systems differentiate. It is related to the fact that legally the physician is responsible for an action taken. A device cannot be made responsible. The physician can, however, only take responsibility for actions that he could in principle justify himself. This discards ANN and DMS systems as knowledge based DSS, because numerical coefficients as such are not human intellegible justifications for decisions. Their regime of decision may be human intellegible - for mathematicians better than for physicians - but the individual decision is not. ML systems tend to deliver sets of rules each of which apperars reasonable. However, the set as a whole does not convey a theory of the domain but a collection of coincidences. CBR systems almost ideally address the known preference of physicians to act experience based. Treating patient B like you treated the similar patient A is appealing and appears to address knowledge, although neither patient A nor the methods to classify him as similar to B may be very well justified. Obviously KBS come closest to a theory of the field and hence to a human intellegible foundation of decision making.

Requirements and practice of medical decision making are moving towards evidence based medicine (EBM) i.e. treatment based on metaanalysis of clinical trials of high biometrical standards. Such analysis leads to guidelines for good clinical practice which are characterized by strict inclusion criteria, clear distinctions among risk groups and clear recommendations for each group. Syntactically they are texts of several pages and may contain flow charts, decision trees etc. Presently they have no legal implications. But apart from the need for local variants required in different hospitals clinical guidelines suggest themselves as kinds of standard operating procedures and as such part of the move towards quality assurance in medicine. In the form they exist now one of their major disadvantages is that in practice the physician does not have the time to read texts of such length. But the advice he would receive if doing so would suit objective and subjective context and would be based on high quality data.

Now, KBS can start from guidelines rather than from individual expertise and by this token avoid some of the disadvantages of KBS alone and of guidelines alone. They remove the need that the pracitioner reads long text and avoid the personal bias of expert authors. Therefore, guideline based KBS are certainly one of the promising present developments.

Guideline based KBS, however, need a match to solve the following problem: Their strength or clear inclusion criteria is also a weakness. Many patients do not satisfy the criteria and hence strictly speaking the guideline cannot be applied. Current practice is still to apply a guideline as long as the deviation is small. Major violations are known by administering pharmaceuticals to children which the guideline only recommends for adults. An alternative and more transparent solution would be to treat patients within the criteria according to the guideline and to collect case bases for CBR systems in order to act experience based for patients outside the criteria. Such hybrid - guideline plus case based - systems are among the interesting challenges of the near future.

Medical Bayes Networks

Basilio Sierra, Iñaki Inza and Pedro Larrañaga

Dept. of Computer Science and Artificial Intelligence, University of the Basque
Country, P.O. Box 649, E-20080 San Sebastián, Spain
e-mail: ccpsiarb@si.ehu.es (Basilio Sierra)
Website: http://www.sc.ehu.es/isg

Abstract. In this paper a succint overview of the Bayesian network
paradigm is presented, in an introductory manner. The reader is not supposed to have knowledge about it, although some notions of probability
must be taken into account. Bayesian networks are used as inference tools
in probabilistic expert systems, being its utilization extended to many
research and application fields. Some examples in the medical world are
presented, as well as the way they can be constructed and used. We do
not emphasize in the calculi to be done; as there are many commercial
and free software packages, they can be used without deep knowledge
about the formulae to be applied.

1   Introduction

The practice of medicine is fraught with uncertainty; rarely are physicians sure of
a diagnosis, which tests to perform, which treatment to select, or what a patient's
prognosis is. Yet, this uncertainty does not prevent us from doing what is right
for a particular patient; that is, patient outcomes are often excellent despite this
uncertainty, because people are adept at managing uncertainty. Traditionally,
medical practice has been guided by empirical observation, whether in the form
of anecdotes, case reports, or well designed clinical trials. As health care has
become more unified under the auspices of health-maintenance organizations
and hospital groups, a new source of population data has become available. The
profileration of these data sources, whether in the form of in-house databases,
clinical trials in the literature, or personal experience, threatens to outstrip our
ability to analyze them. In many cases, large databases are collected outside of
the context of a traditional clinical trial, and thus the data may not have been
collected with a particular question in mind.

Computers have superb memories, but until recently, there has been little
they could do with pieces of text information other than display them. Modern
programs contain detailed clinical information and have the knowledge to help
users to determine how that information should be applied. As computer-based
tools offer this kind of expertise, physicians have begun to consult programs
to obtain reasoned advice about Medical Decision Making processes, while the
ultimate decision-making roles are maintained for provider and patient.

Expert systems, one of the most developed areas in the field of Artificial
Intelligence, are computer programs designed to help or replace humans tasks

R.W. Brause and E. Hanisch (Eds.): ISMDA 2000, LNCS 1933, pp. 4–14, 2000.

where the human experience and knowledge are scarce and unreliable. Although there are domains where tasks can be specifed by logic rules, other domains are characterized by inherent uncertainty. Probability was not taken into account, for some time, as a reasoning method for expert systems trying to model uncertain domains, because the computational requirements were considered too expensive. At the end of the 80s, Lauritzen and Spiegelhalter [14] shown that these difficulties can be overcome by exploiting the modular character of the graphical models associated with the so-called probabilistic expert systems, that in this work we call Bayesian Networks.

The rest of the paper is organized as follows: Bayesian Networks are introduced in Section 2, while section 3 presents the role to be played by Bayesian Networks in the Machine Learning community. Section 4 presents some real applications of Bayesian Networks in medicine. Section 5 introduces an extension of the Bayesian Network paradigm called Influence Diagram, also describing a real application. Section 6 presents a brief summary of the work.

2   Bayesian Networks

Bayesian Networks (BNs) [10], [13], [16] constitute a probabilistic framework for reasoning under uncertainty. From an informal perspective, BNs are directed acyclic graphs (DAGs), where the nodes are random variables and the arcs specify the independence assumptions that must be held between the random variables.

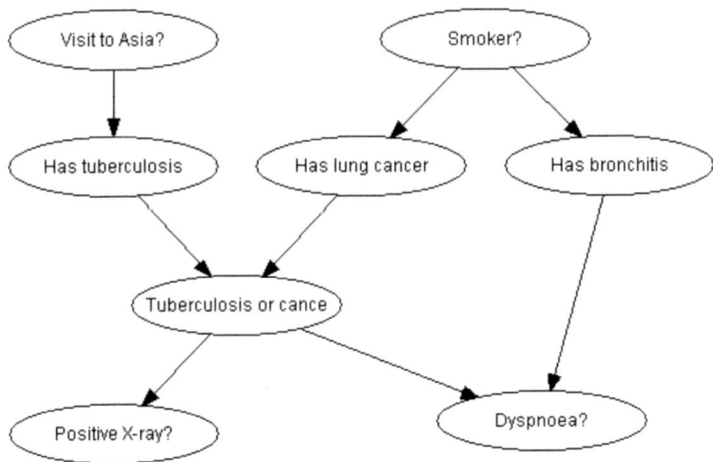

Fig. 1. Typical example of a medical Bayesian network.

Figure 1 presents a classic medical Bayesian Network used to model the lung cancer problem. Each node represents a variable, that can be a symptom or a consequence of some of them. The relations among the variables are expressed by the arcs.

BNs are based upon the concept of conditional independence among variables. This concept makes possible a factorization of the probability distribution of the n-dimensional random variable $(X_1, ..., X_n)$ in the following way:

$$P(x_1, ..., x_n) = \prod_{i=1}^{n} P(x_i|pa(x_i))$$

where x_i represents the value of the random variable X_i, and $pa(x_i)$ represents the value of the random variables parents of X_i.

Thus, in order to specify the probability distribution of a BN, one must give prior probabilities for all root nodes (nodes with no predecessors) and conditional probabilities for all other nodes, given all possible combinations of their direct predecessors. These numbers in conjunction with the DAG, specify the BN completely.

Once the network is constructed it constitutes an efficient device to perform probabilistic inference. This probabilistic reasoning inside the net can be carried out by exact methods, as well as by approximate methods. Nevertheless, the problem of building such a network remains. The structure and conditional probabilities necessary for characterising the network can be either provided externally by experts or obtained from an algorithm which automatically induces them.

Example In order to show how probabilistic reasoning is done, we present in this section a very simple example of our invention. Let suppose **HEADACHE** and **FEVER** variables represent the same name symptoms that are being used to predict whether a patient has **FLU** or not. Be the arcs shown in Figure 2.left-up those which represent the relations among these three variables, and be the numbers shown in Figure 2.right-up the a priori probabilities of each variable.

Probabilistic reasoning is done in the following manner:

1. First of all, the symptoms of the patient have to be collected, and obtained values are given to the Bayesian Network. This step is called *evidence instantiation*.
2. Once evidence has been inserted into the BN, the effect of those values in the rest of nodes must be calculated. This step is called *propagation* in BN nomenclature.

As a result of the previous steps, we obtain the so-called a posteriori probability of the variables corresponding to nodes that have not been instantiated, that is, variables which values are not known by the moment. This can be see in Figure 2.left-down and Figure 2.right-down.

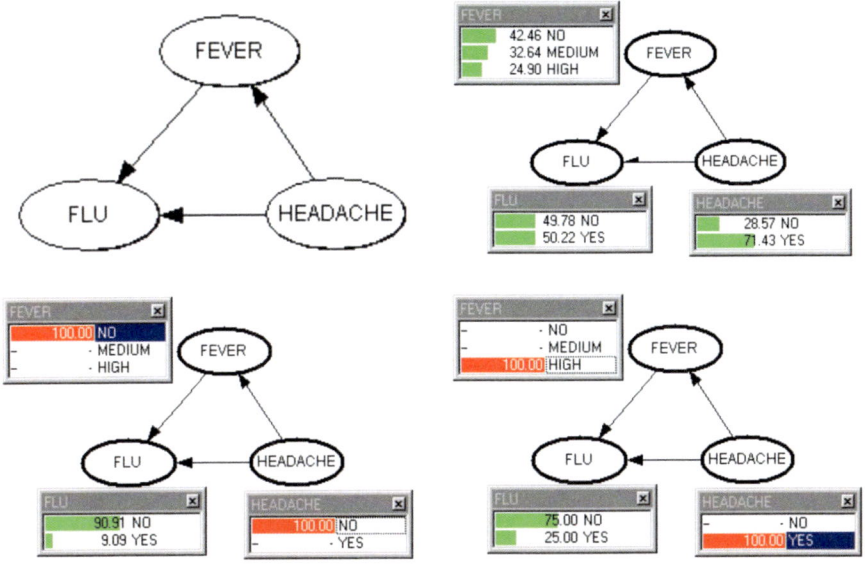

Fig. 2. Probabilistic reasoning with a simple Bayesian Network.

In Figure 2.left-down a patient who has not **FEVER** nor **HEADACHE** is presented to the BN. After propagation of inserted evidence, the a posteriori probabilities of uninstantiated nodes, FLU in this case, are 0.9091 for the **FLU=** NO case and 0.0909 for the YES value. In Figure 2.right-down, a patient with the symptom **HEADACHE** = YES and having HIGH as **FEVER** variable value is presented, obtaining YES = 0.75 and NO = 0.25 as the **FLU** variable a posteriori probabilities.

2.1 Structure Learning in Bayesian Networks

As it could be assumed that the task which has to be carried out to propagate the evidence in BNs is (quasi)-solved, the structure learning problem remains active. In this problem, the main trouble consists in how to stablish the BN structure which better represents the relations existing amongs the variables (nodes) of the problem being taken into consideration.

During the last five years a high number of algorithms with the aim of inducing the structure of the Bayesian Network that better represents the conditional independence relationships in a database of cases have been developed. See Heckerman et al. [8] for a good review.

Cooper and Herskovits [4], Bouckaert [3], Larrañaga et al. [12] and Provan and Singh [17] are some different methods related with the structure learning of a BN.

3   From classification to Bayesian networks in Machine Learning

Machine Learning, ML, represents an emerging Artificial Intelligence technology that has already found its role in many application areas. ML concerns
the automatic acquisition (or adaptation) of knowledge to improve computer
decision-support system performance.

With the aid of ML, the construction of these decision-support systems from
patients databases has longed played an important role in Medical Decision Making (MDM). For example, starting in the early 1960s, researchers investigated
the construction from data of Bayesian diagnostic systems that assume conditional independence of patient features given a disease state [15] [20]. As clinical
information is stored increasingly in computer databases, the opportunities grow
for using ML techniques to help improve MDM.

MDM tasks include prevention, diagnosis, treatment planning, treatment
control and patient follow up. We can state the role of ML in MDM more formally as:

Given: a set of medical records that correspond to a MDM tasks (i.e., diagnosis,
treatment planning, etc.).
Find: descriptions that explain decision making about the selected medical task.

There exist many ML systems that support classification and prediction in
MDM. This area has received much attention from researchers in both ML and
medicine communities, resulting in a large number of classification systems (i.e.,
decision trees, classification rules of IF ... THEN explicit symbolic form, etc.)
and approaches.

However, MDM does not only imply classification. Although BNs can be
used for classification purposes, they do not lead to explicit rule formation,
but they are largely appreciated due to their ability to support explanation
and description of data. To support the MDM process in everyday practice,
physicians need a ML model that is able to explain its decisions: in this way,
BNs can take advantage of their explanation ability in order to be accepted as
a powerful MDM tool.

4   Applications

In the following lines we present several applications of BNs in specific medical
problems:

4.1   The malignant skin melanoma

In spite of the advances achieved in recent years in the treatment of cancer, the
prognosis of patients having developed skin melanoma has changed very little.
The incidence of the disease has continuously grown over the last decade. Annual

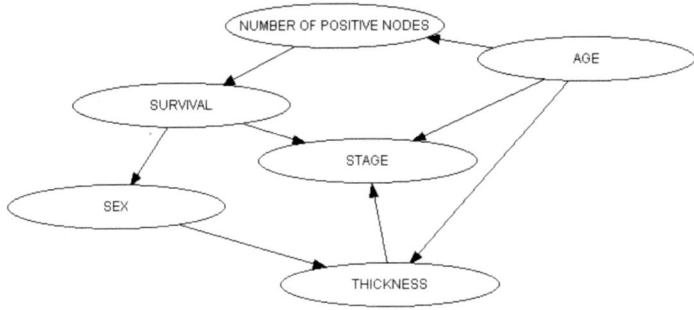

Fig. 3. Bayesian Network used for the Melanoma problem.

incidence has increased and the progressive reduction of the ozone layer, if not stopped, will increase it even more.

Experimental data and the results of epidemiological studies suggest two main risk factors: sun exposure along with phenotype characteristics of the individual. Thus, for example, the continuous sun exposure represents an odds ratio of 9, while the acute intermittent exposition has an associated odds ratio of 5.7. Figure 3 presents the BN structure indueced in this problem by Sierra and Larrañaga [19].

4.2   Promedas: a Bayesian network for anaemia

Promedas (PRObabilistic MEdical Diagnostic Advisory System) [11] is a joint research project by the Foundation of Neural Networks of Nijmegen (The Netherlands) and the University Medical Centre of Utrecht (The Netherlands), and its objective is the development of patient-specific diagnostic support systems. Promedas is based on medical expert knowledge, acquired from the literature by the medical specialists of the research group. Promedas objective is the ranslation of this knowledge into BNs. In this ways, BNs are used as the inference engine of the system to output patient-specific diagnosis, enhancing the system's transparency by explanatory facilities using a graphical user interface (GUI). Promedas target users are physicians seeking diagnostic advice in daily clinical practice. The medical problem covered by Promedas is anaemia diagnosis. Induced Bayesian networks can be used for different purposes:

- to output a diagnostic by instantiation and propagation of the evidences in the network;
- to change the underlying network structure by the addition of new patients that already have a diagnostic.

4.3   A Bayesian network for visual disturbances

A BN for evaluating visual disturbances appears in Herskovits [9]. The network structure can be seen in Figure 4. It is used to help in the diagnosis of three different visual disturbances (Squinting improves vision, Patient complains of poor vision and Undetectable retinal reflex) by the use other three predictive variables.

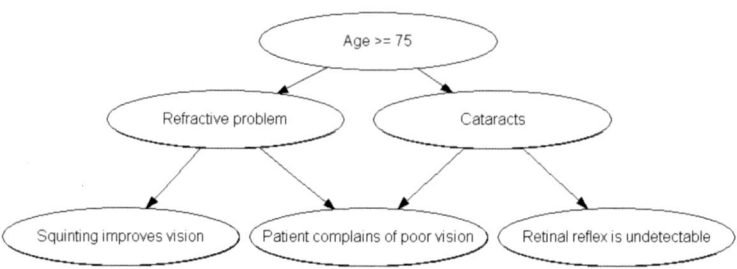

Fig. 4. Evaluation of visual disturbances.

4.4   A Bayesian network for the cervical spinal-cord trauma

The assesment of cervical spinal-cord trauma is tackled by Dagher et al. [6] in a BN framework. The data to induce the network was extracted from the Regional Spinal Cord Injury Center of the Delaware Valley, and each patient case consisted in 7 variables, including motor scores for various muscle groups at the time of injury or at 1 year, and radiological findings. Processing a database of 104 cases the BN of Figure 5 was induced by the a uthors. By inference mechanisms, the induced BN was used to predict the values of two different recovery scores of the patients at 1 year follow-up.

4.5   A Bayesian network for magnetic resonance spectroscopy decision support

Dagher et al. [7] tackle the problem of magnetic resonance spectroscopy decision support by the use of BNs. As magnetic resonance spectroscopy is sensitive to chemical signatures of matter, these signatures, in turn, tend to follow different patterns in various brain disorders. A magnetic resonance dataset which conatained a series of patients that were either normal or had one of five brain disorders was used to induce a BN. The goal of the BN was to predict whether the patient had any specific of five disorders or none of them. The induced network can be seen in Figure 6.

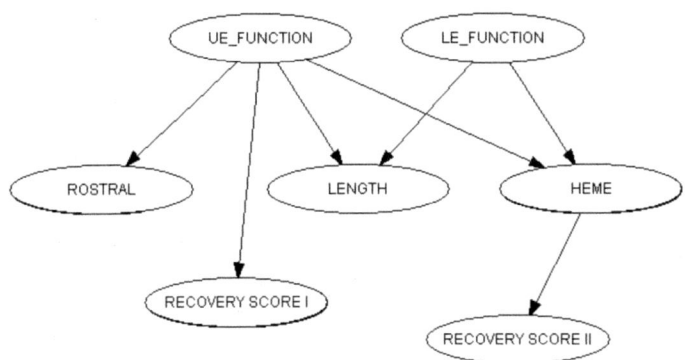

Fig. 5. Bayesian network for the cervical cord trauma database.

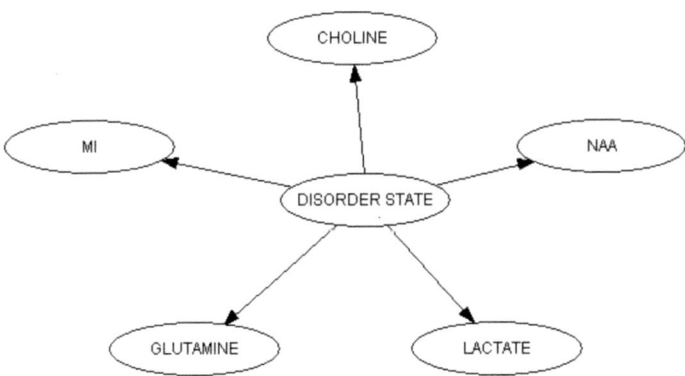

Fig. 6. Bayesian network for magnetic resonance spestroscopy decision support.

5   Influence Diagrams

An influence diagram is a BN extended with decision facilities (decision nodes and utility nodes). An influence diagram cannot contain continuous chance nodes.

An influence diagram should be constructed so that one can see exactly which variables (represented by discrete chance nodes) are known at the point of deciding for each decision node. If the state of a chance node will be known at the time of making a decision, this will (probably) have an impact on what the decision maker should do. Thus, one must add a link from the chance node to the decision node. If the state of a chance node will be known before some given decision, and this chance node has impact on another chance node which is also known before the decision, only the last chance node needs to have a link to the decision node. That is, there only needs to be a directed path from a chance node to a decision node if the chance node is known before the decision is made.

In an influence diagram, there must also be an unambiguous order among the decision nodes. That is, there can be only one sequence in which the decisions are made. In the same way as when defining that a chance node will be known before a decision is made, we add links to show which decisions have already been made when a specific decision is made. Again there only need to be a directed path from one decision node to the next one in the decision sequence.

If the influence diagram is not constructed correctly according to the rules stated above, the calculated expected utilities will (of course) not be correct.

When propagating, you can follow the expected utility of choosing each decision in the next decision node in the decision sequence either in the node list pane or by opening a monitor window for the decision node. The utilities shown in a decision node further down in the decision sequence should not be considered before all previous decisions have been made. This simply makes no sence.

5.1   IctNeo System for Jaundice Management

IctNeo is a complex decision Support System for neonatal jaundice management, a typical medical problem which could be briefly explained as follows:
A few hours after birth, a baby skin and ices may take a yellowish cast. This is called jaundice. It is caused by the breakdown of excess red blood cells, in the baby system which produces a substance called bilirubin. The baby liver is not mature enough to assimilate all the waste products and does not excrete bilirubin into the intestines at a normal rate. This excess bilirubin builds up in the baby bloodstream and tissues, giving the skin the characsteristic yellow color.

A large number of treatments, pathologies and different tests are involved in the jaundice management problem. In this way, Neonatology Service of Gregorio Marañón Hospital in Madrid has applied an influence diagram scheme to tackle this problem [2]. Figure 7 shows an initial approach to construct an influence diagram for the presented task.

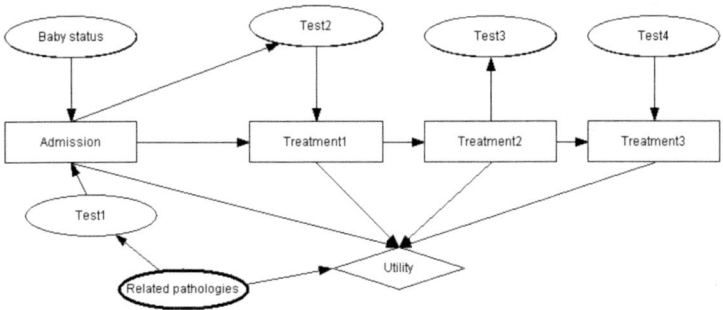

Fig. 7. A generic Influence Diagram for the Jaundice Management problem.

6   Summary

In this paper a resume of the Bayesian network paradigm and several of its relations with the medical decision support task have been presented. The use of BNs and its extensions, such as Influence Diagrams and Gaussian Networks, have augmented in the last years. In this way, many applications of BNs are being used in healthcare worldwide. Some of them are shown in this article, as well as the way probabilistic reasoning could be done.

See Jensen [10], Andersen et al. [1], Ramoni and Sebastiani [18] and Cozman [5] for practical information and software about the construction and evaluation of BNs.

Acknowledgements
This work was supported by the CICYT under grant TIC97-1135-C04-03 and by the grant PI 96/12 from the Gobierno Vasco - Departamento de Educación, Universidades e Investigación.

References

1. Andersen, S.K., Olesen, K.G. Jensen, F.V.: HUGIN - a shell for building Bayesian belief universes for expert systems. Proceedings of the Eleventh International Joint Conference on Artificial Intelligence (1989) 1128-1133
2. Bielza, C. et al.: IctNEO System for jaundice management. Revista de la Real Academia de Ciencias Exactas **4** (1998) 307-315
3. Bouckaert, R.R.: Properties of Bayesian belief networks learning algorithms. Proceedings of the Tenth Annual Conference in Uncertainty in Artificial Intelligence (1994) 102-109
4. Cooper, G.F., Herskovits, E.A.: A Bayesian method for the induction of probabilistic networks from data. Machine Learning **9** (1992) 309-347
5. Cozman, F.G.: JavaBayes. Bayesian Networks in Java User Manual. http://www.usp.br/ fgcozman/home.html. (1999)

6. Dagher, A.P., Herskovits, E.H.: Expert refinement of data derived Bayesian networks for medical diagnosis. American Medical Informatics Association Annual Fall Symposium, Washington DC (1996)

7. Dagher, A.P., Herskovits, E.H.: Decision support software for brain pMRS. American Society of Neuroradiology, Toronto, Canada (1997)

8. Heckerman, D., Geiger, D., Chickering, D.M.: Learning Bayesian networks: The combination of knowledge and statistical data. Technical Report MSR-TR-94-09, Microsoft (1994)

9. Herskovits, E.H.: Computer-Based probabilistic-network generation. PhD thesis, Medical Informatics, Stanford University, CA (1991)

10. Jensen, F. V.: Introduction to Bayesian networks. University College of London (1996)

11. Kappen, H.J. et al.: Promedas: Probabilistic Medical Diagnostical Visory System. http://servius.mbfys.kun.nl/SNN/Research/promedas (1999)

12. Larrañaga, P., Poza, M., Yurramendi, Y., Murga, R., Kuijpers, C.: Structure Learning of Bayesian Networks by Genetic Algorithms: A Performance Analysis of Control Parameters. IEEE Transactions on Pattern Analysis and Machine Intelligence **18** (1996) 912-926

13. Lauritzen, S.L.: Graphical Models. Oxford University Press (1996)

14. Lauritzen, S.L., Spiegelhalter, D.J.: Local computations with probabilities on graphical structures and their application on expert systems. Journal Royal of Statistical Society B **50** (1988) 157-224

15. Miller, M.C., Westphal, M.C., Reigart, J.R., Barner, C.: Medical diagnostic models: A bibliographie. University Microfilms International, Ann Arbor, MI (1977)

16. Pearl J.: Probabilistic Reasoning in Intelligent Systems: Networks of Plausible Inference. Morgan Kaufmann, San Mateo (1988)

17. Provan, G.M., Singh, M.: Learning Bayesian Networks Using Feature Selection. Learning from Data: AI and Statistics V, Lecture Notes in Statistics 112, Springer Verlag (1996) 291-300

18. Ramoni M., Sebastiani S.: BKD: Bayesian Knowledge Discoverer. http://kmi.open.ac.uk/projects/bkd/ (2000)

19. Sierra, B., Larrañaga, P.: Predicting the survival in malignant skin melanoma using Bayesian networks automatically induced by genetic algorithms. An empirical comparison between different approaches. Articial Intelligence in Medicine **1,2** (1998) 215-230

20. Warner, H. R., Toronto, A.F., Veny, L.G., Stephenson, R.: A mathematical approach to medical diagnosis: Application to congenital heart diseases. Journal of American Medicine Association **177** (1961) 177-183

Synchronization Analysis of Bivariate Time Series and Its Application to Medical Data

M. Rosenblum

Potsdam University, Germany
mros@agnld.uni-potsdam.de

A typical problem in time series analysis is to reveal the presence of an interdependence between two (or more) signals. Such an analysis is traditionally done by means of cross-correlation (cross-spectrum) techniques or nonlinear statistical measures.

In our approach we exploit for the analysis of noisy nonstationary bivariate data the concept of phase synchronization. This concept, developed in our theoretical studies, implies the existence of a certain statistical relation between properly introduced phases of interacting complex oscillators.

Synchronization is abundant in live systems; it is encountered on the cell level (synchronization of circadian rhythms in cells, synchronization of cell cycles, neurons firing, etc), on the level of functional units (nephrons, primary and secondary pacemakers of the heart, etc) and physiological systems (cardiovascular and respiratory ones), or even on the level of species (self-synchronization in ensembles of fireflies and crickets, population dynamics, etc). Hence, synchronization analysis is especially useful in biomedical applications.

Generally, we try to access the following problem: suppose we observe a system with a complex structure that is not known exactly, and measure two time series at its outputs. Our goal is not only to find out whether these signals are dependent or not - this can be done by means of traditional statistical techniques - but to extract additional information on the interaction of some subsystems within the system under study.

We illustrate our approach by application to the human posture control data, to multichannel magnetoencephalography records and records of muscle activity of a Parkinsonian patient, and to human heart rate and respiratory data.

We show that our analysis allows to detect weak interaction between physiological subsystems that cannot be done by linear techniques. In particular, our study of pathological brain activity shows that the temporal evolution of the peripheral Parkinsonian tremor rhythms directly reflects the time course of the

R.W. Brause and E. Hanisch (Eds.): ISMDA 2000, LNCS 1933, pp. 15–16, 2000.

synchronization of abnormal activity between cortical motor areas. Moreover, our technique allows to localize the areas of pathological synchronized activity.

References

1. Rosenblum, M.G., Pikovsky, A.S., Schäfer, C., Tass, P., Kurths, J.: Phase Synchronization: From Theory to Data Analysis. to appear in: Handbook of Biological Physics, Elsevier Science, Series Editor A.J. Hoff, Vol. 4, Neuro-informatics, Editors: S. Gielen and F. Moss
2. Schäfer, C., Rosenblum, M.G., Abel, H.-H., Kurths, J.: Synchronization in the Human Cardiorespiratory System. Physical Review E **60** (1999) 857–870
3. Tass, P., Rosenblum, M.G., Weule, J., Kurths, J., Pikovsky, A.S., Volkmann, J., Schnitzler, A., Freund, H.J.: Detection of n:m Phase Locking from Noisy Data: Application to Magnetoencephalography. Physical Review Letters **81** (1998) 3291–3294
4. About this paper: Physics Today. March (1999) 17–19
5. Rosenblum, M.G., Kurths, J., Pikovsky, A.S., Schäfer, C., Tass, P., Abel, H.-H.: Synchronization in Noisy Systems and Cardiorespiratory Interaction. IEEE Eng. in Medicine and Biology Magazin **17**(6) (1998) 46–53
6. Schäfer, C., Rosenblum, M.G., Kurths, J., Abel, H.-H.: Heartbeat Synchronized with Ventilation. Nature **392**(6673) (1998) 239–240
7. Rosenblum, M.G., Pikovsky, A.S., Kurths, J.: From Phase to Lag Synchronization in Coupled Chaotic Oscillators. Physical Review Letters **78** (1997) 4193–4196
8. Rosenblum, M.G., Pikovsky, A.S., Kurths, J.: Phase Synchronization of Chaotic Oscillators. Physical Review Letters **76** (1996) 1804–1807

A Survey of Data Mining Techniques

Victor Maojo and José Sanandrés

Medical Informatics Group. Artificial Intelligence Laboratory.
School of Computer Science. Universidad Politecnica of Madrid.
Boadilla del Monte.28660 Madrid. Spain
vmaojo@fi.upm.es

Abstract. In this short paper we have resumed a keynote speech, to be given at the ISMDA 2000 conference, about data mining research and tools. We state a brief summary of the main concepts associated to data mining and some of the methods and tools used in the scientific world, mainly those that can associated to medical applications. Finally, some practical projects and conclusions are presented.

1. Introduction

According to some assessments the world data volume stored in electronic databases doubles each 20 months [7]. Regarding the medical domain, no one professional can manage more than a minimal part of the knowledge that it is generated and published in the scientific literature, recorded in databases, or made available over the WWW. Thus, a myriad of systems and tools are built to help users to manage such information.

The rapid growth and spread of the WWW has facilitated the exchange of information among researchers and medical professionals. Nevertheless, the huge amount of information that is currently available makes necessary new methods to search, extract, validate, and use it. An example is the induction of models to be used as the knowledge base for decision support systems in domains where there are no available experts, but where there is a great amount of available clinical data from real patients. These data can be stored and accessed at classical or "virtual" databases over Internet.

For instance, a general practitioner, working in an isolated village in any particular country can generate clinical data that can be stored in an electronic medical record. These files and others from remote sites can be gathered and analyzed to extract evidences that can be objectively used by health services researchers, educators, and administrators, to create practice guidelines and health policies.

In the next sections we will review some of the different methods used for data mining, particularly those which can be applied to the medical domain.

2. Data mining

2.1. Concepts

The large number of cases and attributes describing examples, make the database analysis far beyond the human capabilities. The raise from $50

R.W. Brause and E. Hanisch (Eds.): ISMDA 2000, LNCS 1933, pp. 17–22, 2000.
© Springer-Verlag Berlin Heidelberg 2000

millions in 1996 to $800 million of the data analysis market [11] shows the importance of these tools.

The Knowledge Discovery in Databases (KDD) is the process to exploit the possibilities of extracting the knowledge implicit in the collected data. A commonly accepted definition for KDD is [6]: "the nontrivial process of identifying valid, novel, potentially useful, and ultimately understandable patterns in data".

KDD is a process composed by several steps. Perhaps the most popular of them is Data Mining. Sometimes both terms tend to be confused. Data Mining is a step of KDD in which patterns or models are extracted from data by using some automated technique.

The process of data mining depends on the quality and quantity of the available data. Thus, the concept of Data Warehouse (DW) is becoming essential to facilitate the data mining process. The DW is an integrated enterprisewide database designed to input, store, and search a large amount of data derived from multiple (local or remote) sources. If a DW is designed and maintained correctly, the data mining step will be easier.

Other steps, previous to data mining, are preprocessing and transformation. Most prediction methods require that data be in a standard form that can be processed later. Some data features are selected and composed, dealing with missing, time-dependent, or inaccurate values that might be also considered.

2.2. A Data Mining Taxonomy

We can find in the literature several classifications of methods that are used in Data Mining [8,12, 20]. There are several criteria to classify these methods, such as: (1) the kind of patterns discovered: predictive or informative, (2) the representation language: symbolic or subsymbolic, or (3) the data mining goal: classification or regression.

We differentiate three main families, each with several subfamilies: (1) Statistics and Pattern Recognition; (2) Machine Learning (ML), and (3) Neural Networks (NNs)

Statistical methods have been traditionally used , whereas ML and NNs applications have increased in the last years. Solutions offered by all methods can be compared considering performance (classification and prediction accuracy, sensitivity, specificity or learning speed), as well as the comprehensibility and significance of the extracted knowledge [15,13].

Comprehensibility eases the validation and use of the knowledge extracted from a data set. Accuracy and comprehensibility are the most relevant parameters in some domains like medicine. Results presented in comparative studies [20] suggest that accuracy is similar for the three families but comprehensibility is better for ML methods. Weiss points out that decision tree induction is the choice when easily explained solutions are a goal, even though results are slightly weaker than those from other methods [20].

Methods from the three families have been applied in several real and artificial domains [12,1], and their performance have been compared in several studies [14,20]. The main conclusion is that no method is better than the others in all domains [3], because the performance of a method is related to the application domain. We can use the general paradigm for inductive inference [17] to explain this dependency. Within this paradigm, the goal for a DM algorithm is to find from all the possible hypotheses a specific hypothesis, i.e. a description, that is consistent with the set of facts under analysis using some background knowledge.

3 Statistics and Pattern Recognition

Statistical methods rely in having an explicit underlying probability model. This provides a measure of the membership of an example to a class. The application of these methods require human intervention to define models and hypotheses.

Classical methods are based on Fisher's work on linear discrimination. These are the main methods: (1) Linear discriminants. A hyperplane in the space defined by the features is sought to separate the classes minimizing a quadratic cost function; (2) Quadratic discriminant. These are similiar to linear discriminants, but in this case classification regions are separated by quadratic surfaces; (3) Logistic discriminant. They use quadratic surfaces that maximize a conditional likelihood.

Modern methods use more flexible models to provide an estimate of the joint distribution of the features in each class. Since they can be used without knowledge about the form of the underlying densities. The methods in this subfamiliy include Kernel Density Estimation, k-nearest neighbour, Bayesian methods, Alternative Conditional Expectation (ACE), and Multivariate Adaptive Regression Spline (MARS)

4 Machine Learning (ML)

ML is an artificial intelligence research area that studies computational methods for improving performance by mechanizing the acquisition of knowledge from experience [12]. ML algorithms enable the induction of a symbolic model, decision tree or set of rules, of preferably low complexity, but high transparency and accuracy [13]. The most relevant field of ML in DM is inductive learning (IL). IL is a process of acquiring knowledge by drawing inductive inferences from teacher or environment-provided facts [17].

4.1 Case-Based Reasoning

Case-Based or instance-based methods take advantage of previous cases that have been solved. When a problem is presented to the method, it looks for a previous case matching the new one, analyses its solution, and creates an adapted solution to that new case. CBR stores training instances in memory and its performance relies on the indexing scheme and the similarity metric used.

4.2 Decision Trees

Decision trees are a representation of learning from a set of independent instances, with nodes involving tests of a particular attribute. Decision trees can be generated using algorithms such as Quinlan´s ID3 and C4.5 [20], or a recursive partitioning method, such as in CART [2]. ID3 and its successors are very popular methods, although they have several problems to solve, such as: example selection for the training sets; pruning methods; generalization to independent tests sets, and conversion to classification rules.

4.3 Rule Induction

AQ15 [16,18] is a method for learning strong rules, by using constructive induction. That is, it looks for rules with little errors creating new attributes. Moreover, AQ15 has incremental learning facility to use initial hypothesis about the domain being modeled

CN2 [5,4] is a variant of AQ that combines the best features of AQ and ID3 to avoid the problems of AQ when dealing with noisy data. Another drawback of AQ solved by CN2 is the dependency of the order in the training examples. CN2 produces probabilistic rules.

4.4 Inductive Logic Programming

These techniques are used in abstract computational problems, where learning of recursive rules might be needed to address specific problems (e.g., artificial problems that can generate infinite data).

4.5 Genetic Algorithms

The origin of GAs is the study of cellular automata [9,10].GAs simulate the mechanism followed in natural selection. They start with a population of candidates, also called organisms, and grow successive generations by applying crossover and mutations to the organisms. In each generation only the best candidates, according to some evaluation function, survive. GAs are more suited to extract complex concepts from small databases.

Other common methods, not detailed here, are fuzzy sets and rough sets.

5 Neural Networks

NNs are based on models of the brain. They represent knowledge as a network of units, or neurons, distributed in one or several layers that transmits the activation values from the input nodes to the output nodes. There are rules to define the weighting of the transmission, the activation of the nodes and the connection pattern of the network. Different settings of these configuration rules produce different types of NNs. Learning can be supervised or unsupervised by an external entity.

Examples of supervised networks are the classical perceptrons and multi-layer perceptrons, or the radial basis function networks. Unsupervised networks are, for instance, the K-means clustering algorithm, Kohonen networks and learning vectors quantizers, or the RAMnets.

6. Conclusions

During the last years, many scientific conferences have been organized to discuss data mining topics and present research results. Numerous conferences and symposia are organized by the ACM, IEEE, and the AAAI. Within the medical informatics community, special issues of different journals (e.g., Artificial Intelligence in Medicine) have been devoted to data mining applications. The number of contributions to the main general conferences, such as the AMIA Fall Symposium, is also growing up. For instance, during the last 1999 conference, held in Washington,

DC, 9 contributions dealing with data mining were presented.

Numerous public domain and commercial software products for data mining are now currently available to researchers and medical practitioners. E.g., products such as IBM´s Intelligent Miner ©, or MineSet, from Silicon Graphics, and others off-the-shelf software products are used by an increasing number of people and organizations.

Data mining applications in medicine are currently growing up since many organizations and research groups have realized that these techniques are useful to extract knowledge from large databases. In our research group at the Artificial Intelligence Lab, Universidad Politecnica of Madrid, we have carried out various research projects to obtain prediction rules from medical records. First, we have built a system, named ARMEDA, to access and integrate information from heterogeneous remote databases over the WWW. Second, we have analyzed over 1000 paper-based medical records of patients with rheumatoid arthritis and created a electronic database with a selection of around 300 of those records. Applying data mining techniques, such as induction and clustering, we have obtained 6 prediction rules that relate 25 main clinical variables with a few important outcomes, such as death or quality of life; Third, we have implemented a new method to validate rules in a knowledge base, transforming these If...THEN...rules into a logic-algebraic format that can be checked for detecting logical inconsistencies.

Although similar projects are currently being carried out at many organizations, researchers must be careful with the applications they design. Some epidemiological constraints, such as: (1) sample selection; (2) how to avoid various different biases, (3) to perform external validations, and others, must be observed to ensure that the results obtained with these methods can be applied to health populations.

Selected Bibliography

[1]. Ivan Bratko and Stephen Muggleton. Applications of inductive logic programming. *Communications of the ACM*, 38(11):65-70, November 1995.

[2]. L. Breiman, J. Friedman, R.Olshen, and Stone C. *Classification and Regression Trees*. Wadsworth International Group, 1984.

[3]. Carla E. Brodley. Recursive automatic bias selection for classifier construction. *Machine Learning*, 20:63-94, 1995.

[4] P. Clark and R. Boswell. Rule induction with CN2: Some recent improvements. In Y.Kodratoff, editor, *Proceedings of the European Working Session on Learning : Machine Learning (EWSL-91)*, volume 482 of *LNAI*, pages 151-163, Porto, Portugal, March 1991. Springer Verlag.

[5] Peter Clark and Tim Niblett. The CN2 induction algorithm. *Machine Learning*, 3:261, 1988.

[6] Usama M. Fayyad, Gregory Piatetsky-Shapiro, and Padhraic Smyth. *Advances in Knowledge Discovery and Data Mining*, chapter From Data Mining to Knowledge Discovery: An Overview. The MIT Press, March 1996.

[7] W.J. Frawley, G., Piatetsky-Shapiro, and C.J. Matheus. Knowledge discovery in databases: an overview. *AI Magazine*, 13(3):57-70, 1992.

[8] Michael Goebel and Le Gruenwald. A survey of data mining and knowledge discovery software tools. In *SIGKDD Explorations*. ACM SIGKDD, June 1999.

[9] John H. Holland. Escaping brittleness. In *Proceedings Second International Workshop on Machine Learning*, pages 92-95, 1983.

[10]. John H. Holland, J. Holyoak K, R. E. Nisbett, and P. R. Thagard. *Induction: Processes of Inference, Learning, and Discovery*. MIT Press, Cambridge, MA, 1987.

[11]. Meta Group Inc. Data mining: Trends, technology, and implementation imperatives, February 1997.

[12]. Pat Langley and H.A. Simon. Applications of machine learning and rule induction. *Communications of the ACM*, 38(11):55-64, Nov 1995.

[13]. Nada Lavrac, Elpida Keravnou, and Blaz Zupan. *Intelligent Data Analysis in Medicine and Pharmacology*, chapter Intelligent Data Analysis in Medicine and Pharmacology: An Overview, pages 1-13. Kluwer, 1997.

[14]. T.-S. Lim, W.-Y. Loh, and Y.-S. Shih. An empirical comparison of decision trees and other classification methods. Technical Report 979, Department of Statistics, University of Wisconsin-Madison, Madison, WI, June 30 1997.

[15].W.J. Long, J.L. Griffith, H.P. Selker, and R.B D'Agostino. A comparison of logistic regression to decision-tree induction in a medical domain. *Computers and Biomedical Research*, 26:74-97, 1993.

[16]. R. Michalski, I. Mozetic, J.Hong, and N. Lavrac. The AQ15 inductive learning system: an overview and experiments. In *Proceedings of IMAL 1986*, Orsay, 1986. Université de Paris-Sud.

[17]. R S Michalski. A theory and methodology of inductive learning. *Artificial Intelligence*, 20:111-161, 1983.

[18]. Ryszard S. Michalski, Igor Mozetic, Jiarong Hong, and Nada Lavrac. The multi-purpose incremental learning system AQ15 and its testing application to three medical domains. In *Proceedings of the 5th national conference on Artificial Intelligence*, pages 1041-1045, Philadelphia, 1986.

[19]. J.R. Quinlan. *C4.5: Programs for Machine Learning*. Morgan Kaufmann, San Mateo, CA, 1992.

[20] Weiss, S and Indurkhya:. Predictive Data Mining. A Practical Guide.Morgan Kaufmann. San Frncisco, CA. 1998.

Prognoses for Multiparametric Time Courses

Rainer Schmidt, Lothar Gierl

Institut für Medizinische Informatik und Biometrie, Universität Rostock
Rembrandtstr. 16 / 17, D-18055 Rostock, Germany
Email: {rainer.schmidt , lothar.gierl} @medizin.uni-rostock.de

Abstract. In this paper, we describe an approach to utilize Case-Based Reasoning (CBR) methods for trend prognoses for medical problems. Since using conventional methods for reasoning over time does not fit for course predictions without medical knowledge of typical course pattern, we have developed abstraction methods suitable for integration into our Case-Based Reasoning system ICONS. These methods combine medical experience with prognoses of multiparametric courses. We apply them to the monitoring of the kidney function in an Intensive Care Unit (ICU) setting. We generate course-characteristic trend descriptions of the renal function over the course of time. Using Case-Based Reasoning retrieval methods, we search in the case base for courses similar to the current trend descriptions. We present a current course together with similar courses as comparisons and as possible prognoses to the user.

1. Introduction

Up to 60% of the body mass of an adult person consists of water. The electrolytes dissolved in body water are of great importance for an adequate cell function. The human body tends to balance the fluid and electrolyte situation. But intensive care patients are often no longer able to maintain adequate fluid and electrolyte balances themselves due to impaired organ functions, e.g. renal failure, or medical treatment, e.g. parenteral nutrition of mechanically ventilated patients. Therefore physicians need objective criteria for the monitoring of fluid and electrolyte balances and for choosing therapeutic interventions as necessary.

At our ICU, physicians daily get a printed renal report from the monitoring system NIMON [1] which consists of 13 measured and 33 calculated parameters of those patients where renal function monitoring is applied. For example, the urine osmolality and the plasma osmolality are measured parameters that are used to calculate the osmolar clearance and the osmolar excretion. The interpretation of all reported parameters is quite complex and needs special knowledge of the renal physiology.

The aim of our knowledge based system ICONS is to give an automatic interpretation of the renal state to elicit impairments of the kidney function on time and to give early warnings against forthcoming kidney failures. That means, we need a time course analysis of many parameters without any well-defined standards. At first glance, this seemed to be a field to apply statistical methods. However, our good results of experiments with a Case-Based Reasoning approach and our investigations of the difficulties to handle multiparametric time course problems without a medical domain theory revealed that Case-Based Reasoning methods are more applicable in

R.W. Brause and E. Hanisch (Eds.): ISMDA 2000, LNCS 1933, pp. 23–33, 2000.

this field. Although much research has been performed in the field of conventional temporal course analyses in the recent years, none of them is suitable for this problem. Allen's theory of time and action [2] is not appropriate for multiparametric course analysis, because time is represented as just another parameter in the relevant predicates and therefore does not give necessary explicit status [3]. As traditional time series techniques [4] with known periodicities work well unless abrupt changes, they do not fit in a domain characterized by possibilities of abrupt changes and a lack of well-known periodicities at all. One ability of RÉSUMÉ [5] is the abstraction of many parameters into one single parameter and to analyse the course of this abstracted parameter. However, the interpretation of the courses requires complete domain knowledge. Haimowitz and Kohane [6] compare many parameters of current courses with well-known standards. In VIE-VENT [7] both ideas are combined: courses of each quantitativ measured parameter are abstracted into qualitativ course descriptions, that are matched with well-known standards.

However, in the domain of fluid and electrolyte balance, neither a prototypical approach in ICU settings is known nor exists complete knowledge about the kidney function. Especially, knowledge about the behaviour of the various parameters over time is yet incomplete. So we had to design our own method to deal with course analyses of multiple parameters without prototypical courses and without a complete domain theory. Fig.1. shows our method within the Case-Based Reasoning cycle according to Aamodt [8].

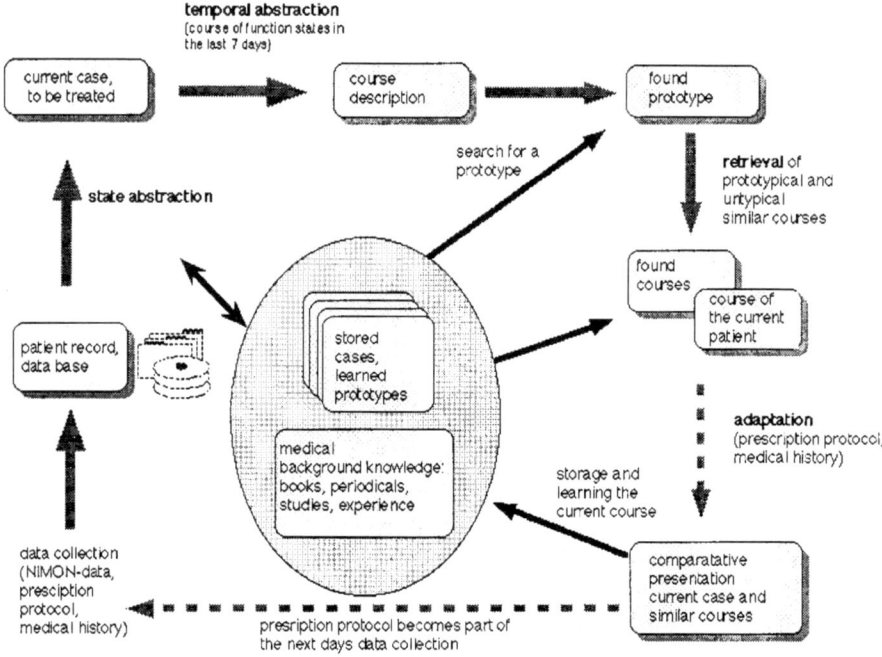

Fig. 1. The Case-Based Reasoning cycle for ICONS

2. Methods

Our procedure to interpretate kidney function courses can be seen in Fig.2. First, the monitoring system NIMON gets 13 measured parameters from the clinical chemistry and calculates 33 meaningful kidney function parameters. To elicit the relationships among these parameters a three dimensional presentation ability was implemented inside the renal monitoring system NIMON. However, complex relations among all parameters are not visible.

We decided to abstract these parameters. For this data abstraction we use states of the renal function which determine states of increasing severity beginning with a normal renal function and ending with a renal failure. Based on these state definitions, we determine the appropriate state of the kidney function per day. Therefore, we present the possible states to the user sorted according to their probability. The physician has to accept one of them. Based on the transitions of the states of one day to the state of the respectively next day, we generate four different trends. These trends, that are abstractions of time, describe the courses of the states. Then we use Case-Based Reasoning retrieval methods [9, 10, 11, 12] to search for similar courses. We present similar courses together with the current one as comparisons to the user, the course continuations of the similar courses serve as prognoses.

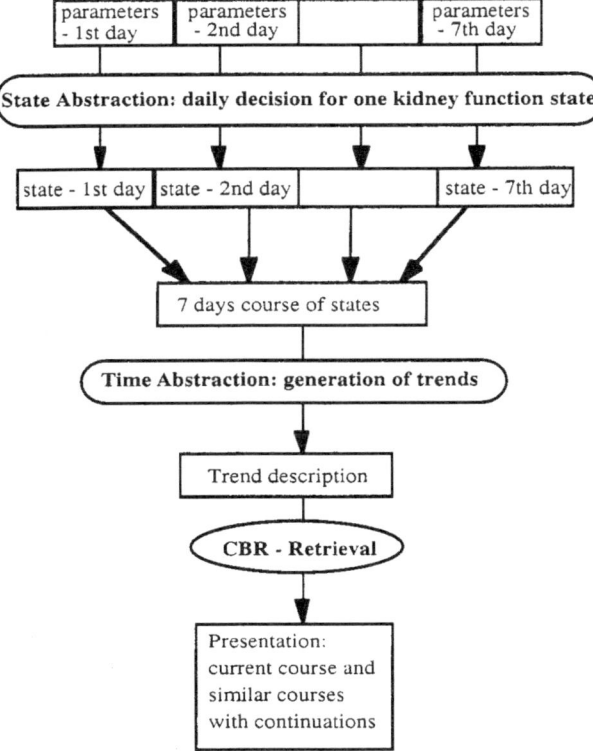

Fig. 2 .Abstractions for Multiparametric Prognoses in ICONS

As the integration of presciption protocols will be part of the next phase of the ICONS project, an adaptation of a similar to a current course is not yet possible. So far ICONS offers only diagnostic and prognostic support, the user has to decide about the relevance of all displayed information. When presenting a comparison of a current course with a similar one, ICONS supplies the user with the ability to access additional renal syndromes and the courses of single parameter values during the relevant time period.

2.1. Determination of the Kidney Function State

Based on the kidney function states, characterized by obligatory and optional conditions for selected renal parameters, first we check the obligatory conditions. For each state that satisfies the obligatory conditions we calculate a similarity value concerning the optional conditions. We use a variation of Tversky 's [9] measure of dissimilarity between concepts. If two or more states are under consideration, ICONS presents these states sorted to the similarity values together with information about the satisfied and not satisfied optional conditions (see Fig. 3.).

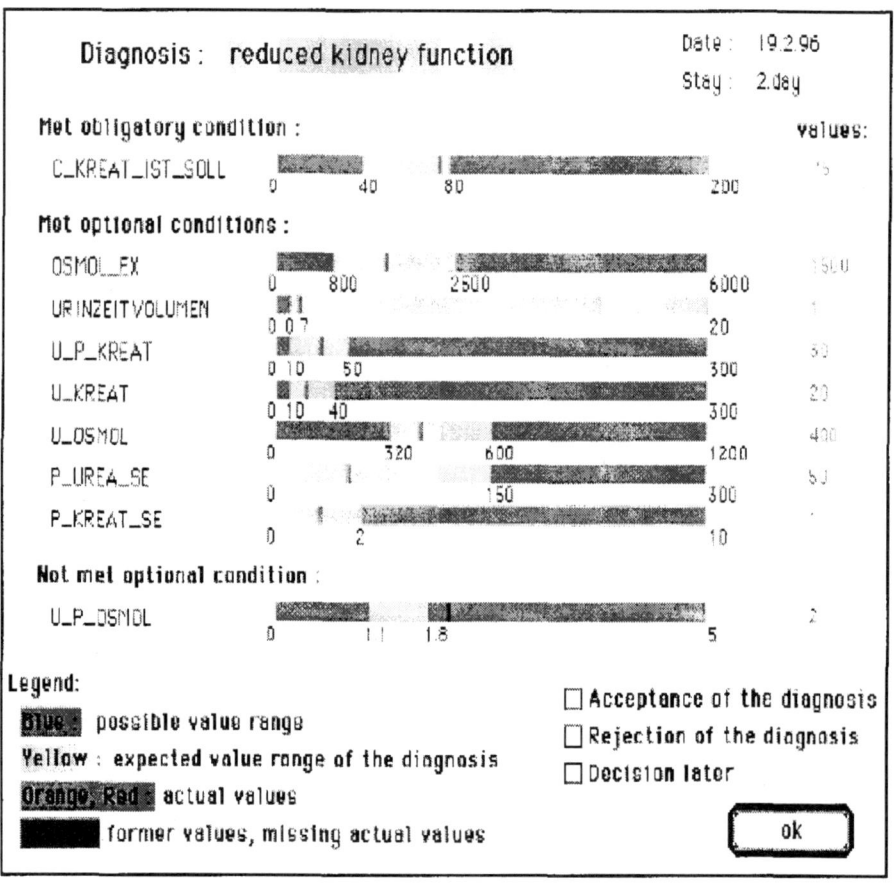

Fig. 3. Presentation of a kidney function state estimated as reduced kidney function

The user can accept or reject a presented state. When a suggested state has been rejected, ICONS selects another state. Finally, we determine the central state of occasionally more than one states the user has accepted. This central state is the closest one towards a kidney failure. Our intention is to find the state indicating the most profound impairment of the kidney function.

When we determine the kidney function states, we abstract all daily measured and calculated quantitative kidney function parameters from the monitoring system NIMON to one single qualitative value. In the next section we describe our course analysis of these qualitative values, which are ordered according to decreasing fluid and electrolyte situations. More than one value can be related to the same severity value.

2.2. Course-characteristic Trend Descriptions

First, we have fixed five assessment definitions for the transition of the kidney function state of one day to the state of the respectively next day. These assessment definitions are related to the grade of renal impairment:

steady: both states have the same severity value.

increasing: exactly one severity step in the direction towards a normal function.

sharply increasing: at least two severity steps in the direction towards a normal function.

decreasing: exactly one severity step in the direction towards a kidney failure.

sharply decreasing: at least two severity steps in the direction towards a kidney failure.

These assessment definitions are used to determine the state transitions from one qualitative value to another. Based on these state transitions, we generate three trend descriptions. Two trend descriptions especially consider the current state transitions.

T1, short-term trend:=	current state transition
T2, medium-term trend:=	looks recursively back from the current state transition to the one before and unites them, if they are both of the same direction or one of them has a "steady" assessment
T3, long-term trend:=	characterizes the whole considered course of at most seven days

For the long-term trend description we introduced in addition to the five former assessment definitions four new ones. If none of the five former assessments fits the complete considered course, we attempt to fit one of these four definitions in the following order:

alternating: at least two up and two down transitions and all local minima are equal.

oscillating: at least two up and two down transitions.

fluctuating: distance of the highest to the lowest severity state value is greater than 1.

nearly steady: the distance of the highest to the lowest severity state value equals one.

Only if there are several courses with the same trend description, we use a minor fourth trend description T4 to find the most similar among them. We assess the whole considered course by adding up the state transition values inversely weighted by the distances to the current day. Together with the current kidney function state, these four trend descriptions form a course depiction, that abstracts the sequence of the kidney function states.

Looking back from a time point t, these four trend descriptions form a pattern of the immediate course history of the kidney function considering qualitative and quantitative assessments.

Why these four trend descriptions?

There are domain specific reasons for defining the short-, medium- and long-term trend descriptions T1, T2 and T3. If physicians evaluate courses of the kidney function, they consider at most one week prior to the current date. Earlier renal function states are irrelevant for the current situation of a patient. Most relevant information is derived from the current function state, the current development and sometimes a current development within a slightly longer time period. That means, very long trends are of no interest in our domain. In fact, sometimes only the current state transition or short continuous or slightly longer developments are crucial.

The short-term trend description T1 expresses the current development. For longer time periods, we have defined the medium- and long-term trend descriptions T2 and T3, because there are two different phenomena to discover and for each, a special technique is needed. T2 can be used for detecting a continuous trend independant of its length, because equal or steady state transitions are recursively united beginning with the current one. As the long-term trend description T3 describes a well-defined time period, it is especially useful for detecting fluctuating trends.

As every abstraction loses some specific information, information about the daily kidney function states is lost in our second abstraction step. The course description contains only information about the current and the start states of the three trend descriptions. The intermediate states are abstracted into trend description assessments.

Example

The following kidney function states (see the current course in Fig. 4.) may be observed in this temporal sequence:

selective tubular damage, reduced kidney function, reduced kidney function, selective tubular damage, reduced kidney function, reduced kidney function, sharply reduced kidney function

So we get these six state transitions:

decreasing, steady, increasing, decreasing, steady, decreasing

with these trend descriptions:

current state: sharply reduced kidney function
T1: decreasing, reduced kidney function, one transition
T2: decreasing, selective tubular damage, three transitions
T3: fluctuating, selective tubular damage, six transitions
T4: 1.23

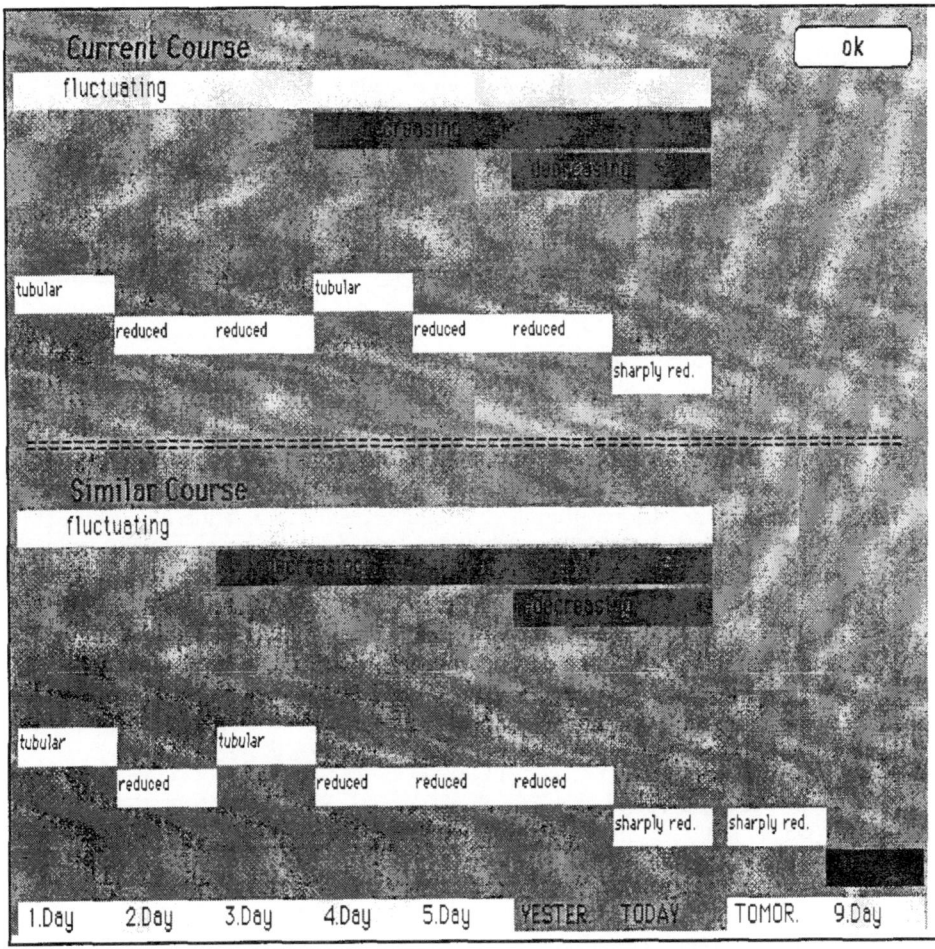

Fig. 4. Comparative presentation of a current and a similar course. In the lower part of each course the (abbreviated) kidney function states are depicted. The upper part of each course shows the deduced trend descriptions.

In this example, the short-term trend description T1 assesses the current state transition as "decreasing" from a "reduced kidney function" to a "sharply reduced kidney function". As the medium-term trend description T2 accumulates steady state transitions, this trend assesses a "decrease" in the last four days from a "selective tubular damage" to a "sharply reduced kidney function". The long-term trend description T3 assesses the whole course of seven days as "fluctuating", because there is only one increasing state transition and the difference between the severity values of a "selective tubular damage" and a "sharply reduced kidney function" equals two.

2.3. Retrieval

We use the parameters of the four trend descriptions and the current kidney function state to search for similar courses. As the aim is to develop an early warning system, we need a prognosis. For this reason and to avoid a sequential runtime search along the whole cases, we store a course of the previous seven days and a maximal projection of three days for each day a patient spent on the intensive care unit.

As there are many different possible continuations for the same previous course, it is necessary to search for similar courses and different projections. Therefore, we divided the search space into nine parts corresponding to the possible continuation directions. Each direction forms an own part of the search space. During the retrieval these parts are searched separately and each part may provide at most one similar case. The similar cases of these parts together are presented in the order of their computed similarity values.

Before the main retrieval, we search for a prototype that matches most of the trend descriptions. Below this prototype the main retrieval starts. It consists of two steps for each part. First we search with an activation algorithm concerning qualitative features. Our algorithm differs from the common spreading activation algorithm [10] mainly due to the fact that we do not use a net for the similarity relations. Instead, we have defined explicit activation values for each possible feature value. This is possible, because on this abstraction level there are only ten dimensions (see the left column of Table 1) with at most six values. The right column of Table 1 shows the possible activation values for the description parameters. E.g. there are four activation values for the current kidney function state: courses with the same current state as the current course get the value 15, those cases whose distance to the current state of the current course is one step in the severity hierarchy get 7 and so forth.

Dimensions	Activation values
Current state	15, 7, 5, 2
Assessment T1	10, 5, 2
Assessment T2	4, 2, 1
Assessment T3	6, 5, 4, 3, 2, 1
Length T1	10, 5, 3, 1,
Length T2	3, 1
Length T3	2, 1
Start state T1	4, 2
Start state T2	4, 2
Start state T3	2, 1

Table 1. Retrieval dimensions and their activation values

Subsequently, we check the retrieved cases with a similarity criterion [11] that looks for sufficient similarity, since even the most similar course may differ from the current one significantly. This may happen at the beginning of the use of ICONS, when there are only a few cases known to ICONS, or when the current course is rather exceptional. Because of the lack of medical knowledge about sufficient similarity, we defined a minimal similarity criterion that may be improved after some experience with ICONS.

If several courses are selected in the same projection part, we use a sequential similarity measure concerning the quantitative features in a second step. So far it is only the single parameter of the trend description T4. This measure is a variation of TSCALE [12] and goes back to Tversky [9].

3. Learning

Prognosis of multiparametric courses of the kidney function for ICU patients is a domain without a medical theory. Moreover, we can not expect such a theory to be formulated in the near future. So we attempt to learn prototypical course pattern. Therefore, knowledge on this domain is stored as a tree of prototypes with three levels and a root node (see Fig. 5.). Except for the root, where all not yet clustered courses are stored, every level corresponds to one of the trend descriptions T1, T2 or T3. As soon as enough courses that share another trend description are stored at a prototype, we create a new prototype with this trend. At a prototype at level 1, we cluster courses that share T1, at level 2, courses that share T1 and T2 and at level 3, courses that share all three trend descriptions. We can do this, because regarding their importance, the short-, medium- and long-term trend descriptions T1, T2 and T3 refer to hierarchically related time periods. T1 is more important than T2 and T3.

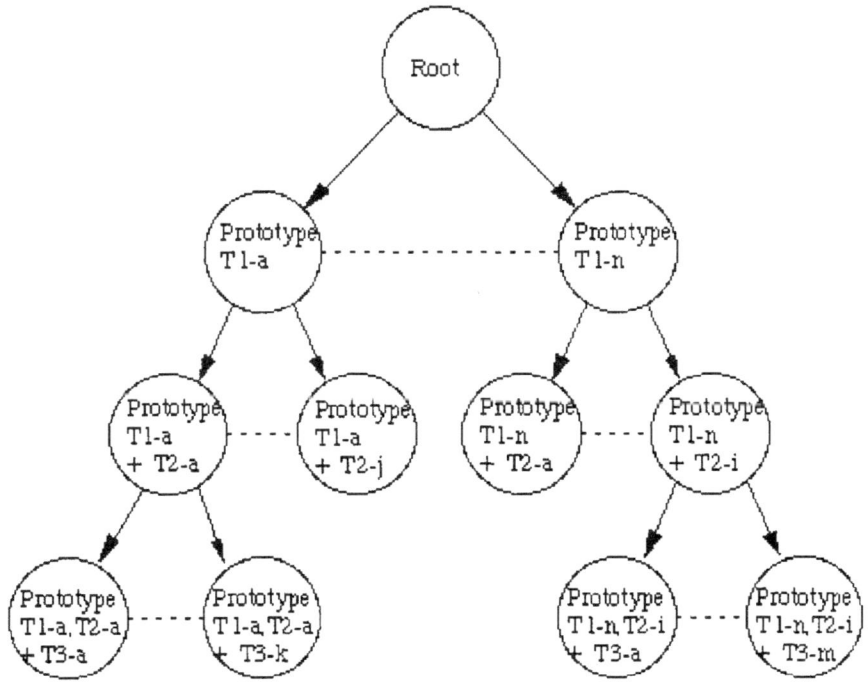

Fig. 5. General structure of the prototype tree

We start the retrieval with a search for a prototype that has most of the trend descriptions in common with the current course. The search begins at the root with a check for a prototype with the same short-term trend description T1. If such a prototype can be found, the search goes on below this prototype for a prototype that has the same trend descriptions T1 and T2, and so on. If no prototype with a further trend in common can be found, we search for a course at the last accepted prototype. If no prototype exists that has the same T1 as the current course, we search at the root node, where all courses are stored that are not related to a prototype.

4. Evaluation

To verify the knowledge base we selected 100 data sets from the NIMON database. The selection was only partly at random, because we wanted adequate representation of all kidney function states. Two physicians experienced with the kidney function were asked to classify the selected data sets according to the concepts, but without knowing ICONS`s obligatory and optional conditions of the kidney function states. We compared the results of the physicians with ICONS`s classifications of the same data sets. The comparison was mostly satisfactory. For 83 parameter sets the classifications of ICONS corresponded to those of the physicians. The 17 deviations are shown in Table 2. In 16 cases ICONS tended more towards the direction of kidney failures. Only once ICONS classified the parameter set as a "reduced kidney function" while the most experienced physician assessed it as a "kidney failure" and the other physician as a "filtration rate reduction due to prerenal impairment". However, as a result of the evaluation we slightly modified the state definition of the "reduced kidney function".

Physicians	ICONS	Quantity
normal kidney function	reduced kidney function	7
normal kidney function	selective tubular damage	3
sharply reduced kidney function	kidney failure	3
selective tubular damage	reduced kidney function	1
selective tubular damage	sharply reduced kidney function	1
reduced kidney function	sharply reduced kidney function	1
kidney failure	reduced kidney function	1

Table 2. Deviating classifications between two experienced physicians and ICONS

5. Conclusion

Our aim is to produce an early warning system that helps to avoid kidney failures. ICONS helps the physicians to abstract from the measured and calculated NIMON parameters to a function state. For time periods up to seven days, we describe courses of function states using four trend descriptions as a second abstraction step. At this double abstraction level, ICONS provides the physicians with courses of other patients with similar developments as potential warnings. As no prototypical courses towards a kidney failure are known, we search for cases with similar courses and present them as possible prognoses. We hope to find some prototypical courses by merging similar courses into prototypes. One advantage of combining temporal course analyses with Case-Based Reasoning is the projection. Without medical knowledge about possibilities and probabilities of future developments ICONS shows future developments of patients with similar courses.

References

1. Wenkebach, U., Pollwein, B., Finsterer, U.: Visualization of large datasets in intensive care. In: Proc Annu Symp Comput Appl Med Care (1992) 18-22
2. Allen, J.P.: Towards a general theory of action and time. *Artificial Intelligence 23*, (1984) 123-154
3. Keravnou, E.T.: Modelling Medical Concepts as Time Objects. In: P. Barahona, M. Stefanelli, J. Wyatt (eds.): Artificial Intelligence in Medicine, Lecture Notes in Artificial Intelligence 934, Springer-Verlag, Berlin Heidelberg New York (1995) 67-78
4. Robeson, S.M., Steyn, D.G.: Evaluation and comparison of statistical forecast models for daily maximum ozone concentrations. *Atmospheric Environment 24 B 2*, (1990) 303-12
5. Shahar,Y., Musen,M.A.: RÉSUMÉ: A Temporal-Abstraction System for Patient Monitoring. *Computers and Biomedical Research 26* (1993) 255-273
6. Haimowitz,I.J., Kohane,I.S.: Automated Trend Detection with Alternate Temporal Hypotheses. In: Bajcsy,R. (ed.): Proceedings of IJCAI-93, Morgan Kaufmann, San Mateo, CA (1993) 146-151
7. Miksch, S., Horn, W., Popow, C., Paky, F.: Therapy Planning Using Qualitative Trend Descriptions. Barahona, P., Stefanelli, M., Wyatt, J. (Eds.) Artificial Intelligence in Medicine, Lecture Notes in Artificial Intelligence 934, Springer-Verlag, Berlin Heidelberg New York (1995) 209-217
8. Aamodt, A.: Case-Based Reasoning : Foundation Issues. *Methodological Variation-and System Approaches, AICOM* 7 (1994) 39-59
9. Tversky, A.: Features of Similarity. *Psychological Review 84* (1977) 327-352
10. Anderson, J.R.: A theory of the origins of human knowledge. *Artificial Intelligence 40*, Special Volume on Machine Learning (1989) 313-351
11. Smyth, B., Keane, M.T.: Retrieving Adaptable Cases: The Role of Adaptation Knowledge in Case Retrieval. First European Workshop on Case-Based Reasoning, EWCBR-93, (1993) 76-81
12. DeSarbo, W.S., Johnson, M.D., Manrei, A.K., Manrai, L.A., Edwards, E.A.: TSCALE: A new multidemensional scaling procedure based on Tversky's contrast model. *Psychometrika 57* (1992) 43-69

Estimation of the Time Delay of Epileptic Spikes by ICA

Aleš Černošek[1], Vladimír Krajča[2], Jitka Mohylová[1], Svojmil Petránek[2],
Miloš Matoušek[3], Karel Paul[4]

[1] Technical University Ostrava
{ales.cernosek, jitka.mohylova}@vsb.cz
[2] Faculty Hospital Bulovka, Prague
{krajca, petranek}@neuro.anet.cz
[3] Psychiatric Center, Prague
[4] Inst. Care Mother and Child, Prague

Abstract. The contribution concentrates on application of Independent Component Analysis (ICA) for the detection of small time delays of epileptic spikes in electroencephalographic (EEG) recordings. The ICA method isolates spike's activity by decomposing the input EEG record into independent components. Some of them contain epileptic spikes. ICA detects the time delay of epileptic spikes between channels by separating the epileptic spikes into two or more components. We propose a method of epileptic focus location by ICA from EEG recordings which contain epileptic spikes. The analysis allows presentation of the results in the form of topographic maps. The method was tested on real EEG background signal with artificially simulated epileptic spikes and on EEG records containing real epileptic activity, obtained in four epileptic patients. The tests were used for a comparison with the results of a visual analysis. The tests confirmed a satisfactory agreement between computerized and visual assessments.

Introduction

The correct location of epileptic foci is of great importance in neurosurgical treatment of epilepsy. To estimate the site of the area in the brain, where the epileptic discharge is initiated, the activity of the brain tissue is derived from a number of electrodes and presented in a form of electroencephalographic (EEG) tracings. Typically, the assessment is done by a visual inspection of the multichannel recordings. The method is elaborious and the results of a visual assessment, although done by an experienced doctor, can be erroneous. Therefore, a great effort has been devoted to the development of the computerized methods to detect and localize the source of the epileptiform activity from the EEG signal. A series of amplitude maps was found to be helpful to detect the foci but the method could be employed only as a supplement to a competent visual analysis.

A promising method seemed to be to measure the small time differences (delays) between the individual activities as recorded from different electrode sites. Of course,

R.W. Brause and E. Hanisch (Eds.): ISMDA 2000, LNCS 1933, pp. 34–42, 2000.

the time delay is too short to be discovered by a visual evaluation of the tracings and the measurement requires an instrumental analysis.

A method which was more successful in practical application used a time-domain analysis to define specific wave shapes in the EEG signal [2]. The next version was based on the EEG spectrum analysis, using a common FFT algorithm to estimate the spectra.

In our paper we chose a different approach based on Independent Component Analysis (ICA). As previously shown by Lee, the method can be applied to isolate epileptic activity in the multichannel EEG recordings [6]. The present study broadens the application of the ICA method, aiming to use the time delay between the EEG channels for a subsequent localization of the epileptic focus. Recently, the technique was also discussed by Kobayashi et al. who proposed the ICA application for the separation of epileptiform discharges from EEG background [5]. Nevertheless, this work concerned only EEG records with focal graphoelements. In contrast, the application in the present study deals with generalized spikes, those with epileptiform activity which is not only limited to the source area, being widely spread in the whole multichannel recording. These types of EEG records with generalized epileptic activity are very difficult to be analyzed by the conventional visual analysis.

Methods and Materials

ICA Data Model

ICA is a technique for the processing of signals which provides a transformation of the multidimensional random vector into mutually independent components. ICA decomposes measured (obtained) signals corresponding with the realization of m-dimensional random vector of the discrete time signal $\mathbf{x}(k)$, $k=1, 2, \ldots$ into components $\mathbf{s}(k)$, $k = 1, 2 \ldots$

The $\mathbf{s}$ components are usually called source or original signals and they are often mutually independent. These signals can be obtained from linearly mixed signals $\mathbf{x}$ by identifying a transformation in which the transformed signals are independent (components).

Let $\mathbf{x} = [x_1, x_2, \ldots, x_m]^T$ denote m-dimensional random vector (measured data) and let $\mathbf{s} = [s_1, s_2, \ldots, s_n]^T$ denote n-dimensional vector of components (source vector). These components are an unknown but mutually independent sources of the signals.

Let us assume the following data model:

$$\mathbf{x} = \mathbf{A}.\mathbf{s},\tag{1}$$

where $\mathbf{A}_{mxn}$ is the constant mixing matrix which is to be set. The source separation can be denoted as:

$$\mathbf{y} = \mathbf{W}.\mathbf{x},\tag{2}$$

where $\mathbf{y} = \hat{\mathbf{s}}$ is estimation of components and $\mathbf{A} \approx \mathbf{W}^{-1}$.

ICA Projection

ICA projection performs mapping of the influence of the individual components on the electrodes located on the scalp of the patient [4], [7]. Therefore, it can be used to determine the contribution of any electrode for the establishment of the relevant independent component s_j.

With respect to the data model (1), it can be said that columns of matrix $\mathbf{A}$, or $\mathbf{W}^{-1}$ denote "the strength of projection" of the respective components onto the individual electrodes. The ICA projection is explained in more detail in Fig. 1. For simplicity we assume that only three electrodes are connected. Using the ICA method we decompose the input EEG signal into three independent components thus obtaining the square matrix $\mathbf{W}_{3x3}$. Columns of the matrix $\mathbf{W}^{-1}$ or $\mathbf{A}$, respectively, represent the respective individual components; rows of the matrix represent the individual electrodes. The influence rate of the specific electrode on the given component is defined by the value of the elements of matrix $\mathbf{A}$. The greater the value of the element, the greater the influence of the electrode. To increase the descriptive value of the projection, we chose a gray scale for the representation of values of the individual elements.

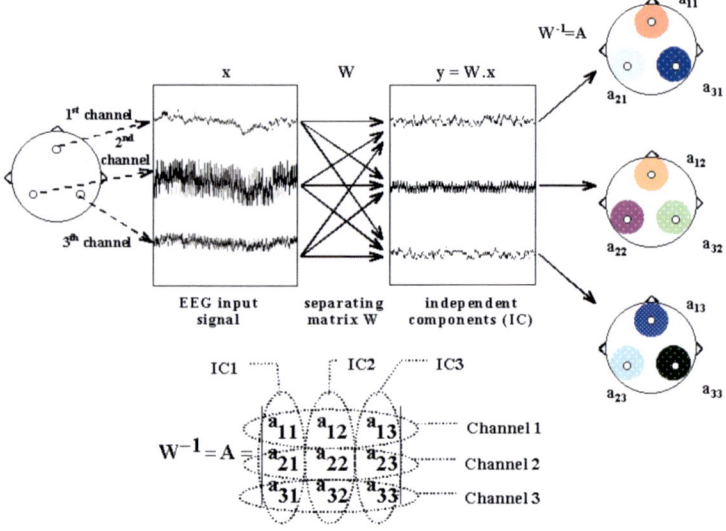

Fig. 1. Schematic illustration of ICA application to EEG record analysis and ICA mapping. Description of rows and columns of matrix A.

Method for Epileptic Focus Location

Assume that we have n-channels EEG record. In the following we describe a new method for epileptic focus location in five steps.

1. The input EEG signal is decomposed, using ICA into n independent components.

2. The epileptic activity is characterized by only a few components from a total of n components called "epileptic components".
3. One component with the smallest time delay of spikes is chosen from all "epileptic components".
4. The ICA projection is performed on the component selected under 3.
5. The epileptic focus is determined from the obtained map (Fig. 6).

EEG Signals Description

The ICA method was applied to two types of input EEG data. The first class contained real EEG record with simulated spikes, the second one contained real EEG record with epileptic activity. In both cases the records were obtained by means of 19 electrodes by using the digital electroencephalograph BrainQuick connected under the international 10-20 system with sampling rate 128 Hz. The EEG data were obtained form Faculty Hospital Bulovka, Prague, Department of Neurology.

In the first case the real EEG record did not contain any spikes. Therefore, we added the artificial spikes into EEG record in order to evaluate the ICA technique's capability of working with well-defined waveforms. Total length of the record was 10 sec and the analysis was performed for the entire length of this record (a segment between the 0th and 4th second is shown in Fig. 2). Artificial spikes, which we created, were added into the EEG record. From several types of artificial spikes we used for the tests those having the following parameters: the duration of one spike 9 samples (70 msec in EEG record with sampling rate 128 Hz). Whenever we added more than one spike to the signal, their frequency was 3 spikes per second.

The second class of input data includes the real EEG record containing genuine epileptic activity. An artifact-free segment of 47 sec length was stored for the analysis. The processing was carried out in 10 sec epochs of the record (a segment between the 3rd and 7th second is shown in Fig. 3).

Analysis

There are several implementations of ICA. In our tests we use Fast Fixed-Point Algorithm (FFPA) [3]. Computing time of FFPA depends on many parameters (e.g. algorithm accuracy, number of channels, sampling rate, type of computer) therefore it cannot be determined exactly. In our tests computing time of FFPA ranged from 5 sec to 15 sec. The algorithm was implemented in C++ programming language in C++ Builder and was tested on PC, CPU Celeron 333 MHz, 64 MB RAM with operating system Windows 95. Detailed information about FFPA, its properties and its comparison with other algorithms are presented in [1].

The ICA method was carried out in various length of the analyzed records (the length ranges from 4 to 10 sec). We introduced only tests with 10 sec-segment analysis. No well-marked differences on the results in relation to the length of analyzed segment were detected (except computing time).

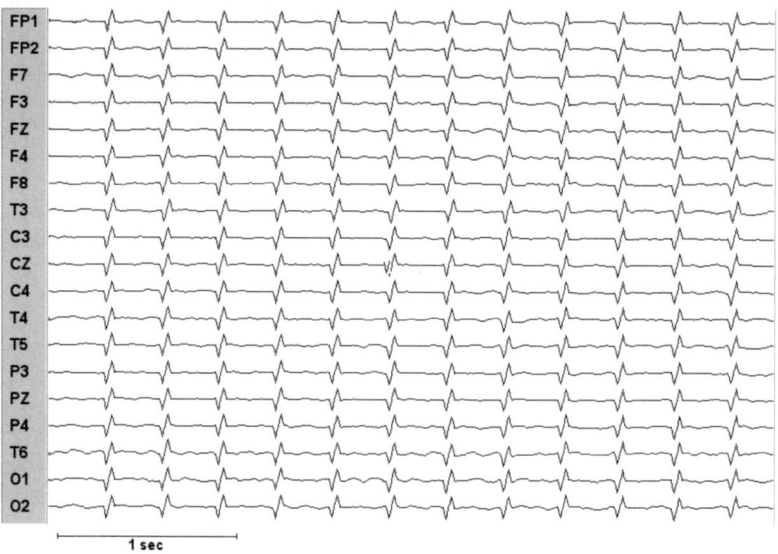

Fig. 2. EEG input record with simulated spikes (19 channels, 4 sec). In channel T3, the spikes have 1 sample delay with respect to the other spikes.

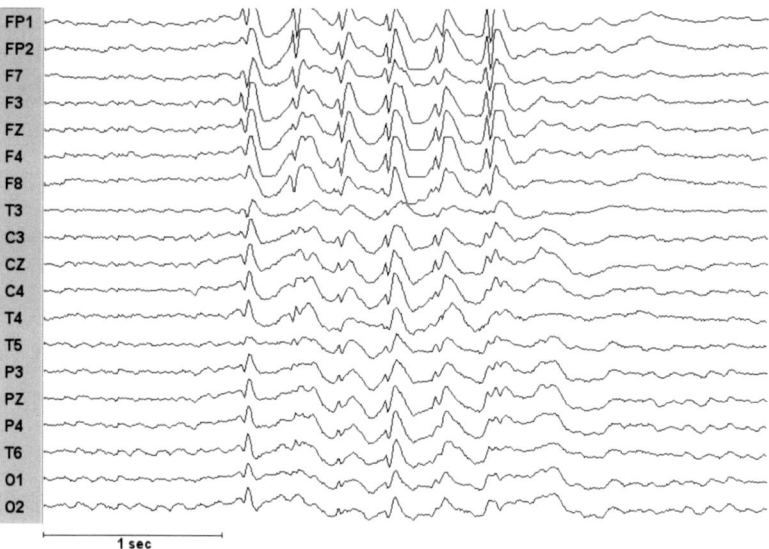

Fig. 3. EEG input record with epileptic activity (4 sec).

Results

Artificial Spikes

The properties of ICA were investigated by performing of 50 tests. The objective of these tests was to evaluate the theoretical assumptions on the behavior of ICA in the analysis of the multidimensional signal containing spikes. Only one test is introduced.

We added 12 spikes to the background activity as recorded in each of the nineteen EEG channels. In the channel T3 the spikes were shifted by 1 sample in regard to the other channels (Fig. 2). After completing the analysis we found out that ICA decomposed the input record into independent components with the spikes detected in two components. The first component corresponded to the spikes which appeared synchronously in all the channels. In contrast, the second component separately reflected those spikes which were shifted in one channel in regard to the other channels. Thus, ICA considered the delayed signals as being what can be called the second source of the spikes Fig. 2 and Fig. 4.

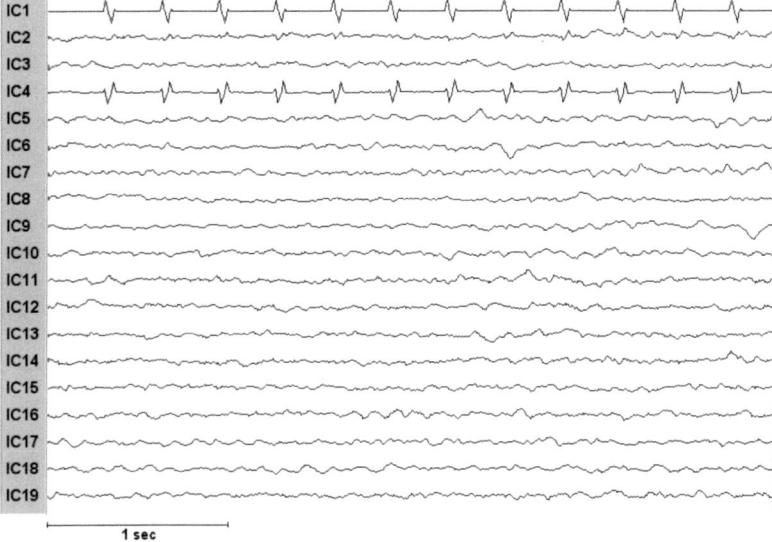

Fig. 4. Independent components obtained by using ICA.

Real Epileptic Spikes

The relevant segment of nineteen independent components obtained by ICA is shown in Fig. 5. Some of these components characterized the epileptic activity and the remaining (majority) part of the components the "residual" EEG activity (point 2 in section "Method for Epileptic Focus Location"). According to the ICA definition [3] some of the estimated components **y** (2) may be multiplied by the coefficient -1 with respect to the original components **s** (1). Therefore, it is necessary to take into account also those components in which the spikes are reversed along the horizontal axis. In our test we included in the analysis the components IC4, IC8 and IC12.

We determined the lowest time delay of spikes among the "epileptic components". We found IC4 to be the component with the lowest time delay (point 3).

Then we performed a mapping for the IC4 (point 4). From a graphic map (Fig. 6) we identified the area with the highest activity of IC4 (point 5). This area is displayed in black. The gray (light) color indicates the areas with the lowest activity. In our test we identified the epileptic focus around the electrodes FP1, FP2, and FZ.

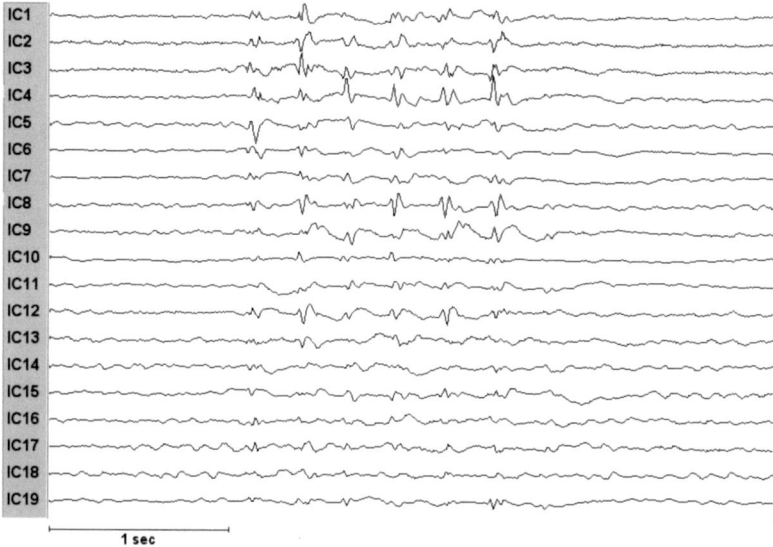

Fig. 5. Independent components obtained by using ICA from input signal with epileptic spikes.

Discussion

This paper proposed a method aimed at localizing the epileptic focus using ICA. The tests were performed both with the EEG records with simulated spikes and with records contained real epileptic spikes. We introduced the theoretical opportunity (simulated spikes) of ICA for epileptic spikes isolation and time delay detection in EEG records. We found out that the epileptic spikes were detected as independent source of signals. Therefore, they were isolated into independent components. The time delay of spikes between two channels was detected by ICA as decomposing the spikes into two different components. The spikes' time appearance in these components is equal as in analyzed record.

Next, we performed tests with real epileptic spikes. Four epileptic patients were tested (the results are introduced only for one patient) and the results obtained by using the ICA method (located epileptic focuses) were in good agreement with physician's opinion. Of course, the material is limited and conclusions on the practical applicability of the material can hardly be done before a sufficient number of analyzed epileptic patients will be available. Thus, this work can be considered as "feasibility study". We would like to increase the number of analyzed patients and improve the suggested method with respect to the evaluation of record by physician in the future.

In any case, the detection of the epileptic focus requires an assistance of the neuro-physiologist. From this point of view, the method does not differ from e.g. phase spectrum analysis. However, the latter is handicapped by certain limiting conditions and this technique cannot always be used correctly (e.g. there is no sense in deter-mining the slope of phase characteristics for frequencies with low coherence). On the other hand, the ICA technique can always be adequately applied to analyze the EEG record and thus to localize the epileptic focus. However, ICA has some disadvantages – low speed of ICA computation, the necessity to define in advance the component characterizing the epileptic activity. The above-mentioned disadvantages of ICA proved that this location of an epileptic focus may not always be precise, so it may be suitable to combine it with another method (e.g. phase spectrum analysis), thus in-creasing the number of correctly analyzed records.

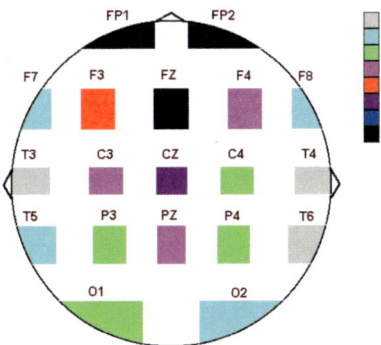

Fig. 6. Results of mapping obtained by computer analysis. The map represents the result ob-tained by using ICA. The probable source of epileptic activity is presented by black color area.

Acknowledgements

This work was supported by grant MŠMT ČR FRVŠ 739, IGA NE6222-3/2000 and NG 14-3.

References

1. Černošek, A., Krajča, V., Petránek, S., Mohylová, J.: Practical experiences with the applica-tion of Independent Component Analysis (ICA) and Principal Component Analysis (PCA) for EEG artifacts elimination. Lékař a Technika (2000) 2:29-36. (In Czech)

2. Gotman, J.: Measurement of small time differences between EEG channels: Method and application to epileptic seizure propagation. Electroenceph. Clin. Neurophysiol. (1983) 56:501-514.
3. Hyvärinen, A., Oja, E.: A Fast Fixed-Point Algorithm for Independent Component Analysis. Neural Computation (1997) 9:1483-1492.
4. Jung, T.P., Makeig, S., Westerfield, M., Townsend, J., Courchesne, E., Sejnowski, T.J.: Analyzing and Visualizing Single-Trial Event-Related Potentials. Advances in Neural Information Processing Systems 11, (1998)
5. Kobayashi, K., James, C. J., Nakahori, T., Akiyama, T., Gotman, J.: Isolation of epileptiform discharges from unaveraged EEG by independent component analysis. Clinical Neurophysiology (1999) 110:1755-1763.
6. Lee, I.K.: Independent component analysis (ICA) of epileptiform discharges. Clinical Neurophysiology, Vol. 110, Supplement 1, (1999) S 127.
7. Makeig, S., Jung, T.P., Bell, A.J., Ghahremani, D., Sejnowski, T.J.: Blind Separation of Auditory Even-related Brain Responses into Independent Components. Proc. Natl. Acad. Sci. USA (1997) 94:10979-10984.

Change-Point Detection in Kinetic Signals

Gerhard Staude and Werner Wolf

Institut fuer Mathematik und Datenverarbeitung
Universitaet der Bundeswehr Muenchen, D-85577 Neubiberg, Germany
gerhard.staude@unibw-muenchen.de

Abstract. A method to precisely determine the onset of voluntary discrete movements in kinetic signals (e.g. joint angle) is presented. The movement onset is identified as an abrupt change in the (time varying) parameters of a statistical process model. An adaptive Kalman whitening filter transforms the digitized kinetic signal into a sequence of innovations which is examined for possible change-points by a generalized log-likelihood-ratio test. The accuracy of the algorithm is assessed by statistical simulations and compared to the accuracy of a standard threshold criterion. Results show that the method provides accurate change time estimates even for weak and highly variable response profiles.

1 Introduction

An important aspect of studying motor control mechanisms in humans is the analysis of reaction time (RT). RT (i.e., the time interval between stimulus presentation and the instant of movement initiation) has usually been measured with mechanical switches or photoelectric devices that indicate the onset of a voluntary motor response. Alternatively, the movement onset may be derived from the digitized kinetic signal by some automatic procedure (e.g., a threshold operation). However, when using simple amplitude threshold methods, particularly weak and abnormal response profiles which are typical for a variety of central motor disorders may introduce high RT variability as well as systematic errors [1]. This paper describes a new method for computerized onset detection which is based on statistical signal processing and includes a priori knowledge on the generator process of kinetic signals.

2 The Process Model

The method is based upon the process model in Fig. 1 which was derived from the nonlinear single-joint model established in [2]. The digitized kinetic signal is approximated by a discrete random process $(Y_k)_k$ which is generated by a Gaussian white noise process $(X_k)_k$ driving a linear filter $H(z)$. The former reflects the discharge timing and recruitment of independent signal sources involved (twitch forces contributed by single motor units), the latter describes the shape of the twitch forces as well as the mechanical properties of the joint. A distortion component $(N_k)_k$ considers measurement errors and "noise" contributed by other biological signal generators. $H(z)$ is modeled by an all-pole representation (autoregressive (AR) model) of order p

$$H(z) = \frac{1}{1 + a_1 z^{-1} + a_2 z^{-2} + \ldots + a_p z^{-p}} . \tag{1}$$

R.W. Brause and E. Hanisch (Eds.): ISMDA 2000, LNCS 1933, pp. 43–48, 2000.

$a_1, a_2, ... a_p$ are the AR parameters and z is the complex frequency of the z-transform. The time-domain representation of the signal generator is

$$X_k = \mu(k) + W_k , \qquad \tilde{Y}_k = -\sum_{i=1}^{p} a_i \tilde{Y}_{k-i} + X_k , \qquad Y_k = \tilde{Y}_k + N_k \qquad (2)$$

where $\tilde{Y}_k$ denotes the undisturbed output signal of the filter. Sequences $(W_k)_k$ and $(N_k)_k$ are uncorrelated zero mean Gaussian white noise signals with constant variances q and r, respectively. As an essential property of the model, the mean $\mu(k)$ of the white noise excitation $(X_k)_k$ is time variant. This yields the motor system the control over the biological signal generator in order to produce a particular movement. Within this framework, the response onset t_0 is defined as an abrupt change between two time varying profiles $\mu_0(k)$ and $\mu_1(k, t_0)$, as illustrated in Fig. 1.

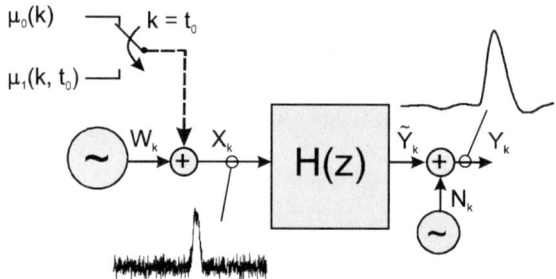

Fig.1 Process model for the kinetic signal of a responding subject.

3   The Algorithm

The properties of the sequence $(Y_k)_k$ are fully described by the (time varying) vector

$$M = \begin{bmatrix} a_1 & a_2 & \cdots & a_p & q & r & \mu(k) \end{bmatrix}^T \qquad (3)$$

comprising the parameters of the process model in Fig. 1. Thus, statistically optimal onset detection can be achieved with the aid of a binary hypothesis test between the two statistical models M_0 and M_1 which describe the signal properties before and after the change, respectively. The method consists of two stages, (i) an adaptive whitening filter $H_w(z)$, and (ii) a statistical decision element, as illustrated in Fig. 2. The whitening filter $H_w(z)$ adapted to the M_0 model transforms the measured signal $(Y_k)_k$ into an uncorrelated („white") sequence $(\varepsilon_k)_k$ of innovations. The new series $(\varepsilon_k)_k$ sensitively reflects deviations of $(Y_k)_k$ from the M_0 model. It is examined by a decision rule based upon the log-likelihood ratio test, which signals a possible change in model parameters (alarm time t_a) and, in addition, computes an estimate $\hat{t}_0$ of the unknown change time t_0.

3.1   The Adaptive Whitening Filter

The properties of $(Y_k)_k$ are determined to a large extend by the transfer function $H(z)$. According to the model, however, the change to be detected predominantly affects the excitation $(X_k)_k$, whereas $H(z)$ remains comparably constant.

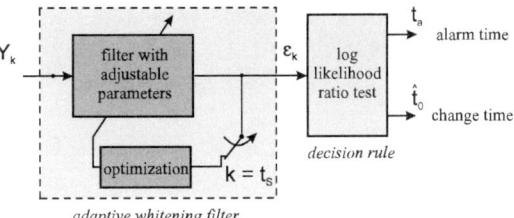

adaptive whitening filter

Fig. 2 Detection scheme for the determination of the response onset

This implies that all the information for event detection available in $(Y_k)_k$ is comprised by the mean profile $\mu(k)$ of the excitation, but the information contained in the AR parameters a_i is not relevant for correct detection of changes. In order to remove this irrelevant component from the signal before it enters the decision stage, an adaptive whitening filter is used. The filter with transfer function

$$H_w(z) = \frac{1 + c_1 z^{-1} + c_2 z^{-2} + \ldots + c_p z^{-p}}{1 + b_1 z^{-1} + b_2 z^{-2} + \ldots + b_p z^{-p}} \tag{4}$$

transforms the measured sequence $(Y_k)_k$ into a new series $(\varepsilon_k)_k$ called „the innovations". The filter coefficients are related to the M_0 model according to

$$c_i = a_i, \qquad b_i = \begin{cases} c_i(1 - l_1) + l_{i+1} & when \ 1 \le i < p \\ c_i(1 - l_1) & when \ i = p \end{cases} \tag{5}$$

where $L = [l_1 \, l_2 \cdots l_p]^T$ is the steady-state Kalman gain vector which depends upon the variances q and r of the process model [3].

Under noise-free conditions ($r = 0$), (4) reduces to a pure moving average (MA) filter

$$H_w(z) = 1 + c_1 z^{-1} + c_2 z^{-2} + \ldots + c_p z^{-p} \tag{6}$$

Thus, for $c_i = a_i$ and $r = 0$, the whitening filter represents an ideal inverse filter $H_w(z) = H^{-1}(z)$ with respect to the transfer function $H(z)$. The excitation $(X_k)_k$ can completely be reconstructed and the detection task reduces to the detection of a change in the dynamic mean $\mu(k)$ of a series of statistically independent Gaussian random variables with variance q. For $r > 0$, the filter still produces an independent Gaussian sequence, but with different mean profile $\mu^*(k)$. Since $\mu^*(k)$ can be obtained by filtering $\mu(k)$ with a filter

$$H_\mu(z) = \frac{1}{1 + b_1 z^{-1} + b_2 z^{-2} + \ldots + b_p z^{-p}}, \tag{7}$$

detection for $r > 0$ can be performed as in the ideal noise-free situation by using the modified (filtered) profile $\mu^*(k)$.

Usually, the parameters of the M_0 model are unknown. In this case, the coefficients b_i and c_i of the whitening filter are individually determined from the pre-stimulus interval $k < t_s$ which, by definition, only contains data produced by the M_0 model. As illustrated in Fig. 2, before stimulus presentation ($k < t_s$), model parameters are subjected to a standard least squares optimization technique [3]. At $k = t_s$, optimization is stopped and a filter with constant parameters is used to compute the innovations $(\varepsilon_k)_k$ for the remaining part of the record.

3.2   The Decision Element

From a statistical point of view, event detection represents a binary testing problem between the null hypothesis H_0 saying "there is no change in the statistical properties of the sequence $\varepsilon_1, \varepsilon_2, \cdots, \varepsilon_k$ actually observed and the mean profile is $\mu_0(i)$ for all times $1 \leq i \leq k$", and the alternate hypothesis H_1 "there is a change in statistical properties at some unknown change time $1 \leq j \leq k$, and the mean profiles are $\mu_0(i)$ before and $\mu_1(i, j)$ after this change". The adequate tool for binary hypothesis testing is the log-likelihood ratio test which compares the logarithm of the ratio between the two joint probability density functions for either hypothesis with a threshold [4]. The implementation of the test depends on the knowledge about $\mu_0(i)$ and $\mu_1(i,j)$.

If the model parameters (except t_0) are exactly known, the test can be efficiently implemented as a CUSUM type decision rule by comparing the cumulative sum

$$S_j^k = \sum_{i=j}^{k} s_i(j) , \qquad s_i(j) = \ln \frac{p_{\mu_1}(\varepsilon_i, j)}{p_{\mu_0}(\varepsilon_i)} \tag{8}$$

of the log-likelihood ratios $s_i(j)$ of the single samples with a threshold h [4]. $p_{\mu_0}(\varepsilon_i)$ and $p_{\mu_1}(\varepsilon_i, j)$ are the probability density functions of the i-th random variable before and after a possible change at j, respectively. Assuming a Gaussian density distribution, the individual log-likelihood ratio is explicitly given by

$$s_i(j) = \frac{\mu_1(i,j) - \mu_0(i)}{\sigma^2} \left[\varepsilon_i - \frac{1}{2} (\mu_1(i,j) + \mu_0(i)) \right] \tag{9}$$

where σ^2 is the (constant) variance of the process, and $\mu_0(i)$ and $\mu_1(i,j)$ denote the mean profiles before and after a change at j, respectively. Since the exact change time in (8) is unknown, it is replaced by its maximum likelihood (ML) estimate, i.e., a maximum operator selects the largest value of the test function with respect to all possible change times $1 \leq j \leq k$. The resulting CUSUM detection rule is

$$t_a = min \left\{ k \geq 1: \max_{1 \leq j \leq k} S_j^k \geq h \right\}, \quad \hat{t}_0 = arg \max_{1 \leq j \leq t_a} S_j^{t_a}$$

$$S_j^k = \sum_{i=j}^{k} \left[\frac{\mu_1(i,j) - \mu_0(i)}{\sigma^2} \left[\varepsilon_i - \frac{1}{2} (\mu_1(i,j) + \mu_0(i)) \right] \right] \tag{10}$$

The data sequence is analysed by a growing observation window which comprises all data points available at time k. A test window with the upper bound k fixed at the current observation and with its lower bound j proceeding reversely in time is applied to the data. For each possible change time j, S_j^k is computed from the observations $\varepsilon_j, \varepsilon_{j+1}, \cdots, \varepsilon_k$ within the test window. If the maximum of S_j^k with respect to all hypothetical change times $1 \leq j \leq k$ exceeds the threshold h, an event alarm is given (alarm time t_a). The time j at which the maximum value is obtained serves as the maximum likelihood estimate $\hat{t}_0$ of the unknown change time t_0.

In case the exact profiles $\mu_0(i)$ and $\mu_1(i,j)$ are unknown, they must be replaced by appropriate estimates. Generally, the mean profiles will depend upon several parameters θ_0 and θ_1 associated with the actual movements before and after the change, respectively. Estimates $\hat{\theta}_0$ of the unknown parameters θ_0 before change can be obtained off-line from the pre-stimulus interval which, by definition, contains signal samples corresponding to the null hypothesis only. During detection, these parameters then are considered to be known. Estimates $\hat{\theta}_1$ of the unknown parameters θ_1 after change, however, must be computed individually for each possible change time $1 \leq j \leq k$, at each time k a new data point is available. In order to avoid the multiple scheme of growing test windows of such a generalized likelihood ratio (GLR) procedure, an approximated GLR decision rule (AGLR) was used, which splits the detection procedure into separate phases of detection and change time estimation. During detection, a sliding window of fixed size L is continuously shifted along the data sequence. For each location of the window, the ML estimate $\hat{\theta}_1$ of the unknown parameter vector θ_1 is determined from the L data points covered by the window, and the corresponding $\hat{S}_{k-L+1}^{k}$ is computed. After a change has been indicated, the exact change time is estimated off-line by a ML procedure from all possible candidates $1 \leq j \leq t_a$. The AGLR decision rule can be summarized as

$$t_a = \min \left\{ k \geq d \colon \hat{S}_{k-L+1}^{k} \geq h \right\}, \qquad \hat{t}_0 = \arg\max_{1 \leq j \leq t_a} \hat{S}_j^{t_a+d^*}$$

$$\hat{S}_j^k = \sup_{\theta_1} \sum_{i=j}^{k} \frac{\mu_1(i,j,\theta_1) - \mu_0(i)}{\sigma^2} \left[\varepsilon_i - \frac{1}{2} \left(\mu_1(i,j,\theta_1) + \mu_0(i) \right) \right] \tag{11}$$

The quantities d and d^* are appropriate dead zones confining parameter estimation to a minimum number of observations.

In this study, the shape $u(i,j)$ of the change in the innovations was assumed to be known but with its exact magnitude unknown, i.e., $\mu_1(i,j,\theta_1) = \theta_1 u(i,j)$. In this case, maximization with respect to θ_1 is explicitly possible, and the log-likelihood ratio in (11) can be written as

$$\hat{S}_j^k = \frac{1}{\sigma^2} \left[\frac{1}{2} \left(\sum_{i=j}^{k} u(i,j)\varepsilon_i \right)^2 \left(\sum_{i=j}^{k} u^2(i,j) \right)^{-1} - \sum_{i=j}^{k} \mu_0(i) \left(\varepsilon_i - \frac{1}{2}\mu_0(i) \right) \right] \tag{12}$$

which facilitates efficient implementation of the test.

4   Simulation Results

The method was tested on 4000 simulated kinetic signals each comprising 1000 data points with known change time $t_0 = 500$. Signals were produced by using pseudo-noise sequences driving an AR system $H(z)$ of order $p = 4$ with narrow band transfer characteristic. The movements were initiated by ramp-like impulses in the mean pattern $\mu(k)$ with randomly varying magnitude and slope. The AGLR method was implemented using a ramp template with unit slope ($u(i,j) = i - j$) and a test window size of $L = 25$ samples. Fig. 3 depicts histograms of the estimation error $\Delta = \hat{t}_0 - t_0$ for several onset detectors. The AGLR method was compared to a simple (adaptive) threshold (ST) criterion. In addition, results of the CUSUM method exactly tuned with the true profiles $\mu_0(i)$ and $\mu_1(i,j)$ are shown as a reference for optimal performance. The ST method employed an adaptive threshold: event alarm occurred when the current sample Y_k exceeded three times the standard deviation of $(Y_k)_k$ estimated from the pre-stimulus period $k < t_s$. The broad shape of the error distribution of the ST method indicates highly variable onset estimates for this standard detection criterion. By contrast, the small error variance of only few samples indicates precise onset estimates of the AGLR method being nearly as accurate as those obtained with the (optimal) CUSUM detector.

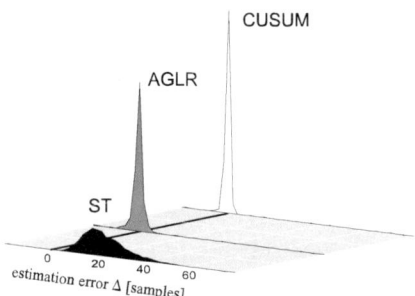

Fig. 3 Histograms of estimation error for different detection methods

5   Discussion

Inclusion of a priori knowledge on the biomechanical generator process of kinetic signals significantly enhances the accuracy of detected movement onsets. When the parameters of the process model are exactly known, the CUSUM detector can serve as a reference criterion, e.g., in order to assess the performance of more „realistic" methods by statistical simulations. When the exact model parameters are unknown, the AGLR method still provides high detection power by computing appropriate estimates of the unknown parameters.

References

1.   Staude, G., Wolf, W., Appel, U., Dengler, R.; Methods for onset detection of voluntary motor responses in tremor patients. IEEE Trans. Biomed. Eng., Vol. 43. (1996) 177-88
2.   Staude, G., Dengler, R., Wolf, W.: The discontinuous nature of motor execution I. A model concept for single-muscle multiple-task coordination. Biol. Cybern., Vol. 82. (2000) 23-33
3.   Goodwin, G.C., Sin, K.S.: Adaptive filtering, prediction and control. Prentice-Hall, Englewood Cliffs, New Jersey. (1984)
4.   Basseville, M., Nikiforov, I.V.: Detection of abrupt changes: Theory and application. Prentice-Hall, Englewood Cliffs, New Jersey. (1993) 29-43

Hierarchical Clustering of Functional MRI Time-Series by Deterministic Annealing[*]

Axel Wismüller[1], Dominik R. Dersch[2],
Bernadette Lipinski[3], Klaus Hahn[1], and Dorothee Auer[3]

[1] Institut für Radiologische Diagnostik,
Ludwig-Maximilians-Universität München,
Klinikum Innenstadt, Ziemssenstr. 1, D-80336 München, Germany
email: Axel.Wismueller@physik.uni-muenchen.de
[2] Integral Energy Corp., Sydney, Australia
[3] Max Planck Institute of Psychiatry, Munich, Germany

A bstract. In this paper, we present a neural network approach to hierarchical unsupervised clustering of functional magnetic resonance imaging (fMRI) time-sequences of the human brain by self-organized fuzzy minimal free energy vector quantization (VQ). In contrast to conventional model-based fMRI data analysis techniques, this deterministic annealing procedure does not imply presumptive knowledge of expected stimulus-response patterns, and, thus, may be applied to fMRI experiments in which the time course of the stimulus is unknown like in spontaneously occurring events, e.g. hallucinations, epileptic fits, or sleep. Moreover, as minimal free energy VQ represents a hierarchical data analysis strategy implying repetitive cluster splitting, it can provide a natural approach to the subclassification task of activated brain regions on different scales of resolution with respect to fine-grained differences in pixel dynamics.

1   Introduction

fMRI experiments induce spatio-temporal patterns of changing imaging properties in the human brain. Interpretation of these patterns as a response to a given experimental stimulus is the key problem of fMRI data analysis. Model-based approaches like cross-correlation techniques are commonly used to perform this task. However, as they imply presumptive knowledge of expected stimulus-response patterns, they may sometimes fail in unveiling complex signal changes, thus discarding valuable information about the fMRI signal. Moreover, in fMRI studies of spontaneously occurring events like hallucinations, epileptic fits, or sleep, even the exact time course of the stimulus is unknown.

Unsupervised clustering techniques offer a powerful strategy to overcome these problems. In this context, different vector quantization (VQ) algorithms have been proposed for a wide scope of biomedical signal processing problems including fMRI data analysis [11]. Here, the time-sequences of pixel grey values

R.W. Brause and E. Hanisch (Eds.): ISMDA 2000, LNCS 1933, pp. 49–54, 2001.
© Springer-Verlag Berlin Heidelberg 2001

obtained from fMRI experiments can be interpreted as feature vectors representing a multidimensional probability distribution. VQ procedures map a data
space onto a finite set of prototypical feature vectors, a so-called codebook. Examples of this class of algorithms are Kohonen's self-organizing maps (SOMs)
[8], minimal free energy VQ [10], [5], [4], [2], and the 'neural gas' algorithm [9].
    The mathematical properties of these algorithms, their motivation from sta-
tistical mechanics, as well as their strengthes and weaknesses in the field of
biosignal analysis have been thoroughly investigated in the literature (see e.g.
[2], [11]). SOMs have already been applied to fMRI data analysis [7]. Minimal free
energy VQ is a deterministic annealing procedure minimizing the free energy of
a multiparticle system in analogy to a canonical ensemble tending towards thermal equilibrium. In contrast to SOMs, this algorithm offers a specific advantage
for practical data analysis problems: it provides a *hierarchical* clustering scheme
on different scales of resolution [2], [3].
    In the field of fMRI time-sequence analysis, this offers a convenient method
for subclassification of activated areas according to similarities in signal time-
sequences. At the same time, heuristic manual merging of pixel clusters belonging
to different codebook vectors like in the SOM approach can be avoided. Merging
into larger meta-clusters can be replaced by back-tracking the codebook hierarchy tree to an earlier stage of the annealing procedure. Thus, the coarse-grained
structure of the data set can be explored in a natural manner.

2   Theory

Let n denote the number of subsequent scans in a fMRI experiment. The dynamics of each voxel i, i.e. the sequence of grey values $x_i(t)$ over all scan acquisition
time spots t can be interpreted as a vector $\boldsymbol{x}_i \in \mathbb{R}^n$ in the n-dimensional feature space of possible fMRI signal time-sequences. Clustering identifies groups
k of pixels with similar dynamics. These groups are represented by prototypical time-sequences called codebook vectors $\boldsymbol{w}_k$. Soft-competing VQ procedures
determine these cluster centers by an iterative adaptive update according to

$$\boldsymbol{w}_k(t+1) = \boldsymbol{w}_k(t) + \epsilon a_k(\boldsymbol{x}_i(t); W(t), \kappa)(\boldsymbol{x}_i(t) - \boldsymbol{w}_k(t)), \tag{1}$$

where ϵ denotes a learning parameter, a_k a so-called cooperativity function
which, in general, depends on the codebook $W(t)$, a cooperativity parameter
κ, and the presented feature vector $\boldsymbol{x}_i$ itself. In the fuzzy clustering scheme
proposed by Rose, Gurewitz, and Fox [10], the cooperativity function a_k reads

$$a_k(\boldsymbol{x}_i; W, \kappa \equiv \rho) = \frac{\exp(-E_k(\boldsymbol{x}_i)/2\rho^2)}{\mathcal{Z}} \tag{2}$$

Here, the 'energy' $E_k(\boldsymbol{x}_i) = \|\boldsymbol{w}_k - \boldsymbol{x}_i\|^2$ measures the distance between the
codebook vector $\boldsymbol{w}_k$ and the data vector $\boldsymbol{x}_i$. $\mathcal{Z}$ denotes a partition function given
by $\mathcal{Z} = \sum_k \exp(-E_k(\boldsymbol{x}_i)/2\rho^2)$ and ρ is the cooperativity parameter of this
model. That so-called 'fuzzy range' ρ defines a length scale in data space and

is annealed to repeatedly smaller values in the VQ procedure. The learning rule
(1) with a_k given by (2) describes a stochastic gradient descent on the error
function

$$F_\rho(W) = -\frac{1}{2\rho^2} \int P(\boldsymbol{x}) \ln \mathcal{Z} d^n x, \qquad (3)$$

which ia a free energy in a mean-field approximation [3]. Here, $P(\boldsymbol{x})$ denotes
the probability density of feature vectors $\boldsymbol{x}_i$. For the minimal free energy VQ
procedure, the codebook vectors mark local centers of this multidimensional
probability distribution. Thus, for the application to fMRI signal analysis, the
codebook vector $\boldsymbol{w}_k$ is the weighted average fMRI signal of all the time-sequences
$\boldsymbol{x}_i$ belonging to group k with respect to a fuzzy tesselation of the feature space.
    In contrast to SOMs, minimal free energy VQ

(i) can be described as a stochastic gradient descent on an explicitly given energy
     function (see (3)), [10],
(ii) preserves the probability density without distortion [5], [6], and, most im-
     portant for practical applications,
(iii) allows hierarchical data analysis on different scales of resolution [4].

    In the beginning of the VQ process, there is only one cluster representing the
center of the whole data set. As the deterministic annealing procedure contin-
ues, phase transitions occur and large clusters split up into smaller ones marking
increasingly smaller regions of the feature space. Tracing this repetitive cluster
splitting through the whole VQ procedure leads to a 'genealogy' of cluster centers, i.e. a resemblance tree of codebook vectors. Thus, the manual merging of
cluster centers into larger meta-clusters like in the SOM approach to fMRI analysis can be avoided. At the same time, the scope of resolution can be adapted
according to the observer's needs. The similarity of different codebook vectors
can easily be derived by back-tracking the clustering tree. The procedure can
be monitored by various control parameters like the free energy, entropy, reconstruction error etc. which allow an easy detection of cluster splitting [5].

3   Methods

Functional imaging was performed on a 1.5 T system (Signa, General Electrics,
Milwaukee) using a GI-EPI sequence (TR/TE = 4,000/66 msec) with 8 slices
and 64 images per experiment. Resolution was 3x3x4 mm, and three periods of
photic stimulation (8 Hz alternating checkerboard, central fixation point) were
interleaved by four control periods (dark background, central fixation point). The
first scan was discarded from analysis for remaining saturation effects. Movement
artifacts were compensated by automatic image alignment (AIR software, [12]).
    Average-corrected time-sequences of each pixel were clustered by minimal
free energy VQ employing 30 codebook vectors. The results were compared with
classical cross-correlation images (e.g. [1]).

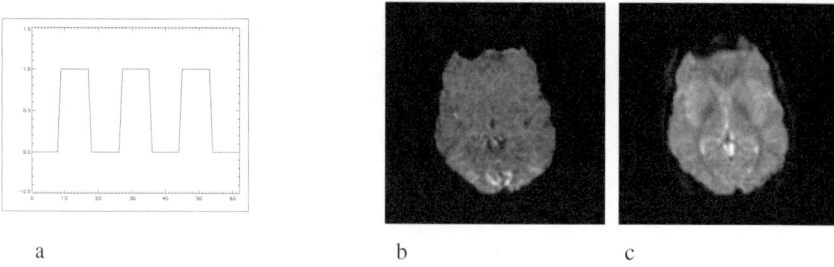

a   b   c

Fig. 1. (a) Stimulus. (b) Cross-correlation image. (c) Anatomical image.

4   Results

Figure 2 shows a part of the hierarchical clustering tree covering two subsequent VQ steps of the deterministic annealing procedure. Figure 2a presents one of 17 cluster centers present at the observed stage of VQ. Note the apparent similarity compared with the stimulus (Fig. 1a). Figure 2d shows all the pixels belonging to this cluster center according to a minimal distance criterion in the metric of the time-sequence feature space. The highlighted regions can be attributed to the visual cortex. They clearly correspond to the activated regions in the cross-correlation image (Fig. 1b).

Now a phase transition occurs in the subsequent VQ step, and the cluster of Fig. 2a splits up into two descendant clusters representing smaller regions of the visual cortex with different pixel dynamics. They are presented in the lower part of Fig. 2. Note that the sum of the activated areas in Fig. 2e and Fig. 2f is greater than the area of the cluster in Fig. 2b. This is based on a reduction in local reconstruction error due to the fact that the new codebook structure better fits the underlying local probability density. Thus, the descendant clusters can take over pixels which formerly were attributed to adjacent codebook vectors.

5   Discussion and Conclusion

The study shows that deterministic annealing by the minimal free energy VQ is a useful strategy for the analysis of fMRI data sets without presumptive knowledge of stimulus-response models or the stimulus function itself. In contrast to Kohonen's SOM algorithm, it realizes a hierarchical clustering procedure unveiling the structure of the data set with gradually increasing resolution. Therefore, heuristic manual merging of pixel clusters belonging to different codebook vectors like in the SOM approach can be avoided. Merging into larger meta-clusters can be replaced by back-tracking the codebook hierarchy tree to an earlier stage of the annealing procedure.

Thus, the structure of the data set can be explored in a natural manner. Therefore, we recommend minimal free energy VQ as an alternative to SOMs for unsupervised fMRI data analysis. Especially, it may be helpful in situations

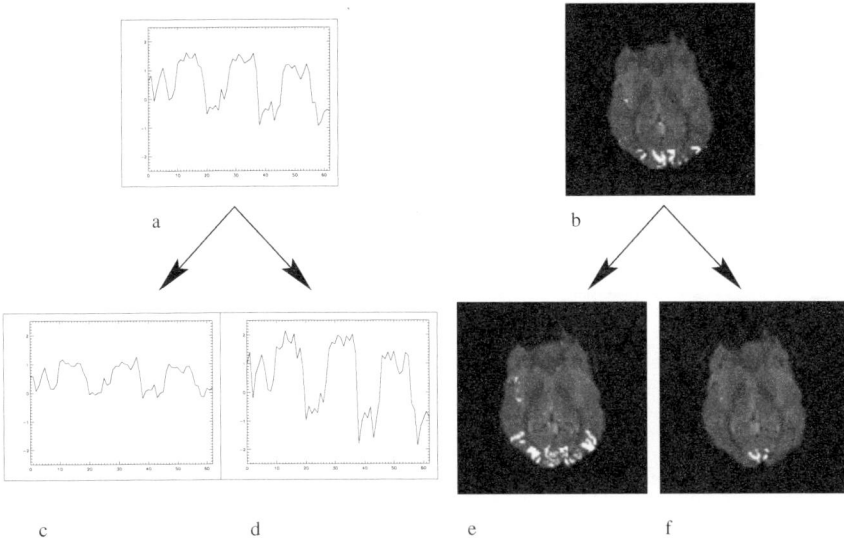

Fig. 2. Part of the hierarchical clustering tree demonstrating cluster separation during deterministic annealing by minimal free energy VQ. (a) Cluster center before phase transition, i.e. cluster separation. (b) Corresponding pixel cluster before phase transition according to a minimal distance criterion. (c,d) Cluster centers after phase transition. (e,f) Corresponding pixel clusters after phase transition.

where subclassification of activated brain regions on different scales of resolution is focused with respect to fine-grained differences in pixel dynamics.

Acknowledgements

This work has been funded by grants from the Hanns-Seidel-Foundation and the German Federal Ministry of Science and Technology (BMBF).

[*)] A similar paper has been presented at ICANN98.

References

1. P.A. Bandettini, A. Jesmanowicz, E.C. Wong, and J.S. Hyde: Processing strategies for time-course data sets in functional MRI of the human brain. Magn. Reson. Med. 30 (1993) 161–173 51

2. D.R. Dersch: Eigenschaften neuronaler Vektorquantisierer und ihre Anwendung in der Sprachverarbeitung. Verlag Harri Deutsch, Reihe Physik, Bd. 54, Thun, Frankfurt am Main (1996) ISBN 3-8171-1492-3 50, 50, 50

3. D.R. Dersch, S. Albrecht, and P. Tavan: Hierarchical fuzzy clustering. In A. Wismüller and D.R. Dersch, editors, Symposion über biologische Informationsverarbeitung und Neuronale Netze – SINN '95, Konferenzband. Hanns-Seidel-Stiftung, München (1996) 50, 51

4. D.R. Dersch and P. Tavan: Control of annealing in minimal free energy vector quantization. In Proceedings of the IEEE International Conference on Neural Networks ICNN'94, Orlando, Florida (1994) 698–703 50, 51

5. D.R. Dersch and P. Tavan: Load balanced vector quantization. In Proceedings of the International Conference on Artificial Neural Networks ICANN, Springer (1994) 1067–1070 50, 51, 51

6. D.R. Dersch and P. Tavan: Asymptotic level density in topological feature maps. IEEE Transactions on Neural Networks 6 (1) (1995) 230–236 51

7. H. Fischer, M. Buechert, and J. Hennig: Assessing the dynamics of fMRI data using self-organizing map clustering. In Proceedings of the 5th SMR meeting (1997) 50

8. T. Kohonen: The self-organizing map. Proceedings of the IEEE 78 (9) (1990) 1464–1480 50

9. T.M. Martinetz and K. Schulten: A 'neural gas' network learns topologies. In Proceedings of the International Conference on Artificial Neural Networks ICANN, Amsterdam, Elsevier Science Publishers (1991) 397–402 50

10. K. Rose, E. Gurewitz, and G.C. Fox: Vector quantization by deterministic annealing. IEEE Transactions on Information Theory 38 (4) (1992) 1249–1257 50, 50, 51

11. A. Wismüller and D.R. Dersch: Neural network computation in biomedical research: chances for conceptual cross-fertilization. Theory in Biosciences 116 (3) (1997) 49, 50

12. R.P. Woods, S.R. Cherry, and J.C. Mazziotta: Rapid automated algorithm for aligning and reslicing PET images. Journal of Computer Assisted Tomography 16 (1992) 620–633 51

Classification of Electro-encephalographic Spatial Patterns

T. Müller[1], T. Ball[2], R. Kristeva-Feige[2], Th. Mergner[2], and J. Timmer[1]

[1] Zentrum für Datenanalyse und Modellbildung,
Universität Freiburg,
Eckerstr. 1, 79104 Freiburg, Germany,
muellert@physik.uni-freiburg.de,
WWW home page: http://www.fdm.uni-freiburg.de
[2] Neurologische Universitätsklinik, Neurozentrum
Breisacher Str. 64, 79106 Freiburg, Germany

Abstract The aim of this study is to describe a general approach to determine important electrode positions in the case when the measured EEG-signal is used for classification. To classify planning of movement of right and left index finger, three different approaches were compared: classification using a physiologically motivated set of four electrodes, a set determined by principal component analysis and electrodes determined by spatial pattern analysis. Spatial pattern analysis enhanced the classification rate significantly from $61.3 \pm 1.8\%$ (with four electrodes) to $71.8 \pm 1.4\%$ whereas the classification rate using the principal component analysis is significantly lower ($65.2 \pm 1.4\%$). Most of the 61 electrodes used had no influence on the classification rate so that in future experiments the setup can be simplified drastically to 6 to 8 electrodes without loss of information.

1 Introduction

In many clinical studies using EEG as a measuring device, it is important to determine which electrodes carry significant information and which do not. Especially when using modern EEG-equipment with 32, 64 or even more electrodes it is often preferable to concentrate on a subset of electrodes. The process of selecting relevant electrode positions is a major problem when classifying single-trail EEG signals in real time to forecast the side of finger movements. With help of the measured time series various physiologically motivated quantities can be calculated which build up a feature vector. Adding the feature vectors of several electrodes, the problem of differentiating brain states is then reduced to the mathematical problem of classifying vectors in a high dimensional space. This paper was aimed at comparing the following approaches: 1) classification with four out of 61 electrodes motivated by physiological considerations, 2) classification with electrodes determined by principal component analysis (PCA) and 3) by spatial pattern analysis introduced by [6]. The general mathematical background and the results of data processing of five subjects are presented and discussed.

R.W. Brause and E. Hanisch (Eds.): ISMDA 2000, LNCS 1933, pp. 55–60, 2000.
© Springer-Verlag Berlin Heidelberg 2000

2 Experimental set-up and data recording

The EEG was measured from 61 equidistant scalp positions on both hemispheres
following the 10-20-system [4] with additional electrodes at the interspaces using
a 64-channel EEG system (NeuroScan).
Since the outer electrodes were distorted
by muscle artifacts, only the 42 inner
electrodes were used for analysis as displayed in Fig.1. The signal was band
pass filtered (0.1 to 40 Hz) and the sampling rate was 125 Hz. For a more detailed discussion see [8]. This procedure
lead to approx. 300 artifact free trials for
each subject, with approx. 150 trials for
left and right index finger movements.

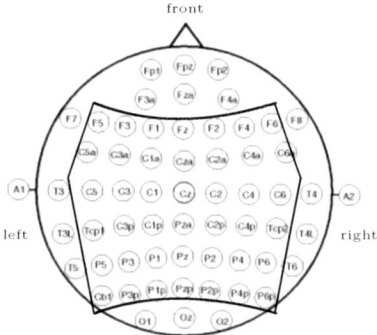

Figure 1: The 61 electrode
setup. The 42 inner electrodes
which are used for classification
are framed.

3 Parameter estimation and feature vector

When differentiating brain states by means of the measured EEG-signal, it is
important to characterize the underlying physiological processes by the recorded
time series. Denoting the measured EEG-signal at any electrode at time t by
$x(t)$, we used the μ-rhythm as the basis of the calculation for the feature vector
$\mathbf{f}$. Characterization of the μ-rhythm was performed by calculating the spectral
power in the frequency range $8 - 13\ Hz$ as proposed by [11]. Other physiological
processes are the readiness potential or the ERD/ERS, see [5,9]. These features
did not enhance classification rates and were therefore discarded, see [8]. The
μ-rhythm feature was calculated at each of the 42 electrode sites in every trial
and classification was done using the widely used multivariate approach, see [1].
Classification rates were estimated with cross-validation (95 % learning vectors,
5 % testing vectors, ten randomly chosen learning/testing sets).

4 Determining the optimal number of electrodes

4.1 The four electrode approach

A first approach is to use physiological information. Since the generator of the μ-
rhythm is located in the somatosensory cortex [2,10], only those electrodes which
are located over the sensorimotor cortex are considered for analysis. Based on
MRI-scans with electrode locations from four of the five subjects of the study,
electrodes of C3, C4, CP3 and CP4 were chosen for analysis.

a) left movements:

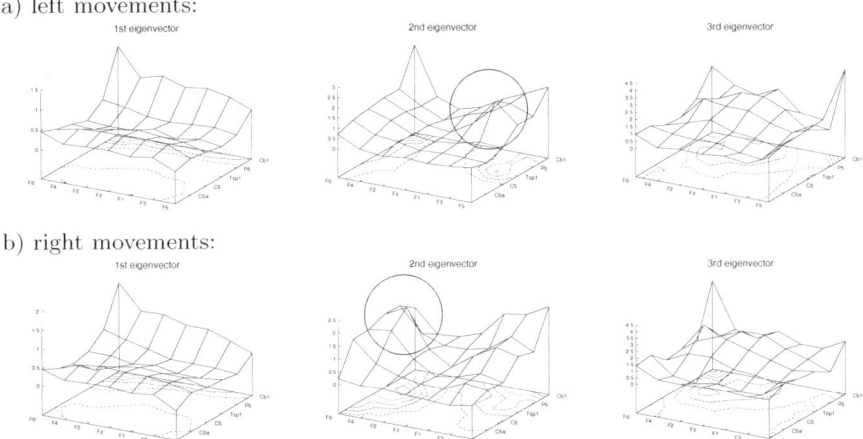

b) right movements:

Figure 3: The first three principal components of the measured EEG signals. The asymmetric behaviour of left- and right-handed movement leads to differences in the second principal component.

4.2 The principal component analysis approach

The second approach is to calculate the principal components of the EEG signals of the left and the right movements and to use only those electrodes which form the eigenvectors with the largest singular values. Given n measurements of the feature vector $\boldsymbol{x}(t_i) \in \mathbb{R}^q$ ($i=1,\ldots,n$, n=number of time points, q=number of electrodes) of left or right movements, the principal component analysis (PCA) determines a signal representation with vectors $\boldsymbol{\phi}_l$ ($l=1,\ldots,n$) so that

$$\mathbf{x}(t_i) = \sum_{l-1}^{q} \xi_{il}\boldsymbol{\phi}_l, \quad \boldsymbol{\phi}_l \in \mathbb{R}^q.$$

When using only some of the eigenvectors for signal representation to reduce the number of electrodes (e.g. the set $\mathbf{C} \subsetneq (1, \ldots, q)$), the least-squares error is

$$\varepsilon^2 = \sum_{i=1}^{n} \left(\mathbf{x}(t_i) - \sum_{l \in \mathbf{C}} \xi_{il}\boldsymbol{\phi}_l \right)^T \left(\mathbf{x}(t_i) - \sum_{l \in \mathbf{C}} \xi_{il}\boldsymbol{\phi}_l \right) = \sum_{l \notin \mathbf{C}} \lambda_l.$$

Therefore, taking the eigenvector with the largest eigenvalue is optimal in the sense of signal representation of each class. It is crucial that it is not optimal in the sense of classification although it seems highly probable that the differentiating signal, due to planning of left or right index finger movement, determines the EEG signal.

(a) spatial pattern of left movements

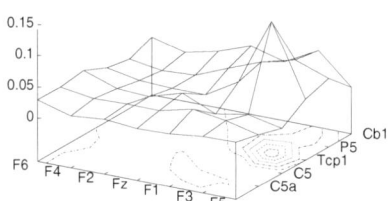

(b) spatial pattern of right movements

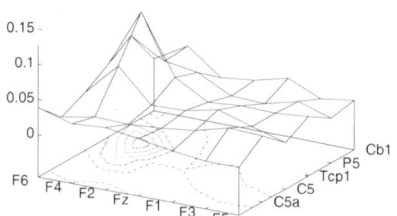

Figure 4: Spatial pattern determined with simultaneous diagonalisation. The electrodes with high impact are in accordance with the physiological information.

4.3   The spatial pattern approach

The third approach to determine the optimal electrodes aims directly at searching the set of vectors which maximizes the classification rate. The signal representation of the feature vectors of both left and right movements has to be done in the same base and we have to look for a base of eigenvectors of both covariance matrices $\mathbf{S}^1$ and $\mathbf{S}^2$ of the feature vectors of both classes. This is the mathematical problem of simultaneous diagonalisation, see [3]. If $\mathbf{S}^j$ $(j = 1, 2)$ are the covariance matrices of both classes and $\mathbf{S}^0 = \mathbf{S}^1 + \mathbf{S}^2$, then there exists an orthogonal matrix $\mathbf{P}$ with $\mathbf{P}\mathbf{S}^0\mathbf{P}^T = \mathbb{1}$ and the following equations for the transformed covariance matrices $\mathbf{T}^j = \mathbf{P}\mathbf{S}^j\mathbf{P}^T$ hold:

$$\mathbf{T}^1 + \mathbf{T}^2 = \mathbf{P}\mathbf{S}^1\mathbf{P}^T + \mathbf{P}\mathbf{S}^2\mathbf{P}^T \quad = \mathbb{1}$$
$$\Leftrightarrow \quad \mathbf{T}^1 = \mathbb{1} - \mathbf{T}^2. \tag{1}$$

If ϕ_l^j and λ_l^j are the eigenvectors and eigenvalues of the transformed and whitened covariance matrices $\mathbf{T}^j$, we get with eq. 1:

$$\mathbf{T}^2\phi_l^2 = \overset{\bullet}{\mathbb{1}} - \mathbf{T}^1{}^{\bullet}\phi_l^2 \quad = \lambda_l^2\phi_l^2$$
$$\Leftrightarrow \quad \mathbf{T}^1\phi_l^2 = (1 - \lambda_l^2)\,\phi_l^2,$$
$$\text{thus} \qquad \phi_l^1 = \phi_l^2 =: \phi_l, \quad \lambda_l^1 = (1 - \lambda_l^2). \tag{2}$$

Equation (2) means that the eigenvector with the largest eigenvalue of the transformed covariance matrix of class one equals the eigenvector with the smallest eigenvalue of the transformed covariance matrix of class two and vice versa. This ensures a minimum least-squares error when the signals of both classes are represented by a subset of eigenvectors with large and small eigenvalues. After calculating the common eigenvectors of the transformed matrices by simultaneous diagonalisation and after whitening the matrices, the new coefficients of the feature vector can be computed.

(a) Four electrodes   (b) PCA   (c) Spatial pattern

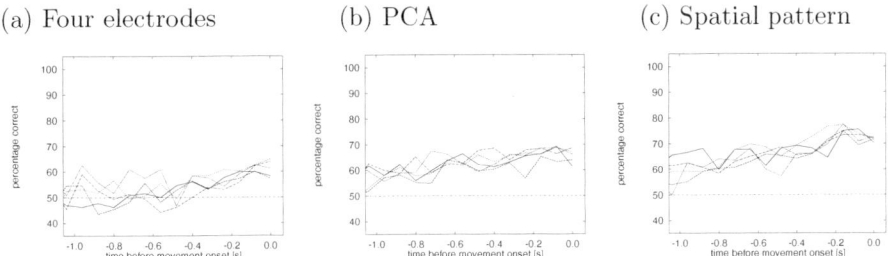

Figure 5: Time courses of the classification rates of all five subjects with the three different approaches. Movement onset is at $0.0s$.

5   Results

Fig.3 shows the first three principal components and the respective weight of each electrode of left and right movements of subject 5 determined with PCA. It is obvious that the principal components with the largest and the third largest singular value of both classes (left and right index finger movements) resemble each other. The principal components with the second largest singular value indicate the expected asymmetry due to the underlying physiological processes of left and right index finger movement. Fig.4 shows the spatial pattern of subject 5 determined with simultaneous diagonalisation. It follows from Fig. 4 that, like in the physiological approach, electrodes C3P and C4P are selected. In contrast to this approach electrode C3 has no weight at all and weight of electrode C4 is the same as of electrode P4, an electrode not considered by the first approach. To rate the three different approaches, the temporal evolution of the classification rates in the interval $[-250ms, 0ms]$ before movement onset are compared. Fig.5 shows the temporal evolution of the classification rates of every subject for the three different approaches. As expected, the classification rate at 1 s before the actual movement is 50% and no classification information can be drawn from the data. To compare the classification ability of the three different approaches we calculated the mean classification rate in the interval $[-250ms, 0ms]$. This yields a final classification rate of $61.3 \pm 1.8\%$ for the four electrode approach, $65.2 \pm 1.4\%$ for PCA and $71.8 \pm 1.4\%$ for spatial pattern analysis.

6   Discussion

Although planning of movement of left and right index finger leads to a distinguishable signal, the measured EEG time series are still dominated by physiological processes which are found at both left and right movements. Classification with help of the principal components is therefore inevitably leading to a low classification rate. This confirms the results of [7] who studied PCA as a feature extraction tool in a two electrode setting. In contrast to the PCA the spatial pattern method is able to determine the signal which is caused by the differences in the planning of movement of left and right index finger. In addition it improves the classification rate significantly and facilitates the experimental setup considerably. For every subject an optimal electrode setup can be determined.

7   Acknowledgement

We thank Johannes Müller-Gerking for valuable discussion on the analysis. This study was partly supported by DFG grant KR 1392/7-1.

References

1. R. O. Duda and P. E. Hart. *Pattern Classification and Scene Analysis.* John Wiley & Sons, New York, 1973.
2. B. Feige, R. Kristeva-Feige, S. Rossi, V. Pizzella, and PM. Rossini. Neuromagnetic study of movement-related changes in rhythmic brain activity. *Brain Research,* 734:252–260, 1996.
3. K. Fukunaga. *Introduction to statistical pattern recognition.* Academic Press, Boston, 1990.
4. H. Jasper. *Handbook of Electroencephalography and Clinical Neurophysiology 3, Appendix III: The 10-20 electrode system of the International Federation.* Elsevier, Amsterdam, 1974.
5. J. Kalcher, D. Flotzinger, Ch. Neuper, S. Gölly, and G. Pfurtscheller. Graz brain-computer interface II: towards communication between humans and computers based on online classification of three different EEG patterns. *Med. & Biol. Eng. & Comput.,* 34:382–388, 1996.
6. Z. Koles, M. Lazar, and S. Zhou. Spatial patterns underlying population differences in the background EEG. *Brain Topography,* 2(4):275–284, 1990.
7. K. Lugger, Flotzinger D., Schlögl A., Pregenzer M., and Pfurtscheller G. Feature extraction for on-line EEG classification using principal components and linear discriminants. *Med. Biol. Eng. Comput.,* 36:309–314, 1998.
8. T. Müller, T. Ball, R. Kristeva-Feige, T. Mergner, and J. Timmer. Selecting relevant electrode positions for classification tasks based on the electro-encephalogram. *Med. & Biol. Eng. & Comp.,* 38:62–67, 2000.
9. G. Pfurtscheller and A. Aranibar. Evaluation of event-related desynchronisation (ERD) preceding and following voluntary self-paced movement. *Electroenceph. Clin. Neurophysiol.,* 46:138–146, 1978.
10. R. Salmelin and R. Hari. Spatiotemporal characteristics of sensorimotor neuromagnetic rhythms related to thumb movement. *Neuroscience,* 60(2):537–550, 1994.
11. W. Storm van Leeuwen, G. Wieneke, P. Spoelstra, and H. Versteeg. Lack of bilateral coherence of mu rhythm. *Electroenceph. Clin. Neurophysiol.,* 44:140–146, 1977.

Detection and Classification of Sleep-Disordered Breathing Using Acoustic Respiratory Input Impedance and Nasal Pressure

Holger Steltner[1], Richard Staats[2], Michael Vogel[2], Christian Virchow[2], Heinrich Matthys[2], Josef Guttmann[3], and Jens Timmer[1]

[1] Center for Data Analysis and Modeling, University of Freiburg,
Eckerstr. 1, 79104 Freiburg, Germany,
{steltner, jeti}@fdm.uni-freiburg.de
[2] Department for Pneumology, University Hospital Freiburg,
Hugstetter Str. 55, 79106 Freiburg, Germany,
{staats, vogel, virchow, matthys}@med1.ukl.uni-freiburg.de
[3] Section for Experimental Anaesthesiology, University Hospital Freiburg,
Hugstetter Str. 55, 79106 Freiburg, Germany,
guttmann@ana1.ukl.uni-freiburg.de

Abstract. We are developing an algorithm for off-line detection and classification of sleep-disordered breathing based on time series analysis of nasal mask pressure and acoustic respiratory input impedance measured by forced oscillation technique at a frequency of 20 Hz throughout the night. A first version of the algorithm was applied to a data set consisting of full-night measurements on 5 subjects. The data set had a total duration of 34 hours and contained 577 respiratory events (hypopneas, obstructive and central apneas) recognized by the staff physicians of an accredited sleep laboratory. The algorithm detected 455 (79 %) of these events and 138 events that had not been marked by the physicians. 75 % of the congruently detected events were also concordantly classified. After further optimization and evaluation, this approach might be useful when implemented into a device designed to screening or treatment control of sleep-related breathing disorders at home.

1 Introduction

Sleep-related breathing disorders represent a major public health problem. They are characterized by recurrent episodes of reduced or absent respiratory airflow during sleep. Consequences are, e.g., excessive daytime sleepiness and an increased risk for cardiovascular diseases. Epidemiologic studies have estimated that 4 % of middle-aged men and 2 % of middle-aged women have symptomatic sleep apnea syndrome [1]. Furthermore, 80 % to 90 % of persons with obstructive sleep apnea are likely not to have received a clinical diagnosis [2].

One important aspect of the diagnosis of sleep-disordered breathing (SDB) with respect to the choice of an appropriate therapeutic method is the detection

R.W. Brause and E. Hanisch (Eds.): ISMDA 2000, LNCS 1933, pp. 61–66, 2000.
© Springer-Verlag Berlin Heidelberg 2000

and distinction of different kinds of respiratory events: Central apneas are characterized by the absence of both breathing flow and respiratory effort. During obstructive apneas, there is no airflow although the respiratory effort and the corresponding thoracoabdominal movements persist; the upper airways are occluded due to reduced activity of the pharyngeal dilator muscles.Hypopneas are periods of reduced respiratory flow.

Diagnosis of sleep-related breathing disorders is usually performed by polysomnographic examinations during at least one night in a sleep laboratory. Polysomnography (PSG) includes the measurement and recording of numerous signals used to analyze sleep and breathing. While PSG is currently the gold standard for the diagnosis of SDB, it is relatively expensive, and waiting periods are often up to several months. Different portable devices dedicated to the diagnosis of SDB in a home setting have been proposed, however, they either do not allow for the distinction between obstructive and central apneas [3] or rely on a multitude of sensors that have to be thoroughly fixed by the patient [4].

Acoustic respiratory input impedance measured by forced oscillation technique (FOT) and nasal pressure are currently not part of standard PSG. However, nasal pressure has been shown to be a sensitive indicator of sleep-disordered breathing [5]. Acoustic respiratory input impedance reflects diameter and patency of the upper airways [6–8] and has been applied to the detection and distinction of apneas with open and obstructed airways [9, 10]. We are developing an algorithm that retrospectively detects and distinguishes respiratory events by analyzing these two signals which are simultaneously accessible via a nasal mask.

2   Materials and Methods

2.1   Data Acquisition

PSG was performed using a SIDAS-GS device (Stimotron-Respironics, Gießen, Germany) and included recording of two EEG channels, submental and tibial EMG, left and right EOG, ECG, and body position. Furthermore, a pulse oximeter monitored oxygen saturation (Sa_{O_2}), oronasal airflow (Flow) was obtained from a thermistor, thoracic and abdominal movements (Thor, Abdo) from strain gauges and snoring sounds (Snor) from a microphone.

The modulus of acoustic respiratory input impedance ($|Z|$) was measured via a nasal mask by a FOT device (ODS-Messbox, Weinmann, Hamburg, Germany) at a frequency of 20 Hz. The nasal mask was connected to a continuous positive airway pressure (CPAP) device (SOMNOTRON 4, Weinmann, Hamburg, Germany) which is used to treat obstructive sleep-related breathing disorders. In our setting, it provided a subtherapeutic pressure of 4 mbar to allow the awake subject to breathe normally by compensating for the resistance of the mask and by avoiding rebreathing of CO_2. $|Z|$ and nasal mask pressure p_m were stored at respective sampling rates of 10 Hz and 25 Hz together with the standard polysomnographic data.

2.2   Visual Analysis

Visual analysis of the polysomnographic records with respect to SDB events was carried out by the staff physicians of the sleep laboratory in the Department for Pneumology at Freiburg University Hospital according to the following definitions adapted from [11]:

All events have to last 10 seconds or longer.

hypopnea: $> 50\,\%$ decrease from baseline in the amplitude of thermistor signal (Flow) or mask pressure (p_m); or a clear amplitude reduction not reaching the above criteria but associated with an oxygen desaturation of $> 3\,\%$ or an arousal. Baseline is the mean amplitude of stable breathing and oxygenation in the two minutes preceding onset of the event or the mean amplitude of the three largest breaths in the two minutes preceding onset of the event (the latter for individuals without a stable breathing pattern).

obstructive apnea: Zero Flow and constant p_m with persisting thoracoabdominal movements.

central apnea: Zero Flow and constant p_m without thoracoabdominal movements.

Five subjects with SDB of different kinds and severities were examined by PSG including measurement of $|Z|$ and p_m. The data were divided into a training set (duration 1.5 hours) containing 29 hypopneas, 19 obstructive apneas and 7 central apneas and a test set (duration 34 hours) with 419 hypopneas, 134 obstructive and 24 central apneas.

2.3   Acoustic respiratory input impedance during respiratory events

Obstructive respiratory events are characterized by upper airway narrowing. As a consequence, they are always associated with a higher baseline of $|Z|$ than during normal breathing (see Fig. 1). Variations of $|Z|$ within a breathing cycle are less pronounced during obstructive apneas than during hypopneas.

During central apneas with open airways, $|Z|$ is low (see Fig. 2 a). However, upper airway narrowing can also come along with central apneas. In this case, oscillations reflecting the heart beat can be used to distinguish central and obstructive apneas (Fig. 2 b). These cardiac oscillations have frequently been observed in respiratory signals during central apneas, but never in the course of obstructive events [12].

2.4   Algorithm for the Detection and Classification of SDB Events

The automatic detection of respiratory events is based on the definition for hypopneas applied to the nasal mask pressure signal: For each breathing cycle, a threshold $c_{p,\mathrm{ev}}$ is derived from the pressure amplitudes of the preceding two minutes. If the current amplitude falls below this threshold and stays low for at least 10 s, the respective times are stored as onset and end point of a respiratory event.

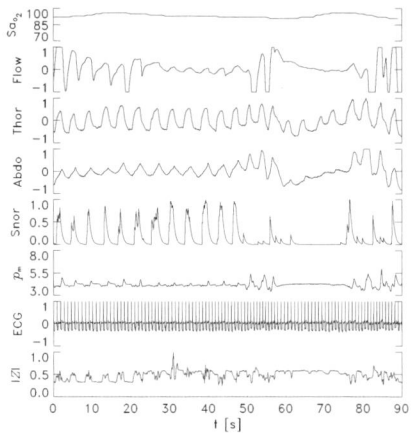

Fig. 1. Sequence of polysomnographic recording including a hypopnea (between $t = 25\,$s and $t = 50\,$s) and an obstructive apnea (between $t = 60\,$s and $t = 75\,$s. Sa_{O_2} is in %, p_m in mbar, the other signals are in arbitrary units.

Thresholds $c_{p,\text{ah}}$ for mask pressure and $c_{|Z|,\text{ah}}$ for acoustic respiratory input impedance are calculated on the basis of the three breaths preceding and following the event. If the amplitudes of p_m and $|Z|$ are below these values for at least 10 s during the event, it is considered to be an apnea, otherwise a hypopnea.

When dealing with an apnea, threshold $c_{|Z|,\text{oc}}$ for the baseline of $|Z|$ is computed using the three breaths preceding and following the event. If the median of $|Z|$ during the event is less than $c_{|Z|,\text{oc}}$, it is classified as a central apnea. If it is higher, the autocorrelation function $\text{ACF}_{|Z|}$ of normalized $|Z|$ is computed for segments of 5 s duration during the apnea. Examples for such patterns of $\text{ACF}_{|Z|}$ during central and obstructive apneas are depicted in Fig. 3. If the first maximum of $\text{ACF}_{|Z|}$ falls within a time interval $[t_{\text{ACF1}}, t_{\text{ACF2}}]$ and if its value is higher than c_{ACF} for one of these segments, the event is classified as a central apnea, otherwise as an obstructive apnea.

Appropriate parameters and thresholds for a first version of the algorithm were determined on the basis of the training set. This algorithm was then applied to the test set, the results were compared to the outcome of the visual analysis.

3 Results

The algorithm detected 455 (79 %) of the visually recognized respiratory events and 138 events that had not been marked by the physicians. 75 % of the congruently detected events were also concordantly classified. In particular, only 4 obstructive apneas were classified as central apneas by the algorithm, and none of the central apneas was classified as obstructive.

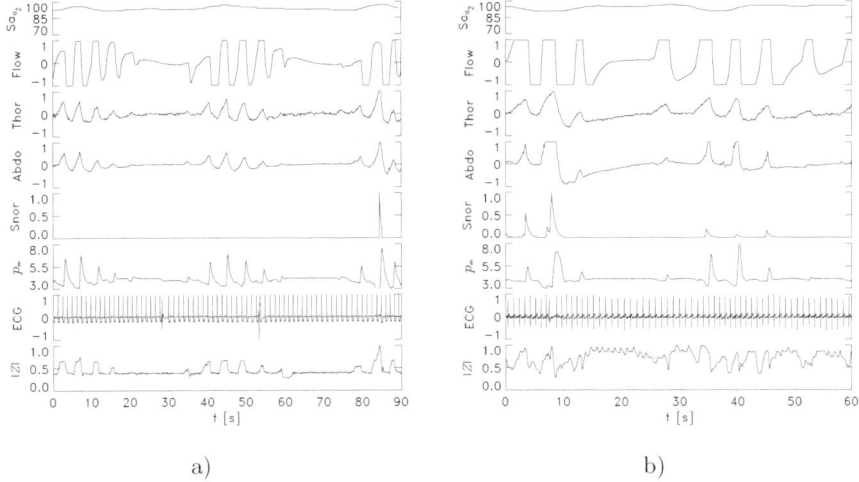

a)   b)

Fig. 2. Sequences of polysomnographic recording including central apneas with (a) low $|Z|$ and (b) high $|Z|$ as well as cardiac oscillations during the apnea. Sa_{O_2} is in %, p_m in mbar, the other signals are in arbitrary units.

4   Discussion

The first version of the described algorithm for retrospective detection and classification of respiratory events provides results comparable to the visual analysis of polysomnographic recordings carried out by human sleep experts. Discrepancies between visual and automatic analysis are mainly due to different opinions concerning the duration of particular events and the presence or absence of respiratory airflow. A more rigorous interpretation of the definitions for apneas and hypopneas might further improve the accordance. In some cases, however, the algorithm can not be expected to produce the same results as a human scorer because of the limited information: For the sake of practical applicability, neither oxygen saturation nor the thermistor signal are used for automatic analysis. Furthermore, a human scorer can use his knowledge about arousals and sleep stages deduced from EEG and EMG signals.

All these aspects considered, the preliminary results are very promising. After further optimization and evaluation using a higher number of data sets, this approach might be useful when implemented into a diagnostic device designed to screening or treatment control of sleep-related breathing disorders.

References

1. Young, T., Palta, M., Dempsey, J., Skatrud, J., Weber, S., Badr, S.: The Occurrence of Sleep-Disordered Breathing among Middle-Aged Adults. N. Engl. J. Med. **328** (1993) 1230–1235

66   H. Steltner et al.

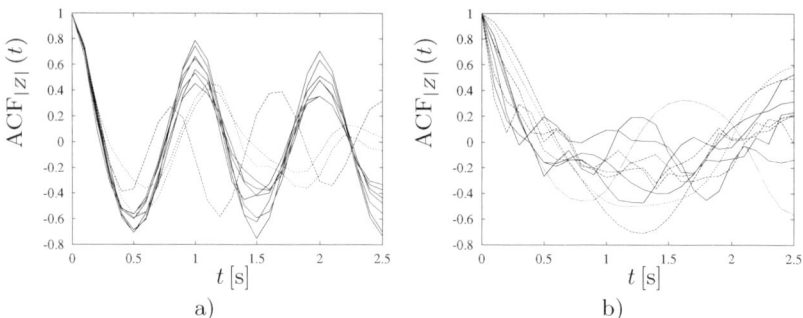

Fig. 3. Autocorrelation function of ten segments of $|Z|$ measured during central apneas with cardiac oscillations (a) and obstructive apneas (b). Each linestyle represents a different patient.

2. Young, T., Evans, L., Finn, L., Palta, M.: Estimation of the Clinically Diagnosed Proportion of Sleep Apnea Syndrome in Middle-Aged Men and Women. Sleep **20** (1997) 705–706
3. Baltzan, M. A., Verschelden, P., Al-Jahdali, H., Olha, A. E., Kimoff, R. J.: Accuracy of Oximetry with Thermistor (OxiFlow) for Diagnosis of Obstructive Sleep Apnea and Hypopnea. Sleep **23** (2000) 61–69
4. Mykytyn, I. J., Sajkov, D., Neill, A. M., McEvoy, R. D.: Portable computerized polysomnography in attended and unattended settings. Chest **115** (1999) 114–122
5. Norman, R. G., Ahmed, M. M., Walsleben, J. A., Rapoport, D. M.: Detection of Respiratory Events During NPSG: Nasal Cannula/Pressure Sensor Versus Thermistor. Sleep **20** (1997) 1175–1184
6. Farré, R., Peslin, R., Rotger, M., Navajas, D.: Inspiratory Dynamic Obstruction Detected by Forced Oscillation during CPAP: a Model Study. Am. J. Respir. Crit. Care Med. **155** (1997) 952–956
7. Reisch, S., Schneider, M., Timmer, J., Geiger, K., Guttmann, J.: Evaluation of forced oscillation technique for early detection of airway obstruction in sleep apnea: a model study. Technol. Health Care **6** (1998) 245–257
8. Reisch, S., Steltner, H., Timmer, J., Renotte, C., Guttmann, J.: Early detection of upper airway obstructions by analysis of acoustical respiratory input impedance. Biol. Cybern. **81** (1999) 25–37
9. Yen, F.-C., Behbehani, K., Lucas, E. A., Burk, J. R., Axe, J. R.: A Noninvasive Technique for Detecting Obstructive and Central Sleep Apnea. IEEE Trans. Biomed. Eng. **44** (1997) 1262–1268
10. Badia, J. R., Farré, R., Montserrat, J. M., Ballester, E., Hernández, L., Rotger, M., Rodriguez-Roisin, R., Navajas, D.: Forced oscillation technique for the evaluation of severe sleep apnoea/hypopnoea syndrome: a pilot study. Eur. Respir. J. **11** (1998) 1128–1134
11. Sleep-Related Breathing Disorders in Adults: Recommendations for Syndrome Definition and Measurement Techniques in Clinical Research. The Report of an American Academy of Sleep Medicine Task Force. Sleep **22** (1999) 667–689
12. Ayappa, I., Norman, R. G., Rapoport, D. M.: Cardiogenic Oscillations on the Airflow Signal During Continuous Positive Airway Pressure as a Marker of Central Apnea. Chest **116** (1999) 660–666

Some Statistical Methods in Intensive Care Online Monitoring – A Review

Roland Fried[1], Ursula Gather[1], Michael Imhoff[2], and Marcus Bauer[1]

[1] University of Dortmund, Department of Statistics, Vogelpothsweg 87,
D-44221 Dortmund, Germany
{Fried, Gather}@statistik.uni-dortmund.de
http://www.statistik.uni-dortmund.de/sfb475/sfb475.htm
[2] Community Hospital Dortmund, Surgical Department, Beurhausstr. 40,
D-44137 Dortmund, Germany
mike@imhoff.de

Abstract. Intelligent alarm systems are needed for adequate bedside decision support in critical care. Clinical information systems acquire physiological variables online in short time intervals. To identify complications as well as therapeutic effects procedures for rapid classification of the current state of the patient have to be developed. Detection of characteristic patterns in the data can be accomplished by statistical time series analysis. In view of the high dimension of the data statistical methods for dimension reduction should be used in advance. We discuss the potential of statistical techniques for online monitoring.

1 Introduction

In intensive care, today clinical information systems (CIS) acquire and store all physiological and device parameters online every minute. Currently a physician can be confronted with more than 200 variables of the critically ill patient during a typical morning round. However, even an experienced physician is not able to develop a systematic response to any problem involving more than seven variables [1] nor is he able to judge the degree of relatedness between more than two variables [2]. Thus electronic bedside decision support offers huge potential benefit. On the other hand, the technological progress achieved in the electronic patient record during the last ten years [3] bears new challenges for statistical methodology. Techniques of statistical data analysis have to be automated and adapted to the online-monitoring context.

Existing alarm systems based on fixed thresholds produce a large number of false alarms due to measurement artefacts or patient movements [4]. Usually changes of a variable with time are more important than a single pathological value at the time of observation. Hence, the online detection of qualitative patterns such as outliers, level changes or trends in physiological variables is important for assessing the patient's state. Qualitative data abstraction has been developed using deviations of the measurements from the target range [5], so-called trend templates [6], or robust adaptive control charts [7]. However, they

R.W. Brause and E. Hanisch (Eds.): ISMDA 2000, LNCS 1933, pp. 67–77, 2000.
© Springer-Verlag Berlin Heidelberg 2000

do not consider temporal correlations or they demand predefinition of expected behaviour, which is hard to specify in advance because of the irregular patterns found in critical care.

Statistical time series modelling has been proven useful for retrospective analysis of physiologic variables. It leads to interpretable descriptions of complex underlying dynamics, provides forecasts, gives confidence bounds and allows the assessment of the clinical effects of therapeutic interventions [8, 9, 10, 11]. For pattern detection in single variables, techniques such as multiprocess models, dynamic linear models, ARIMA-models, and phase space models have already been applied.

Pattern detection in multivariate time series of several physiologic variables is much more difficult than in univariate series. Furthermore, in high dimensions the computational effort can exceed any available computational power [12]. This problem becomes even more severe in the online monitoring context where fast and robust algorithms are needed. The demand for robustness against disturbances like sequences of patchy outliers arises because of their negative effects on correct pattern classification. In consequence, reliable procedures for analysing multivariate physiologic time series have to be developed and validated with real data. Statistical methods like graphical models, sliced inverse regression, principal component analysis and factor analysis can be applied for dimension reduction.

In the following we discuss statistical methods for time series analysis and for dimension reduction. We explore how they can be combined for achieving suitable bedside decision support and report our experiences w.r.t. analysing the hemodynamic system, i.e. variables such as blood pressures, heart rate, pulse, blood temperature and pulsoximetry.

2   Statistical Time Series Analysis

Subsequent measurements of the same variable typically show autocorrelated behaviour, i.e., subsequent observations are often positively related. Statistical methods for time series allow to consider such autocorrelations in the data analysis. Particularly we aim at the online detection of patterns such as level changes, artefacts and trends in physiologic time series. The reliable distinction between these patterns is difficult since often combinations of several patterns occur (see Figure 1).

2.1   Dynamic Linear Models

In one of the first attempts to apply statistical time series analysis to online monitoring data, Smith and West [13] used a multiprocess dynamic linear model to monitor patients after renal transplantation. In dynamic linear models (DLMs) [14] the observation X_t at time t is considered as a linear transformation of an unobservable vector of state parameters. These states are assumed to change

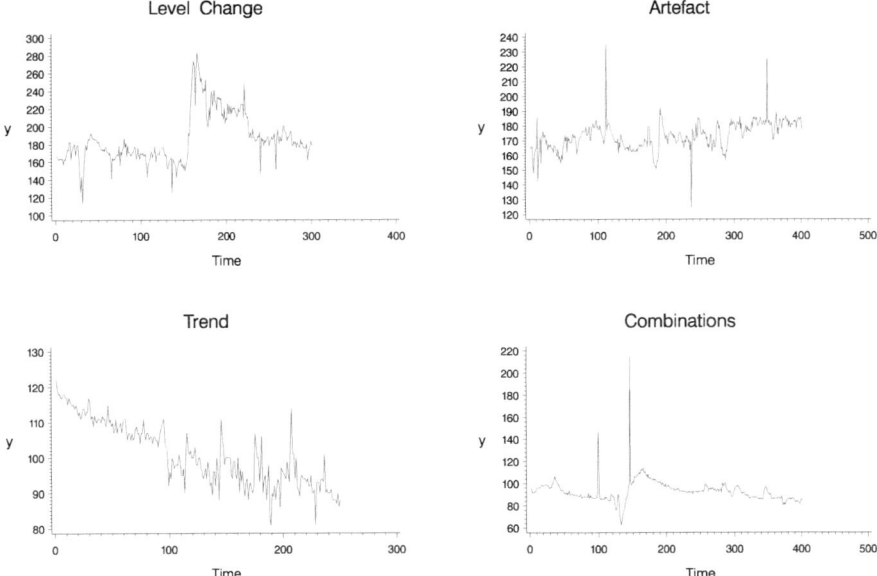

Fig. 1. Patterns of change in univariate physiologic time series. Combinations of several patterns, which usually occur in practice, may cause problems for any identification rule

dynamically in time according to a simple regression model. The linear growth model

$$X_t = \mu_t + \epsilon_t$$
$$\mu_t = \mu_{t-1} + \beta_{t-1} + \delta_{t,1}$$
$$\beta_t = \beta_{t-1} + \delta_{t,2}$$

is very appealing for describing hemodynamic variables. Here, μ_t is the unknown process level and β_t is the unknown slope at time t. In the multiprocess version used by Smith and West different variances of the random observation error ϵ_t and the random change in evolution $\delta_{t,j}$ at time t are assumed for describing the steady state, outliers, level changes and trends. For pattern classification they calculated the posterior probabilities of these states in a Bayesian framework using a multiprocess Kalman filter. In related work time series from anaesthesia were analysed [15].

Routine application of these models has not been practiced yet because of their very strong sensitivity against misspezification of the hyperparameters and their insensitivity against moderate level shifts.

The computational effort can significantly be reduced by using a single-process model. Pattern detection can be accomplished by assessing the influence of recent observations on the parameter estimates. This can be done via influence statistics [16] which compare estimates of the state parameters calculated with and without the most recent observations. When an outlier occurs the current level is supposed to be far from the current observation, while for a level change and a trend the recent observations should have a large influence on the estimate of the level and slope parameter respectively.

While this technique was successfully applied for retrospective analysis [17, 18], online detection of patterns by influence statistics has difficulties with little variability during the estimation period, with level changes occuring stepwise and with patterns of outliers in short time lags. Little variability during the estimation period causes the detection of outliers and level changes to be too sensitive subsequently. Stepwise level changes are hard to detect since the smoothed level parameter adjusts step by step, so that the influence statistics do not have significant values at any time. Several close outliers may either mask each other or be mistaken for a level change. Nevertheless, all kind of patterns in hemodynamic time series could correctly be identified in most cases [19].

2.2 ARMA Models

An autoregressive moving average (ARMA(p, q)) model [20] for a time series formally resembles a multiple regression, where the observation X_t is assumed to be a linear transform of p past observations $X_{t-1}, \ldots, X_{t-p}$ and q unobserved past shocks $\epsilon_{t-1}, \ldots, \epsilon_{t-q}$

$$X_t = \phi_1 X_{t-1} + \ldots + \phi_p X_{t-p} + \theta_1 \epsilon_{t-1} + \cdots \theta_q \epsilon_{t-q} + \epsilon_t, t \in \mathbb{Z},$$

where $\phi_1, \ldots, \phi_p, \theta_1, \ldots, \theta_q$ are unknown weights. The unobserved shocks ϵ_t are assumed to form a sequence of uncorrelated variables from a fixed distribution with mean zero and time invariant variance. This model describes the autocorrelations within a time series in a tractable way and results in simple computational formulas for parameter estimation, prediction and confidence intervals for predictions.

Pattern detection can be accomplished by comparing the incoming observations to confidence intervals for the predictions (PI). Time series segments can be classified into the several patterns according to the number of values outside the PI. Following medical reasoning we can classify observations as outliers if less than 5 consecutive observations are outside the PI, while a level change can be identified by 5 or more consecutive observations outside the PI [21].

In practice, a suitable model order has to be determined first. This can be done by analysing a preliminary estimation period of, say, 60 minutes. Either one could use the autocorrelation and partial autocorrelation function of these observations, or model selection criteria such as the Akaike information criterion [22] could be used to specify a suitable model order for this estimation period. However, this is time-consuming and needs some statistical experience. Moreover, in practice sampling variation makes this task difficult, particularly in the online monitoring context where estimation intervals have to be rather short. Hence, an extensive model selection process is not possible in online monitoring and has to be avoided.

Online application of ARMA models can be simplified significantly by using the same model order for all patients. Analysis of hemodynamic time series provided evidence that autoregressive models (AR(p), i.e. ARMA(p,q)-models with $q = 0$) of order two may be suitable to describe the autocorrelations within the data in most cases [11, 23, 24], while choosing higher model orders results in minor differences only [21]. Therefore, choosing an overparameterized autoregressive model could be suitable.

Adaptive control limits corresponding to the current state of the patient can be achieved by moving a time window through the data for estimation. Prediction intervals for the incoming observations are calculated using the parameter estimates from the observations measured within the last hour for instance. If the incoming observation lies within the prediction interval, then the time window is moved one step ahead, otherwise the incoming observation is replaced by its prediction.

Trend detection cannot appropriately be achieved in an online manner by AR-models, while both outliers and level shifts can be detected reliably. The level chosen for the PI has to be adjusted in case of very high or low variability during the estimation period.

2.3   Phase Space Models

In phase space models the dynamical information of a time series $x_1, \ldots, x_N$ is transformed into a geometric information in an m-dimensional Euclidean space. For this purpose the phase space vectors

$$\boldsymbol{x}_t := \left(x_t, x_{t+1}, \ldots, x_{t+(m-1)}\right)' \in \mathbb{R}^m$$

are constructed, where m can be chosen similarly to the order of an AR-model [25]. Figure 2 visualizes the transformation of a time series into a 2-dimensional space.

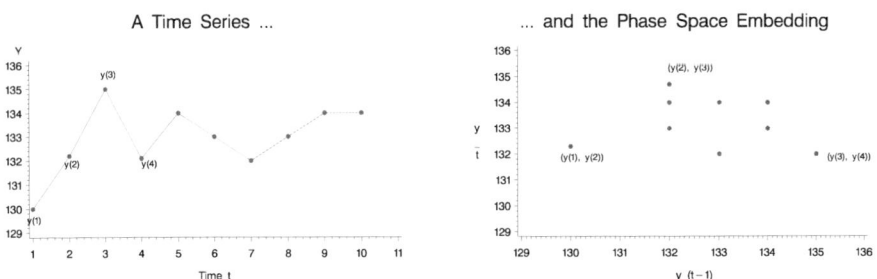

Fig. 2. Two-dimensional phase space vectors from a time series

In the steady state the phase space vectors arising from a linear Gaussian process form an m-dimensional elliptic cloud. A control ellipsoid can be estimated using classical or robust estimators of the mean and the autocovariances of a time series. The position of the phase space vectors w.r.t. this control ellipsoid gives information about their deviation from the steady state. If all observations are inside the estimated ellipsoid, it can be said that the patient is in a steady state. Disturbances can be detected by the movement of the affected vectors in the phase space outside the control ellipsoid [26].

In this way, outliers and level shifts can reliably be detected. A trend, however, can only be detected by looking at the shape of the vector ellipsoid, which is a relatively insensitive method for the detection of slight trends. For achieving adaptive control limits corresponding to the current state moving window techniques can be applied as described above.

3   Dimension Reduction

In critical care a multitude of variables is measured in the course of time. Figure 3 shows a nine-dimensional time series consisting of the heart rate, the pulse, the central venous, the arterial, and the pulmonary arterial pressures of a patient measured during about four hours.

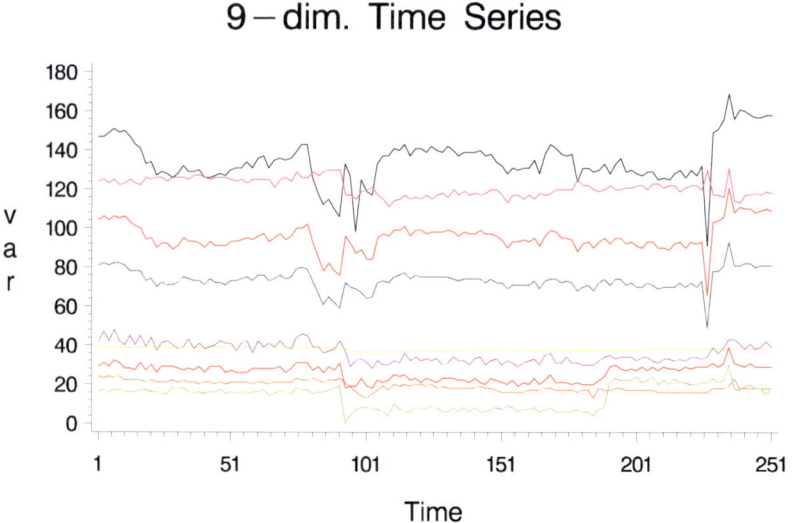

Fig. 3. Multivariate time series representing the hemodynamic system of a patient measured during about four hours. Some patterns of change occur simultaneously in several variables, while others seem to occur in distinct variables in short time lags or in a single variable only

For the reason of interpretability we should reduce the dimension of the data on which decisions are based. This can be achieved either by selecting a subset of the most important variables or by searching for combinations of the observed variables which contain as much information as possible.

3.1   Graphical Models

In clinical practice physicians first select a subset of the monitored variables to get a manageable number of variables. For instance, they neglect the arterial diastolic pressure and the arterial systolic pressure and restrict attention to arterial mean pressure since it is closely related to the other arterial pressures.

Graphical models [27] allow to investigate the associations in multivariate data by statistical analysis. Dahlhaus [28] extended this concept recently to multivariate time series by means of correlation analysis in the frequency domain, where time series are considered as combinations of waves with different harmonic periodicities. This allows to assess the linear, possibly time-lagged relationships between the variables.

The practical value of this new technique for medical data analysis could already be appraised in a clinical study [29]. Known associations within the hemodynamic system could reliably be reidentified by graphical models calculated for critically ill patients. Separate analysis of different clinical states even resulted in characterisations of the states by distinct association structures.

3.2   Sliced Inverse Regression

Sliced inverse regression (SIR) [30] is a powerful statistical instrument for dimension reduction in linear regression. Starting from a regression problem with d covariables a subspace of dimension $k < d$ is calculated which is sufficient to describe the relationships between the dependent variable and the covariables.

SIR can be applied to multivariate time series from intensive care regressing each variable on the others. This allows to calculate the minimal number k of linear combinations of the other variables which is needed to substitute the dependent variable. If k is large a variable has to be considered as important.

When SIR is applied to multivariate time series one should take the dynamical structure of the data into account. This can be done rather easily when we augment the observation space with time lagged measurements.

In most cases the inclusion of lagged observations allowed a large dimension reduction. Furthermore, we obtained different values of k for different clinical states. These findings confirm the results derived with graphical models.

3.3   Principal Component Analysis

While graphical models and SIR analyse the associations between a single variable and the remaining ones, principal component analysis aims at finding a parsimonious joint description for all variables. Those directions (principal components) within the data space are searched for, which contribute most to the variability in the data. Principal component analysis consists of a stepwise search for the direction which explains most of the variability among all directions which are uncorrelated to the previous ones.

First applications of principal component analysis to the hemodynamic system showed, that the first three principal components capture almost all variability. Patterns found in the hemodynamic variables were also visible in the principal components. Thus, the number of variables and the computational effort could significantly be reduced by concentrating on the principal components. The series of the first principal components corresponding to the nine-dimensional time series shown in Figure 3 are provided in Figure 4. The series has been differenced since our phase space procedure for pattern detection is based on the differenced series. The important structural changes in the original series are still obvious in the series of the differenced principal components.

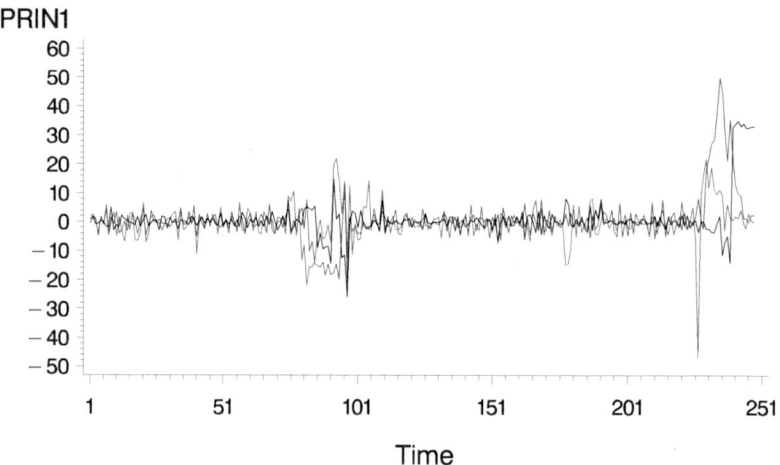

Fig. 4. Time series of the three principal components of a nine-dimensional time series representing the hemodynamic system. The important patterns of change in the original series are also obvious in the series of the principal components

3.4   Factor Analysis

Factor analysis aims just like principal component analysis at the reduction of the dimension of multivariate data by searching suitable linear combinations of the variables. However, factor analysis assumes that there are a few, say q, latent variables (factors) which actually drive the series and cause the correlations between the observable variables. For achieving good interpretability the factors found in the analysis can be rotated in the q-dimensional space.

In view of the good results obtained for three principal components, one can try to describe the hemodynamic system with three latent factors. When the factors are calculated for the whole series they are interpretable by pathophysiologic knowledge. Moreover, we found factors not to vary considerably between patients. However, when factors are determined from short estimation periods, the factors may vary markedly. This would present a serious problem for any automatic analysis based on the time series of extracted factors.

4 Conclusion

Patterns in univariate physiological time series can be identified using models from statistical time series analysis with corresponding detection rules. AR-models and phase space models reliably detect outliers and level changes, but both approaches have problems with trend patterns. For AR-models sometimes manual adjustment of the confidence level is necessary. DLMs allow online trend detection, but they are not as reliable as the other approaches. Hence, a combination of the procedures might give the best results.

All approaches to monitoring of univariate series were found to be more sensitive than clinically relevant. This could be overcome by using an automatically adjusted level. This has already been included into the phase space procedure and has lead to significant improvements. For DLMs robust Kalman filter procedures, which are less sensitive against outliers, might improve the classification.

Statistical methods for dimension reduction offer large potential for the joint monitoring of several variables. Graphical models and SIR explore the associations between the variables and facilitate the choice of a suitable subset of the variables. Principal component and factor analysis result in a set of linear combinations of the variables which could be monitored. Factor analysis could be more suitable than principal component analysis for online monitoring since the results are better interpretable for physicians. However, both approaches suffer from the problem that in any dynamic system both the factors and the principal components may vary over time.

Methods for automatic online analysis of physiological variables give an option for a more reliable evaluation of the individual treatment. Statistical methods could be employed to construct intelligent alarm systems, which are more reliable than simple threshold alarms. Adequate bedside decision support could be achieved by combining the statistical techniques proposed here with methods of artificial intelligence [31].

References

1. Miller, G.: The Magical Number Seven, Plus or Minus Two: Some Limits to Our Capacity for Processing Information. Psychol. Rev. **63** (1956) 81-97
2. Jennings, D., Amabile, T., Ross, L.: Informal Covariation Asessments: Data-Based Versus Theory-Based Judgements. In: Kahnemann, D., Slovic, P., Tversky, A. (eds.): Judgment Under Uncertainty: Heuristics and Biases. Cambridge University Press, Cambridge (1982) 211-230

3. Imhoff, M.: One Year Experience with a UNIX-based Clinical Information System (CIS) on a SICU. In: Lenz, K., Metnitz, P.G.H. (eds.): Patient Data Management in Intensive Care, Springer-Verlag, Wien (1993) 107-114

4. O'Carrol, T.M.: Survey of Alarms in an Intensive Therapy Unit. Anaesthesia **41** (1986) 742-744

5. Miksch, S., Horn, W., Popow, C., Paky, F.: Utilizing Temporal Abstraction for Data Validation and Therapy Planning for Artificially Ventilated Newborne Infants. Art. Int. Med. **8** (1996) 543-576

6. Haimowitz, I.J., Kohane, I.S.: Managing Temporal Worlds for Medical and Trend Diagnosis. Art. Int. Med. **8** (1996) 299-321

7. Daumer, M.: Adaptive Drifterkennung und Intelligente Alarmsysteme. In: Biomedizinische Technik. Ergänzungsband. Schiele und Schoen (2000) to appear

8. Hill, D.W., Endresen, J.: Trend Recording and Forecasting in Intensive Care Therapy. Br. J. Clin. Equipment **1** (1978) 5-14

9. Gordon, K., Smith, A.S.M.: Modeling and Monitoring Biomedical Time Series. J. Am. Stat. Assoc. **85** (1990) 328-337

10. Hepworth, J.T., Hendrickson, S.G., Lopez, J.: Time Series Analysis of Physiological Response During ICU Visitation. West J. Nurs. Res. **16** (1994) 704-717

11. Imhoff, M., Bauer, M., Gather, U., Löhlein, D.: Time Series Analysis in Intensive Care Medicine. Applied Cardiopulmonary Pathophysiology **6** (1997) 263-281

12. Huber, P.J.: Massive Datasets Workshop: Four Years After. J. Comp. Graph. Stat. **8** (1999) 635-652

13. Smith, A.F.M., West, M.: Monitoring Renal Transplants: an Application of the Multiprocess Kalman Filter. Biometrics **39** (1983) 867-878

14. West, M., Harrison, J.: Bayesian Forecasting and Dynamic Models. Springer-Verlag, New York (1989)

15. Daumer, M., Falk, M.: On-line Change-Point Detection for State Space Models Using Multi-process Kalman Filters. In: O'Leary, D. (ed.): Proceedings of the International Linear Algebra Society Symposium on Fast Algorithms for Control, Signals and Image Processing. Elsevier, Amsterdam (1998) 125-135

16. Cook, R.D.: Detection of Influential Observations in Linear Regression. Technometrics **19** (1977) 15-18

17. Peña, D.: Influential Observations in Time Series. J. Business & Economic Statistics **8** (1990) 235-241

18. De Jong, P., Penzer, J.: Diagnosing Shocks in Time Series. J. Americ. Statist. Assoc. **93** (1998) 796-806

19. Gather, U., Fried, R., Imhoff, M.: Online Classification of States in Intensive Care. Technical Report 15/2000, SFB 475, University of Dortmund, 44221 Dortmund, Germany.

20. Box, G.E.P., Jenkins, G.M., Reinsel, G.C.: Time Series Analysis. Forecasting and Control. Third Edition. Prentice Hall, Englewood Cliffs (1994)

21. Imhoff, M., Bauer, M., Gather, U., Fried, R.: Pattern Detection in Intensive Care Monitoring Time Series: Influence of the Model Order. Preprint, SFB 475, University of Dortmund, 44221 Dortmund, Germany

22. De Gooijer, J.G., Abraham, B., Gould, A., Robinson, L.: Methods for Determining the Order of an Autoregressive-moving Average Process: a Survey. Int. Stat. Rev. **55** (1985) 301-329

23. Imhoff, M., Bauer, M.: Time Series Analysis in Critical Care Monitoring. New Horizons **4** (1996) 519-531

24. Lambert, C.R., Raymenants, E., Pepine, C.J.: Time-Series Analysis of Long-Term Ambulatory Myocardial Ischemia: Effects of Beta-Adrenergic and Calcium Channel Blockade. Am. Heart J. **129** (1995) 677-684

25. Bauer, M., Gather, U., Imhoff, M.: The Identification of Multiple Outliers in Online Monitoring Data. Technical Report 29/1999, SFB 475, University of Dortmund, 44221 Dortmund, Germany

26. Bauer, M., Gather, U., Imhoff, M.: Analysis of High Dimensional Data from Intensive Care Medicine. In: Payne, R., Green, P. (eds.): Proceedings in Computational Statistics. Springer-Verlag, Berlin (1999) 185-190

27. Cox, D.R., Wermuth, N.: Multivariate Dependencies. Chapman & Hall, London (1996)

28. Dahlhaus, R.: Graphical Interaction Models for Multivariate Time Series. Metrika (2000) to appear

29. Gather, U., Imhoff, M., Fried, R.: Graphical Models for Multivariate Time Series from Intensive Care Monitoring. Preprint, SFB 475, University of Dortmund, 44221 Dortmund, Germany

30. Li, K.C.: Sliced Inverse Regression for Dimension Reduction. J. Americ. Statist. Asoc. **86** (1991) 316-342

31. Morik, K., Imhoff, M., Brockhausen, P., Joachims, T., Gather, U.: Knowledge Discovery and Knowledge Validation in Intensive Care. Art. Int. Med. (2000) to appear

Entropy Measures in Heart Rate Variability Data

Niels Wessel[1], Agnes Schumann[2], Alexander Schirdewan[3],
Andreas Voss[2], Jürgen Kurths[1]

[1] University of Potsdam, Am Neuen Palais 10, PF 601553,
D-14415 Potsdam, Germany
{niels, jkurths}@agnld.uni-potsdam.de
[2] University of Applied Sciences Jena, Carl-Zeiss-Promenade 2, PF 100314
D-07745 Jena, Germany
voss@fh-jena.de, schumann@fvk-berlin.de
[3] Franz-Volhard-Hospital, Humboldt-University, Berlin,
Wiltbergstr. 50, D-13125 Berlin, Germany
schirdewan@fvk-berlin.de

Abstract. Standard parameters of heart rate variability are restricted in measuring linear effects, whereas nonlinear descriptions often suffer from the curse of dimensionality. An approach which might be capable of assessing complex properties is the calculation of entropy measures from normalised periodograms. Two concepts, both based on autoregressive spectral estimations are introduced here. To test the hypothesis that these entropy measures may improve the result of high risk stratification, they were applied to a clinical pilot study and to the data of patients with different cardiac diseases. The study shows that the entropy measures discussed here are useful tools to estimate the individual risk of patients suffering from heart failure. Further, the results demonstrate that the combination of different heart rate variability parameters leads to a better classification of cardiac diseases than single parameters.

1 Introduction

An accurate identification of patients who are at high risk of sudden cardiac death is an important and challenging problem. Heart rate variability (HRV) parameters, calculated from the time series of beat-to-beat-intervals, have been used to predict the mortality risk in patients with structural heart diseases [1,2]. Linear parameters only provide limited information about the underlying complex system, whereas nonlinear descriptions often suffer from the curse of dimensionality. This means that there are not enough points in the time series to reliably estimate these nonlinear measures. Therefore, we favour measures of complexity which are able to characterise quantitatively the dynamics even in rather short time series [3-5]. Recently we could demonstrate that a multivariate approach including these nonlinear as well as linear parameters significantly improves the results of risk stratification [6]. Entropy measures have been used widely in HRV analysis with encouraging results. Most

R.W. Brause and E. Hanisch (Eds.): ISMDA 2000, LNCS 1933, pp. 78–87, 2000.

frequently the 'approximate entropy' ApEn is used which was firstly applied to heart rate data in [7,8]. Promising applications of ApEn to HRV data are given for example in [9-13]. Other interesting entropy measures are the 'tone entropy' [14], the 'conditional entropy' [15], the 'pattern entropy' [16], the 'Kolmogorov entropy' [17] and the entropy measures based on symbolic dynamics [3,4].

In this contribution we introduce two entropy measures based on periodograms of cardiac beat-to-beat intervals. Both measures - the renormalised and the amplitude adjusted entropy - are calculated from the autoregressive spectral estimation of the time series. The basic idea of these methods is to determine the complexity of cardiac periodograms, however, the renormalised entropy needs and the amplitude adjusted entropy does not need a reference distribution. In this study we investigate the ability of both entropy measures to distinguish between healthy persons and cardiac patients in a clinical pilot study. For the distinction between different kinds of cardiac diseases it is assessed in a multivariate approach whether the amplitude adjusted entropy contributes significantly to other traditional heart rate variability measures.

2   Methods

Applications of renormalised entropy to heart rate data based on the Fast Fourier Transform were previously introduced in [3,4]. To overcome the potential lack of reproducibility and time instability of this measure, the autoregressive method RE_{AR} was developed. Additionally, to avoid the problem of reference selection, the amplitude adjusted entropy AE_{AR} is introduced here. Figure 1 gives two examples of tachograms, i.e. the time series of the beat-to-beat intervals and the corresponding autoregressive spectral estimations.

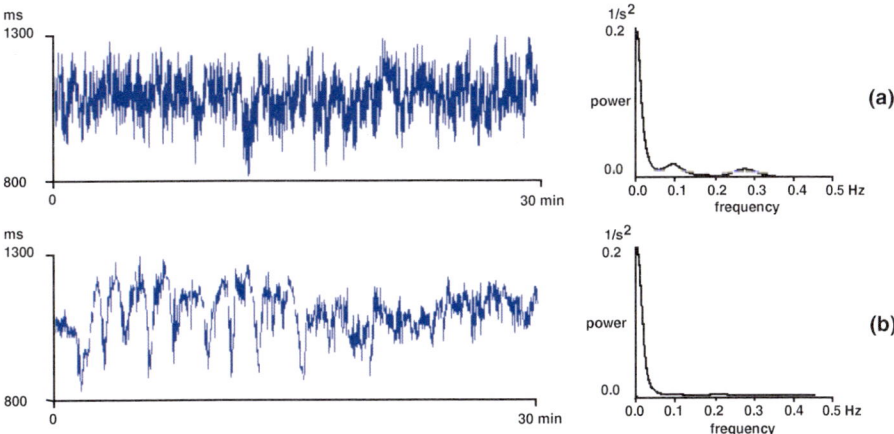

Fig. 1. Tachograms and autoregressive spectral estimations (a) of a healthy person with normal low and high frequency modulations and (b) of a cardiac patient with a single dominant peak in the very low frequency domain – low and high frequency modulations are absent

The low and high frequency oscillations (0.05-0.4 Hz) are rather low in comparison to the very low frequency peak (<0.05 Hz). An autoregressive spectral estimation is useful to emphasise the different spectral domains, the amplitude adjustment guarantees the comparability of different spectral distributions.

2.1 Renormalised Entropy RE_{AR}

To compare the degree of complexity of one distribution in relation to a given reference distribution, the latter one is renormalised to a fixed energy. Considering two tachograms with density estimates $f_0(x)$ and $f_1(x)$ and using the estimate $f_0(x)$ as a reference, the renormalised density distribution $\bar{f}_0(x)$ of $f_0(x)$ is defined as:

$$\bar{f}_0(x) := \frac{f_0(x)^T}{\int f_0(x)^T dx} \tag{1}$$

where the parameter T is the solution of the integral equation

$$\int \ln f_0(x)^{(\bar{f}_0(x)-f_1(x))} dx = 0. \tag{2}$$

The solution of (2) has to be determined numerically. The renormalised entropy RE_{AR} of the distribution $f_1(x)$ is defined by the following interchanging algorithm; where $S(f)$ is the Shannon-entropy of distribution f , that is

$$S(f) = -\int f(x) \cdot \ln f(x) dx . \tag{3}$$

I.   Calculating of $\Delta_1 = S(f_1) - S(\bar{f}_0)$ with the distribution $f_0(x)$ as the reference ($f_0(x)$ is renormalised). The value of T is denoted $T_1 = T$.

II.   Calculating of $\Delta_2 = S(f_0) - S(\bar{f}_1)$ with the distribution $f_1(x)$ as the reference ($f_1(x)$ is renormalised). The resulting T value is denoted $T_2 = T$.

III.   If $T_1 > T_2$, the distribution $f_0(x)$ is found to be the more disordered one (in the sense of renormalised entropy - i.s.r.e.) and the renormalised entropy is defined as $RE_{AR} = \Delta_1$. Otherwise ($T_1 < T_2$) $f_1(x)$ is the more disordered distribution (i.s.r.e.) and the renormalised entropy is $RE_{AR} = -\Delta_2$.

Calculating the renormalised entropy requires estimating the tachogram distributions. Here we use an autoregressive spectral estimation of the filtered and interpolated tachogram. To overcome bias problems a sinusoidal oscillation with a fixed amplitude and frequency was added to the time series. The amplitude of 40 msec was chosen to obtain a dominant peak in the spectral estimation and the frequency was set to 0.4 Hz, which is the upper limit of the high frequency band [18]. A spectral density estimation in the interval [0,0.42] Hz was used to include all physiological modulations and the calibration peak. Using a reference tachogram from a healthy subject with normal low and high frequency modulations the RE_{AR} method is designed so that either a decreased HRV or a pathological spectrum leads to positive values of renormalised entropy.

2.2 Amplitude Adjusted Entropy AE_{AR}

The technique described in the last section requires determining a reference state. This can be done easily by finding the most disordered spectrum of all data sets from a given control group. But, when analysing new data sets, the problem arise, which distribution should be selected for reference. The most disordered from all control group data sets or should we select for each study an own reference state? The latter choice could lead to an incomparability between different studies. The motivation for designing the amplitude adjusted entropy, therefore, was to find a method which is able to estimate the complexity of a given periodogram independently from a reference state. How can this be done?

One main objective in assessing spectral estimations is to determine phases with a decreased heart rate variability, therefore, the amplitude adjustment described above was adopted. A sinusoidal oscillation with an amplitude of 40 msec and a frequency of 0.4 Hz was superimposed to the original time series. In this way we obtained comparable variability values since they refer to the uniform superimposed variability. A second objective in HRV analysis is the determination of pathological spectra with only singular dominant peaks, since the spectral distributions of healthy persons normally have several peaks due to different cardiovascular modulations. To quantify the intensity of these modulations, the Shannon entropy of the amplitude adjusted spectrum is calculated, i.e. the amplitude adjusted entropy AE_{AR} is given by

$$AE_{AR} = S(\hat{f}) = -\int \hat{f}(x) \cdot \ln \hat{f}(x) dx \qquad (4)$$

where $\hat{f}(x)$ is the spectral estimation of the time series superimposed by a uniform sinusoidal oscillation. Correspondingly the Shannon entropy of the original (not amplitude adjusted) periodogram is denoted by E_{AR}.

3 Results

3.1 Clinical Pilot Study

In a clinical pilot study the renormalised entropy RE_{AR} and the amplitude adjusted entropy AE_{AR} were applied to data of 18 cardiac patients and 23 healthy subjects. The cardiac patient group consisted of patients after myocardial infarction with documented life threatening ventricular arrhythmias. From the group of healthy subjects, the most disordered tachogram (i.s.r.e.) was determined as the reference for

RE$_{AR}$ calculation (*RE$_{AR}$* =0 for healthy person no. 16). The results of this clinical pilot study are shown in Figure 2. The Renormalised entropy *RE$_{AR}$* correctly recognised 15 of 18 high risk patients (with the classification rule: greater zero or under the dotted line at –0.33). The Kolmogorov–Smirnov-Z test showed clearly significant differences between both distributions (p<0.001). Due to the bimodal distribution of *RE$_{AR}$* in the cardiac patient group, however, no statistical significance could be achieved with the two-tailed t-test for equality of means.

The classification based on the amplitude adjusted entropy reaches a comparable sensitivity at the 100%- specificity level. 11 of 18 cardiac patients were recognised by the classification rule *AE$_{AR}$*<3.34 (3.34 is the minimum of *AE$_{AR}$* in the healthy group, compare Fig. 3). The t-test for the equality of means, however, was highly significant (4.34±0.49 for the healthy vs. 2.85±1.65 for the high risk group, p<0.001) because of the unimodal distribution of *AE$_{AR}$* in both groups.

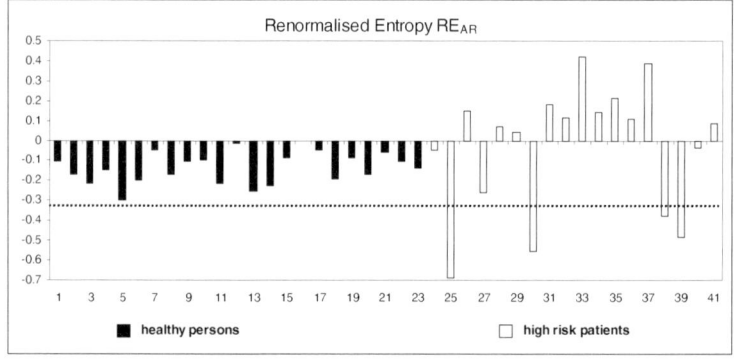

Fig. 2. Results of renormalised entropy *RE$_{AR}$* in a clinical pilot study, black bars represent the control group whereas white bars refer to the cardiac patients

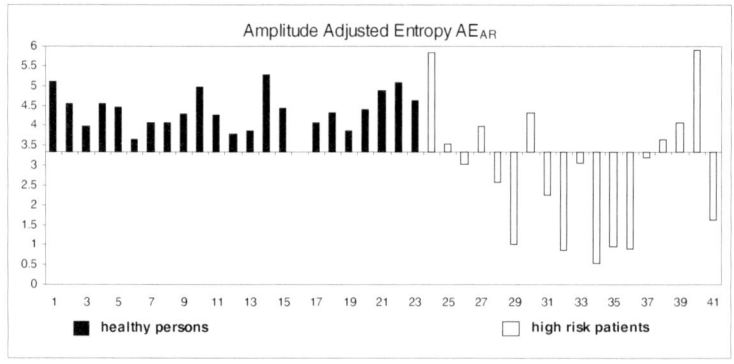

Fig. 3. Results of amplitude adjusted entropy *AE$_{AR}$*, black bars represent the control group whereas white bars refer to the cardiac patients

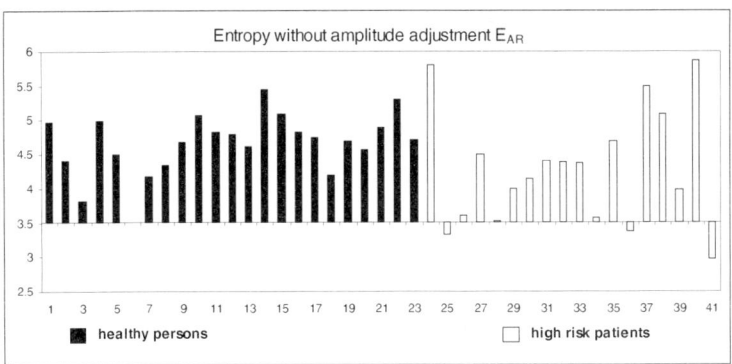

Fig. 4. Results of the Shannon entropy without amplitude adjustment E_{AR}, black bars represent the control group whereas white bars refer to the cardiac patients

Figure 4 demonstrates the effect of leaving the amplitude adjustment out: The entropy values of the healthy and the control group highly overlap. The t-test for equality of means showed no significant differences (4.66 ± 0.45 for the healthy vs. 4.29 ± 0.85 for the high risk group).

3.2 Multiparametric Study

The task of separating different cardiac patient groups on the basis of HRV parameters is a demanding problem. If there are differences, it might be possible to find non-invasive marker for specific cardiac diseases. Or, is there even a potential to estimate the severity of cardiac diseases non-invasively? We studied, whether the HRV behaviour of patients suffering from dilated cardiomyopathy (DCM, 41 male, 9 female, age 52 ± 10 years) and patients which have survived an acute myocardial infarction (MI, 42 male, 8 female, age 58 ± 9 years) can be distinguished. So, standard HRV parameters from time and frequency domain were derived from the whole 24h-time series as well as mean values of 5-minute-segments (see table 1). Additionally, the amplitude adjusted entropy values were calculated to assess, whether they provide new information which is not contained in the standard parameter set. The renormalised entropy was not regarded in this study to avoid the problem of reference selection. Since the variability characteristics of both patient groups highly overlap in all individual features a multiparametric approach is pursued. Correlation analysis reveals that the amplitude adjusted entropy calculated from the whole time series is not highly correlated with any standard parameter (pearson correlation coefficient < 0.5). This is not true for the short term amplitude adjusted entropy which exhibits correlations above 0.7 with the Shannon and Renyi entropy of the original time series, and with LF, RMSSD and pNN50. Linear discriminant analysis is used to distinguish between the two different patient groups, since this technique is able to construct a linear class boundary which is optimally adjusted to correlations between parameters. To assess the class separability of different parameter sets, cross-

Table 1. Standard parameters used in the multiparametric study. For a precise definition see [4,18].

Long term parameters	meanNN	- mean duration of NN
	sdNN	- standard deviation of NN
	sdaNN5	- standard deviation of NN averaged over 5 min
	rmssd	- root mean square of successive NN differences
	pNN50	- the percentage of NN differences > 50 msec
	Shannon	- Shannon entropy of the histogram
	ULF, VLF, LF, HF	- frequency components of the power spectrum
Short term parameters	Shannon	- Shannon entropy of the histogram
	Renyi	- Renyi entropy of the histogram (order 0.25)
	VLF, LF, HF	- frequency components of power spectrum
	LF/HF	- proportion of frequency components

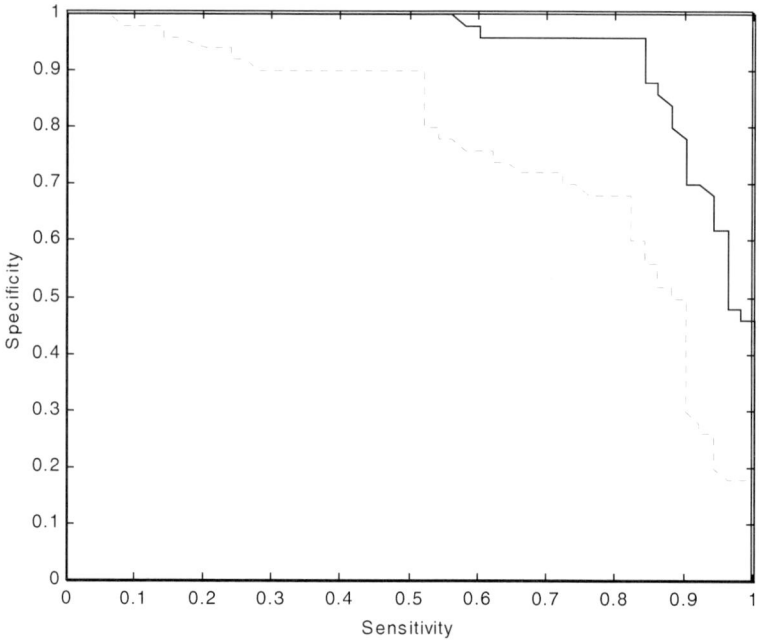

Fig. 5. Receiver operator characteristics achieved with the amplitude adjusted entropy (solid line) and without it (dotted line)

validated recognition rates were calculated providing nearly unbiased estimates of the performance [19-21]. Then all possible parameter sets consisting of 4 parameters were ranked.

It turned out, that the entropy measure AE_{AR} contributes significantly to the classification performance between the two cardiac diseases. The combination of short and long term AE_{AR} with meanNN and sdaNN yields a crossvalidated recognition rate of 89 %. Leaving the amplitude adjusted entropy out of consideration, a maximum separation of 75 % could be achieved with a parameter set consisting of all Shannon and Renyi entropies of the histogram combined with the normalised very low frequency component between 0.0033Hz and 0.04Hz. The improvement is demonstrated in Figure 5 where the receiver-operator-curves of both parameter sets are compared. For each sensitivity value a larger value of specificity can be obtained using AE_{AR}. The Parameters meanNN and sdaNN5 achieve a higher significance value in the t-test than AE_{AR}, but classifying only on these two standard parameters leads to a significantly reduced performance of only 67%. Thus, the amplitude adjusted entropy provides important additional information for cardiac disease classification in this study.

4 Discussion

The renormalised entropy RE_{AR} is designed in such a way that tachograms with a normal variability and typical periodograms have negative values of RE_{AR}. Either a decreased HRV or pathological spectra (dominant ULF, VLF or LF peaks) lead to positive values of RE_{AR}. The results of the clinical pilot study confirmed that in general, healthy persons have negative while most high risk patients have positive renormalised entropy values. The results did not achieve statistical significance in comparing the group mean values, however, in an extensive clinical study RE_{AR} already demonstrated the usefulness for risk stratification [22]. A high statistical significance between survivors of an acute myocardial infarction who survived a two year follow-up and those who died could be shown. Considering these results and the results of the amplitude adjusted entropy AE_{AR} in the clinical pilot study, the application of AE_{AR} to such a large data base seems to be very promising.

For the distinction of DCM and MI patients, which is a more difficult problem than the distinction of cardiac patients and healthy subjects, a multiparametric approach is taken to gain from the information augmentation provided by several parameters. To avoid the problem of selecting a reference spectrum only the amplitude adjusted entropy together with standard parameters from time and frequency domain are considered. It could be shown that the combination of the amplitude adjusted entropy measures with standard HRV parameters leads to better classification results in comparison to the results achieved only with standard parameters. In this study, we got an improvement of more than 10%. This implies that the amplitude adjusted entropy measures contain additional information which is not provided by the standard parameters considered. This suggests further that a multivariate approach using potent

HRV parameters together with clinical parameters may be promising in risk stratification tasks.

Calculating renormalised entropy assumes a fixed reference distribution. In this study, the reference distribution was selected using the interchanging algorithm applied to the data of 23 healthy persons. With the amplitude adjusted entropy, a new method is introduced which does not need a reference distribution. It has to be validated, whether the amplitude adjusted entropy has the same or better properties in the classification of patients after acute myocardial infarction. In summary, both entropy methods RE_{AR} and AE_{AR} seem to be potent for risk stratification of patients after myocardial infarction.

References

1. Kleiger, R.E., Miller, J.P., Bigger, J.T., Moss, A.: Decreased heart rate variability and its association with increased mortality after acute myocardial infarction. Am J Cardiol 59 (1987) 256-262
2. Tsuji, H., Larson, M.G., Venditti, F.J. Jr, Manders, E.S., Evans, J.C., Feldman, C.L., Levy, D.: Impact of reduced heart rate variability on risk for cardiac events. The Framingham Heart Study. Circulation 94 (1996) 2850-2855
3. Kurths, J., Voss, A., Witt, A., Saparin, P., Kleiner, H.J., Wessel, N.: Quantitative analysis of heart rate variability. Chaos 5 (1995) 88-94
4. Voss, A., Kurths, J., Kleiner, H.J., Witt, A., Wessel, N., Saparin, P., Osterziel, K.J., Schurath, R., Dietz, R.: The application of methods of non-linear dynamics for the improved and predictive recognition of patients threatened by sudden cardiac death. Cardiovasc Res 31 (1996) 419-433
5. Wessel, N., Ziehmann, Ch., Kurths, J., Meyerfeldt, U., Schirdewan, A., Voss, A.: Short-term Forecasting of Life-threatening Cardiac Arrhythmias based on Symbolic Dynamics and Finite-Time Growth Rates. Phys Rev E 61 (2000) 733-739
6. Voss, A., Hnatkova, K., Wessel, N., Kurths, J., Sander, A., Schirdewan, A., Camm, A.J., Malik, M.: Multiparametric Analysis of Heart Rate Variability Used for Risk Stratification Among Survivors of Acute Myocardial Infarction. Pacing Clin Electrophysiol 21 (1998) 186-192
7. Pincus, S.M., Gladstone, I.M., Ehrenkranz, R.A.: A regularity statistic for medical data analysis. J Clin Monit 7 (1991) 335-345
8. Pincus, S.M., Viscarello, R.R.: Approximate entropy: a regularity measure for fetal heart rate analysis. Obstet Gynecol 79 (1992) 249-255
9. Pincus, S.M., Goldberger, A.L.: Physiological time-series analysis: what does regularity quantify? Am J Physiol 266 (1994) H1643-1656
10. Makikallio, T.H., Seppanen, T., Niemela, M., Airaksinen, K.E., Tulppo, M., Huikuri, H.V.: Abnormalities in beat to beat complexity of heart rate dynamics in patients with a previous myocardial infarction. J Am Coll Cardiol 28 (1996) 1005-1011
11. Palazzolo, J.A., Estafanous, F.G., Murray, P.A.: Entropy measures of heart rate variation in conscious dogs. Am J Physiol 274 (1998) H1099-1105

12. Vikman, S., Makikallio, T.H., Yli-Mayry, S., Pikkujamsa, S., Koivisto, A.M., Reinikainen, P., Airaksinen, K.E., Huikuri, H.V.: Altered complexity and correlation properties of R-R interval dynamics before the spontaneous onset of paroxysmal atrial fibrillation. Circulation 100 (1999) 2079-2084

13. Van Leeuwen, P., Lange, S., Bettermann, H., Gronemeyer, D., Hatzmann, W.: Fetal heart rate variability and complexity in the course of pregnancy. Early Hum 54 (1999) 259-269

14. Oida, E., Moritani, T., Yamori, Y.: Tone-entropy analysis on cardiac recovery after dynamic exercise. J Appl Physiol 82 (1997) 1794-1801

15. Porta, A., Baselli, G., Liberati, D., Montano, N., Cogliati, C., Gnecchi-Ruscone, T., Malliani, A., Cerutti, S.: Measuring regularity by means of a corrected conditional entropy in sympathetic outflow. Biol Cybern 78 (1998) 71-78

16. Zebrowski, J.J., Poplawska, W., Baranowski, R.: Entropy, pattern entropy and related methods for the analysis of data on the time intervals between heart beats from 24h electrocardiograms, Phys Rev E 50 (1994) 4187-4205

17. Guzzetti, S., Signorini, M.G., Cogliati, C., Mezzetti, S., Porta, A., Cerutti, S., Malliani, A.: Non-linear dynamics and chaotic indices in heart rate variability of normal subjects and heart-transplanted patients. Cardiovasc Res 31 (1996) 441-446

18. Heart rate variability: standards of measurement, physiological interpretation and clinical use. Task Force of the European Society of Cardiology and the North American Society of Pacing and Electrophysiology. Circulation 93 (1996) 1043-1065

19. Fukunaga, K., Introduction to statistical pattern recognition. Academic Press, New York-London (1974)

20. Duda, R.D., Hart, P.E.: Pattern Recognition and Scene Analysis. Wiley, New York (1973)

21. Fahrmeir, L., Hamerle, A.: Multivariate statistische Verfahren. Walter de Gruyter, Berlin-New York (1984)

22. Wessel, N.: Komplexe Analyse nichtlinearer Phänomene in kardiologischen Datenreihen. Dissertation, University of Potsdam (1998)

Determinism and Nonlinearity of the Heart Rhythm

Laura Cimponeriu and Anastassios Bezerianos

Department of Medical Physics, University of Patras, Greece
{laura, tasos}@heart.med.upatras.gr

Abstract. The interaction between sympathetic and parasympathetic nerve activities at the level of sinus node play a dominant role in the magnitude and time course of heart rate fluctuations. The analysis of short-term heart rate variability provides measures of the response of the sinus node to autonomic neural control in different patho-physiological states of the cardiovascular system functioning. Diminished variability, as a result of an ANS control dysfunction is often attended by profound changes in dynamics that cannot be characterized by simple linear measures of the global variability. Our interest regards the predictability and nonlinearity of the heart rhythm and their relation with the state of neural control of the heart. In the present study, we analyze the nonlinear predictability of the RR interval time series in two different states of neural regulation: normal function and pharmacological blockade, by means of atropine and propanolol.

1 Introduction

Harmonic and non-harmonic components of heart rate variability (HRV), both have a physiological origin. Different time constants of the sympathetic and parasympathetic activity reflect in oscillatory components of the heart rhythm at different frequencies. The high-frequency part of the spectrum (HF: 0.15:0.4 Hz) is mediated by the vagus nerve activity, while both ANS components activity contributes to the low frequency part (LF: 0.004 –0.015 Hz) [1]. Aside from the neural regulation, other control mechanisms including thermoregulation and humoral factors account for the multiple scale fluctuations of the heart rhythm, all embedded in a 1/f-like spectral distribution [4]. It is still not complete understood what is the relative contribution of each regulatory component to the HRV and what is the relation between all these rhythms and the level of ANS control.

Linear system analysis techniques applied on short-term HRV data can provide useful measures of the response of the sinus node to autonomic neural control, in various patho-physiological conditions [5]. Deterministic components associated with the autonomic cardiac control are essentially contained in the LF and HF spectral components. However, linear and spectrum-based methods overlook the possible presence of nonlinear correlations in the data that can also contribute to their deterministic properties.

The presence of intrinsic nonlinearities in cardiovascular system functioning (e.g. the nonlinear coupling between vagus and sympathetic at the sinus node) and the rich spectra of dynamics displayed by the heart rhythm, motivates a nonlinear

R.W. Brause and E. Hanisch (Eds.): ISMDA 2000, LNCS 1933, pp. 88–96, 2000.

deterministic framework of analysis. It is also known that, simple (low-dimensional) nonlinear deterministic systems can generate apparently random behavior, similar to that manifested by physiological time series. There have been many attempts to describe the heart rate time series as chaotic, using the methods of nonlinear dynamics. The presence of nonlinear and deterministic structures and whether they reflect some physiological information is of fundamental importance for validation of nonlinear deterministic models. We have approached this issue by exploring the predictability of heart rate time series in two opposite states of ANS functioning, i.e. the normal versus pharmacologically blockade condition.

There are many sources of predictability in any physiological time series, and one of the best-understood is the linear correlations. In a stochastic description of the generating process, autoregressive or moving average models provide the tools to build optimal linear predictors, based on the approximation of each observation as a linear combination of the preceding ones. Aside from the linear correlations, an alternative origin of the predictability is the nonlinear determinism. Predictive models constructed by local approximation of the dynamics in the reconstructed phase space have been proved very useful in capturing the nonlinear and deterministic dynamical structures.

In the present study, nonlinear phase-space predictors have been constructed from the data by local linear approximation of the reconstructed dynamics in the proxy state-space. To test for the presence of nonlinearities, the surrogate data method approach has been involved. The prediction accuracy has been compared to that obtained from surrogated data, i.e. time series that share only the linear properties with the original data, otherwise being random. In this way, we have tested the amount of determinism captured by this predictive models, beyond that reflected by simple linear correlations.

2 Materials and Methods

2.1 Data Acquisition

The data were provided by 10 healthy subjects, before and after administration of propanolol for 5 minutes (0.013 mg/kg/min) followed by atropine for 5 minutes (0.008 mg/kg/min), resulting in both sympathetic and parasympathetic activities blockade. The subjects were placed in the supine position in a quiet surrounding to minimize external influences and to achieve almost stationary data recordings. The ECG was recorded for 10 minutes: before drug injection (control) and immediately after drug injection (blockade) using a CASE 15 MARQUETTE system. The ECG signal was sampled at 256 Hz then consecutive QRS complexes (RR intervals - RRI) were extracted off line from the ECG. A total of 800 data points (RRIs) were extracted from each recording set.

2.2 Nonlinear Prediction Approach

Building nonlinear deterministic models from time series involves the reconstruction and the approximation of their underlying dynamics.   The initial step is the embedding of the scalar data in a higher dimensional space, where the reconstructed dynamics can be considered a faithful representation of the original one. Regarding the dynamics reconstruction from RRI data, a few remarks have to be made. The RRIs data represent inter-event (the occurrence of the R wave peak on the ECG) timings, and not a real time series in the sense required by the embedding methodology. Several studies [6] have reanalyzed the concepts of embedding and nonlinear predictability applied on this data, and the possibility of reconstructing deterministic dynamics from such data has been revealed.

Following the time-delay embedding approach [4], the coordinates of the reconstructed phase space are time-delayed versions of the scalar time series RRI_i, (i=1:N). A point that describes the current state is a vector:

$$x_i = (RRI_i, RRI_{i-\tau}...RRI_{i-(m-1)\tau}) \tag{1}$$

with m being the embedding dimension and τ the time lag. Tests for deterministic structures in the reconstructed dynamics encompass various nonlinear prediction techniques, whose predictive power depends on the quality of the reconstructed dynamics as well as on the dynamics themselves. High dimensional dynamics, or the presence of noise (observational or dynamical) restrict on the ability to capture the deterministic structure, independently of the modeling approach involved. However, local phase-space modeling methods have been proved useful in detecting weak deterministic dynamical components. The predictive model

$$x_{n+1} = F(x_n) \tag{2}$$

built from the data will capture its deterministic component by establishing a functional relationship between the current state x_n and the future state x_{n+1}. Then, trajectories of the dynamical system are obtained by iterating the reconstructed map (2). An effective way to reach F is obtained by locally linear approximation of the dynamics [1], deriving neighborhood relations in the phase space and mapping them forward in time. Thus, in a linear approximation:

$$x_{n+1} = Ax_{n,U} + B \tag{3}$$

where A and B are determined by a least square fit using vectors $(x_{n,U})$ from a small neighborhood U of x_n, and their images. The numbers of neighbors (k) is usually chosen larger than the number of parameters in the linear approximation, that is k>m+1. This will ensure the stability of the solution [2]. The maximum value of k is given by the total number of available delay-vectors, that forms the basis on which the predictive model is built. As k increases from k_{min} to k_{max}, the predictor model becomes more global. The performance of the predictor model is evaluated by computing the normalized mean square error (E) over the range of values (T) in the prediction interval:

$$E = \max(\sum_{i \in T}(\hat{x}_i - x_i)^2) / \sum_{i \in T}(\bar{x}_i - x_i)^2, \sum_{i \in T}(\hat{x}_i - x_i)^2) / \sum_{i \in T}(x_{i-1} - x_i)^2) \qquad (4)$$

By definition, perfect predictions result in E=0. If the value of E is less than 1, the model capture time dependencies that reflect in an improved prediction over that of the trivial predictor (E>1). Whether values of E<1 correspond to linear or nonlinear phase space structures captured by the predictive model, has to be further evaluated.

2.3 Surrogate data analysis

The significance of non-linearity on the predictability has been evaluated by testing against the null hypothesis that the data stem from a linear stochastic process, transformed by a static non-linearity. In this way, predictability that may be accounted for by linear correlations or static nonlinearities induced by the measurement function, is excluded. The surrogate data method was used, where new sets of data are built from the original series, after removing the possible nonlinear structures. 10 separate realizations of Gaussian–scaled surrogates were constructed [8], and analyzed in the same manner as the original data. Then, the significance of the difference in predictability between the original and the surrogate data is evaluated by:

$$S = (E_{original} - \langle E_{surrogates} \rangle) / SD_{surrogates} \qquad (5)$$

where $\langle E_{surogates} \rangle$ and $SD_{surrogates}$ denote the mean and standard deviation of the distribution of the surrogate predictabilities. An S value greater than 3 is considered here as statistically significant. For S>3, the predictability of the original data is statistically different from the predictability of surrogates. This provides indirect evidences about the presence of nonlinear structures captured by the predictive model used.

3 Results

The RRIs recorded in the two experimental conditions and a first image of the linear dependencies revealed by their auto-correlation function and simple return plots are shown in Fig. 1. The markedly reduced variability after blockade coupled with an increased amount of linear correlations (decreased rate of information dissipation with time) are features of a more regular dynamics and smaller complexity of the RRIs fluctuations. The shape of the cloud of points in the return plots reveals complex dependencies between successive data points.

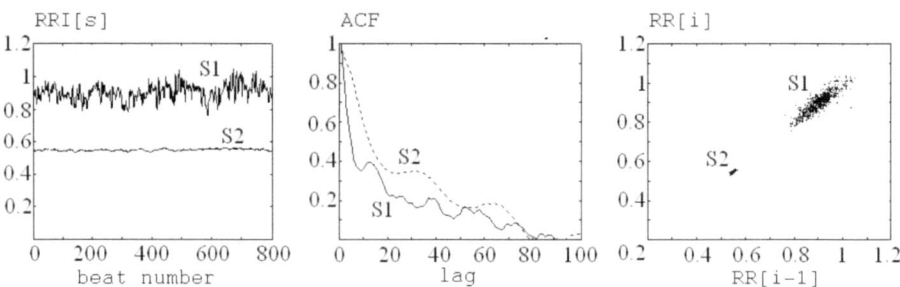

Fig. 1. Representative RRIs in one subject and the two states examined (S1- control and S2- blockade) (*left*), the autocorrelation function (*middle*) and return plots (*right*)

However, if the dimensionality of the dynamics is high, such simple 2D plots cannot provide any information about the type of correlations in the data. For the subsequent analysis, all the data sets were normalized to unit variance and zero mean. A time delay of one has been used for reconstruction of the dynamics, and an optimum embedding dimension has been selected according to our nonlinear measure explored. The nonlinear prediction method briefly summarized above, has been applied on each data set and 10 surrogates consistent with the null hypothesis addressed. The local linear approximation of the dynamics was performed on the first 500 points of each time series, and the remainder segment was used for evaluating the prediction accuracy. In this way, we are provided with an out-of-sample measure of predictability. The one-step nonlinear predictability has been explored for various parameters settings (m and k= the neighborhood size). To note that for $k=k_{max}$ the predictor model is nothing but an autoregressive model of the order of embedding dimension. This allows evaluating the efficiency in terms of predictability, of the local linear approach. The choice of $\tau =1$ has provided the smallest prediction errors in all the dimensions (m=1:15) and neighborhood sizes (k=1:k_{max}) explored. Fig. 2 illustrates the behavior of the E one-step ahead in time, as function of m.

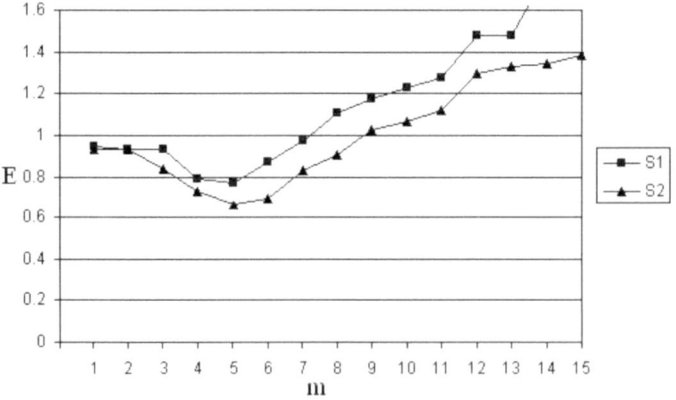

Fig. 2. Plot of E=f(m) corresponding to the same data, as presented in Fig. 1

The optimum value of m=5, has been selected for the further analysis and comparison of our data sets. Regarding the dependence E = f(k) (Fig. 3) in the two state examined, several observations can be done. As the neighborhood size used for the fit of the predictor model increases, the prediction errors decreases and levels off at k = ~ 25, for RRIs corresponding to the S2-state. Therefore, the prediction accuracy is not improved over that of a global (k=k$_{max}$) linear predictor.

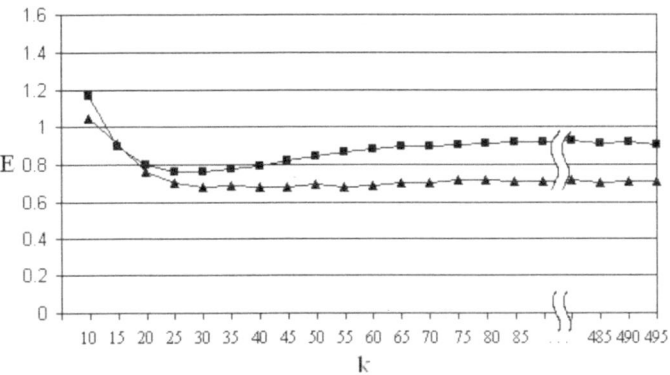

Fig. 3. Plot of E=f(k), k=10:k$_{max}$

This is a first indication that nonlinear dynamical components might be absent in RRIs data corresponding to the S2-state, or cannot be disclosed by this modeling approach. In the S1-state, a small improvement in terms of predictability is gained by locally (k=25-30) linear approximation of the dynamics and this suggests the presence of nonlinearity that has been captured by the predictor model. For all the RRI data analyzed, the predictability is significantly reduced in the S1-state in comparison with the S2-state (see Table 1). In addition, only in 6 out of the 10 data sets (S1 state), the values obtained for E are lower than 1. The failure of the nonlinear predictability on the rest of the data sets suggests the existence of high dimensional dynamical components and the lack of sufficient data to resolve them by using this approach.

Table 1. The one-step prediction errors (E)

Subject	S1	S2
1	0.705	0.563
2	0.923	0.735
3	0.808	0.780
4	1.101	0.652
5	0.872	0.569
6	0.901	0.683
7	1.051	0.582
8	0.778	0.6301
9	1.081	0.644
10	1.032	0.813

We have subjected to the surrogate data analysis all the data sets where values of E lower than 1 has been reported. The surrogate data, consistent with the null hypothesis tested (linearly correlated noise transformed by a static nonlinearity) has been analyzed in the same manner as the original data. The prediction errors have been compared using the S statistic (5). The results are shown in Table 2.

Table 2. The significance of the difference in predictability between the original and the surrogate data

Subject	S1	S2
1	4.269	1.254
2	3.156	1.508
3	3.103	0.292
4	-	0.448
5	3.647	2.128
6	3.014	0.619
7	-	1.457
8	4.578	0.624
9	-	2.014
10	-	1.025

Additional evidences of nonlinearity have been obtained in the data recorded in the S1-state, as the null hypothesis tested could be rejected at the level of confidence corresponding to S values greater than 3. In contrast, the predictability of RRIs disclosed in S1-state could not be distinguished from that of the surrogate data.

Figure 4,5 presents the typical behavior of the predictions errors from original (S1-state) and surrogate data, for different sizes of the neighborhood used for fitting the local linear predictor. For small values of k, the predictability of the surrogates is significant decreased in comparison to that of obtained from the original data, only from the data corresponding to S1-state.

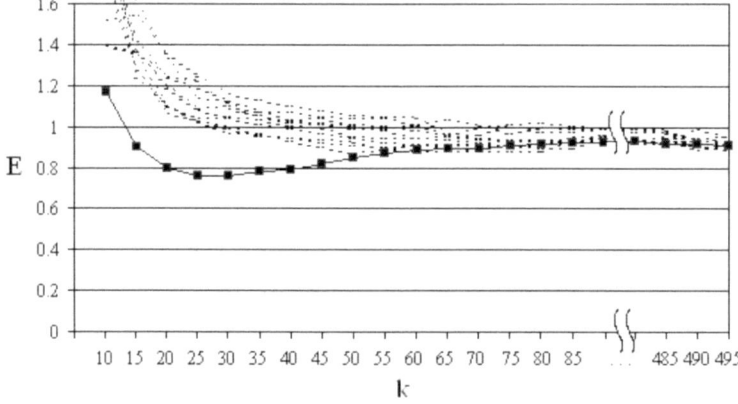

Fig. 4. Plot of E=f(k) - original data (solid line) and surrogates (dashed line), S1- state

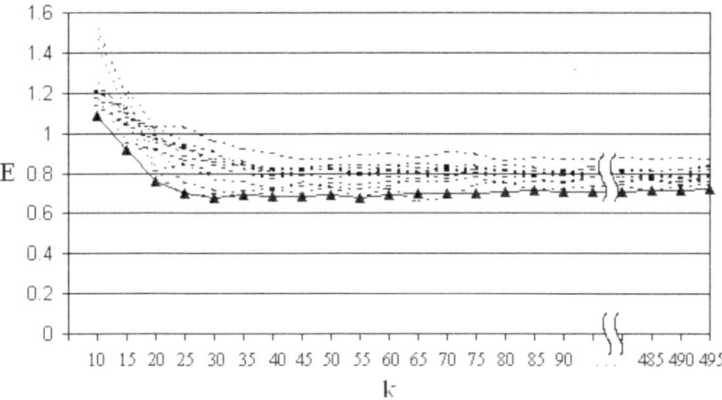

Fig. 5. Plot of E=f(k) - original data (solid line) and surrogates (dashed line), S2- state

4 Discussions

Beat-to-beat variability in the heart rhythm shows both deterministic and stochastic components. The relevance of RR interval time series analysis from the viewpoint of their predictability is related to the assignment of a physiological meaning to the type of time dependencies that account for their deterministic properties. With the autonomous nervous system as the main regulatory component of the heart rhythm, changes in the state of neural control reflect on both deterministic and nonlinear properties of the RRI data.

We have analyzed the RRIs data corresponding to two opposite states of neural regulation: normal and pharmacologically blockade. Using the nonlinear predictability and surrogate data analysis, we have explored the type of correlations that contribute to the nonlinear deterministic structures of our data.

RRIs data recorded in the normal state of ANS functioning display diminished predictability, in comparison with the blockade state. In 4 out of the 10 data sets the nonlinear predictability did not outperform the prediction results of the trivial predictor. This behavior can result from high- dimensional dynamics or noise contamination. Analyzing short length data (800 data points), only low dimensional dynamics can be reliably characterized, independently of the nonlinear measure used. The rest of data recorded in the normal state reports values of the prediction errors smaller than 1, and they can be distinguished from that of the corresponding surrogates. Therefore, there are evidences of nonlinear correlations that contribute to the predictability displayed by these data. Despite of an increased predictability subsequent to the ANS blockade approach, no evidence of nonlinearity could be established in RRIs data, as no statistically significance has been obtained in comparison with surrogate data. Moreover, a global linear model provides similar predictive performance, as that obtained by local linear approximation. These observations are consistent with a stochastic dynamics with strong linear components that generate the RRIs data obtained in the blockade-state.

Based on the assessment of nonlinear predictability of the RRIs, and on comparison with surrogate data, we found evidences of nonlinearity only in the data corresponding to the normal state of cardiovascular functioning and neural control regulation. Predictability, albeit enhanced subsequent to the pharmacologically ANS blockade, could not be distinguished by that of a stochastically forced linear system with the same power spectrum.

Acknowledgement

This study was supported in part by the PENED program (project 99ED146) of the Greek Secretariat of Research and Technology and by the State Scholarships Foundation (S.S.F.) of Athens - Greece who provided the financial support to L. C.

References

1. Akselrod, S., Gordon, D., Ubel, F.A., Shannon, D.C., Berger, A.C., Cohen, R.J.: Power spectrum analysis of heart rate-fluctuations: a quantitative probe of beat-to-beat cardiovascular control. Science 213 (1981) 220-222
2. Farmer, J.D., Sidorowich, I.J.: Predicting Chaotic Series. Phys. Rev. Lett. 59 (1987) 845-848
3. Kobayashi, M., Mysha, T.: 1/f fluctuation of heart beat period. IEEE. Tran. Biomed. Eng. 29 (1982) 456-457
4. Packard, N., Crutchfield, J., Farmer, J.D., Shaw, R.: Geometry from a time series. Phys. Rev. Lett. 45 (1980) 712-716
5. Pagani, M., Lombardi, F., Guzzetti, S., Rimoldi, O., Furlan R., Pizzinelli, P., Sandrone, G., Malfatto, G., Dell'Orto, S., Piccaluga, E., Turiel, M., Baselli, G., Cerutti, S., Malliani, A.: Power spectral snalysis of heart rate and arterial pressure variability as a marker of sympatho-vagal interaction in man and conscious dog. Circ. Res. 59 (1986) 178-193
6. Sauer, T.: Reconstruction of dynamical systems from interspike intervals. Phys. Rev. Lett. 72 (1994) 3811-3814
7. Sugihara, G., May, R.M.: Nonlinear forecasting as a way of distinguishing chaos from measurement error in the time series. Nature 344 (1990) 734-741
8. Theiler, J., Galdrikia, B., Longtin, A., Eubank, A., Farmer, J.D.: Testing for nonlinearity in time series: the method of surrogate data. Phys. D 58 (1992) 77-94
9. Task Force of the European Society of cardiology and the North American Society of Pacing and Electrophysiology: Hear Rate Variability. Circulation. 93 (1996) 1043-1065

Feature Subset Selection Using Probabilistic Tree Structures. A Case Study in the Survival of Cirrhotic Patients Treated with TIPS

Iñaki Inza[1], Marisa Merino[2], Pedro Larrañaga[1], Jorge Quiroga[3], Basilio Sierra[1], and Marcos Girala[3]

[1] Department of Computer Science and Artificial Intelligence, P.O. Box 649, University of the Basque Country, E-20080 Donostia - San Sebastián, Spain
{ccbincai,ccplamup,ccpsiarb}@si.ehu.es
http://www.sc.ehu.es/isg

[2] Basque Health Service - Osakidetza, Comarca Gipuzkoa - Este, Avenida Navarra 14, E-20013 Donostia - San Sebastián, Spain
mmerino@chdo.osakidetza.net

[3] Facultad de Medicina, University Clinic of Navarra, E-31080 Pamplona - Iruña, Spain
jquiroga@unav.es

Abstract. The transjugular intrahepatic portosystemic shunt (TIPS) is an interventional treatment for cirrhotic patients with portal hypertension. In the light of our medical staff's experience, the consequences of the TIPS are not homogeneous for all the patients and a subgroup of them dies in the first six months after the TIPS placement. Actually, there is no risk indicator to identify this group, before treatment. An investigation for predicting the survival of cirrhotic patients treated with TIPS is carried out using a clinical database with 107 cases and 77 attributes. Naive-Bayes, C4.5 and CN2 supervised classifiers are applied to identify this group. The application of several Feature Subset Selection (FSS) techniques has significantly improved the predictive accuracy of these classifiers and considerably reduced the amount of attributes in the classification models. Among FSS techniques, FSS-TREE, a new randomized algorithm inspired on the EDA (Estimation of Distribution Algorithm) paradigm, has obtained the best accuracy results.

1 Introduction

Portal hypertension is a major complication of chronic liver disease. By definition, it is a pathological increase in the portal venous pressure which results in formation of porto-systemic collaterals that divert blood from the liver to the systemic circulation. This is caused by both an obstruction to outflow in the portal flow as well as increased mesenteric flow. In the western world, cirrhosis of the liver accounts for approximately 90% of all patients.

Of the sequelae of portal hypertension (i.e. varices, encephalopathy, hypersplenism, ascites), bleeding from gastro-oesophageal varices is a significant cause of early mortality (approximately $30 - 50\%$ at the first bleed) [2] [29].

R.W. Brause and E. Hanisch (Eds.): ISMDA 2000, LNCS 1933, pp. 97–110, 2000.

Many efforts have been made over the past decades in the treatment of portal hypertension. This has resulted in an increasing number of randomized trials and publications but, unfortunately, therapeutic decision is not easy [8].

The Transjugular Intrahepatic Portosystemic Shunt (TIPS) is an interventional treatment resulting in decompression of the portal system by creation of a side-to-side portosystemic anastomosis. Since its introduction over 10 years ago [27] and despite the large number of published studies, many questions remain unanswered. Taking survival into account, the results of the randomized trials should be interpreted with caution, as the studies were not designed to detect differences in survival [28].

Our medical staff has found that a subgroup of patients dies in the first six months after TIPS placement. Actually, there is no risk indicator to identify this group, before treatment.

Traditionally, Pugh's modification of the Child-Turcotte score (referred to as the Child-Pugh score) has been used to assess risk in patients undergoing portosystemic shunt surgery [25]. Although it is a classic score to assess the level of seriousness of a patient's liver disease, it has inherent problems when applied to patients undergoing TIPS and it cannot be used to predict which patients will die within a certain period of time and which patients will survive that period. The several difficulties and innacuracies in applying the Child-Pugh score to predict survival periods have been detailed by Conn [6].

In this situation, the testing of Machine Learning techniques for TIPS indication or contraindication is an interesting research way. At first, we tested the Naive-Bayes, C4.5 and CN2 classifiers in the prediction of the survival of cirrhotic patients for the first six months after the placement of the TIPS. A period of six month is chosen because our physicians think that beyond that period, factors such as stenosis of the shunt and possible variceal rebleeding as a consequence, would compound the analysis. Furthermore, a critical criteria for choosing this period is that the average waiting time on a list for a liver transplantation at the University Clinic of Navarra is approximately six months.

At this point, in our medical staff's opinion, the obtained predictive accuracies were good enough. However, the used database had a large set of measured attributes and some of them seemed to be irrelevant or redundant. It is well known that the accuracy of Machine Learning classifiers is not monotonic with respect to the amount of attributes [17]: irrelevant or redundant attributes, depending on the specific characteristics of the classifier, may degrade the accuracy of the classification model. In this sense, given the entire set of attributes, we want to select the attribute subset with the best predictive accuracy for a certain classifier. This problem is known in the Machine Learning community as the Feature Subset Selection (FSS) problem and it has been tackled with success in different medical areas [9] [14]. A reduction in the number of variables is of interest as classification models with a smaller number of variables may be more quickly and easily used by clinicians, since those models would require a lesser data input [7]. Models with relatively small number of variables may be more readily converted into paper-based models that could be used widely in current medical practice. Other interesting effects of the dimensionality reduction are the decrease in the cost of adquisition of the data and the rise in the interpretability and comprehensibility of the classification models.

In this work four classic and well known FSS algorithms are applied, obtaining a considerable reduction in the amount of attributes needed by Naive-Bayes, C4.5 and CN2 classifiers, as well as a significant predictive accuracy improvement regarding the models with the whole set of attributes. Coupled with these algorithms, a new randomized method, called FSS-TREE (Feature Subset Selection by TREE structure learning) and inspired in the EDA [19] (Estimation of Distribution Algorithm) paradigm, has obtained the best accuracy results for Naive-Bayes, C4.5 and CN2.

The work is organized as follows: the next section presents the study database. Section 3 presents the Naive-Bayes, C4.5 and CN2 classifiers and their results using the whole set of attributes. Section 4 presents four classic well known FSS techniques and the new approach for feature subset selection, FSS-TREE. The experimental results of the exposed FSS techniques over Naive-Bayes, C4.5 and CN2 are presented in the fifth section. We finish the work with a brief summary and some ideas for future work.

2   Patients. Study database

This study includes 127 patients with liver cirrhosis who underwent TIPS from May 1991 to September 1998 in the University Clinic of Navarra, Spain. The diagnosis of cirrhosis was based in liver histology in all cases. The indications for TIPS placement were: prophylaxis of rebleeding (68 patients), refractory ascites (28 patients), prophylaxis of bleeding (11 patients), acute bleeding refractory to endoscopic and medical therapy (10 patients), portal vein thrombosis (9 patients) and Budd-Chiari syndrome (1 patient).

Statistical analysis includes 107 patients because 20 underwent liver transplantation the first six months after TIPS placement. The follow-up of these transplantationated patients was censored on the day of the transplantation. This censoring was done to remove the effect of transplantation when modeling the six-months survival of patients who undergo TIPS. If these patients were not censored, deaths due to surgical mortality related to transplantation might have influenced the selection of variables that are prognostic for the TIPS procedure. On the other hand, transplantation may prolong survival compared with patients who do not undergo TIPS. It is predictably found that survival in patients who undergo transplantation is significantly improved compared with those who do not undergo transplantation [21].

For each patient 77 attributes were measured before TIPS placement (see Table 1). The problem has two different categories, reflecting whether the patient died in the first six months after the placement of the TIPS or not. In the first six months after the placement of the TIPS 33 patients died and 74 survived for a longer period, thus reflecting that the utility and consequences of the TIPS were not homogeneous for all the patients.

The study was approved by the local Ethics Committe, and informed oral consent was obtained from all patients.

Table 1. Attributes of the study database.

History findings:		
Number of hepatic encephalopathies	Gender	Height
Prophylactic therapy with popranolol	Etiology of cirrhosis	Indication of TIPS
Bleeding origin	Number of bleedings	Weight
Previous sclerotherapy	Restriction of proteins	Age
Type of hepatic encephalophaty	Ascites intensity	Number of paracenteses
Volume of paracenteses	Dose of furosemide	Dose of spironolactone
Spontaneous bacterial peritonitis	Kidney failure	Organic nephropathy
Diabetes mellitus		
Laboratory findings:		
Hemoglobin	Serum conjugated bilirubin (mg/dl)	White blood cell count
Serum sodium	Urine sodium	Serum potassium
Urine potassium	Plasma osmolarity	Urine osmolarity
Urea	Plasma creatinine	Urine creatinine
Creatinine clearance	Fractional sodium excretion	Diuresis
GOT	GPT	GGT
Alkaline phosphatase	Serum total bilirubin (mg/dl)	Hematocrit
Serum albumin (g/dl)	Plateletes	Prothrombin time (%)
Parcial thrombin time	PRA	Proteins
FNG	Aldosterone	ADH
Dopamine	Norepineohrine	Epinephrine
Gamma-globulin		
CHILD score		
PUGH score		
Doppler sonography:		
Portal size	Portal flow velocity	Portal flow right
Portal flow left	Spleen lenght (cm)	
Endoscopy:		
Size of esophageal varices	Gastric varices	Portal gastropathy
Acute hemorrhage		
Hemodinamic parameters:		
Portosystemis venous pressure gradient	Heart rate (beats/min)	Cardiac output (l/min)
Free hepatic venous pressure	Wedged hepatic venous pressure	Central venous pressure
Hepatic venous pressure gradient	Arterial pressure (mm Hg)	Portal pressure
Angiography:		
Portal thrombosis		

3   Application of three Machine Learning classifiers to solve the problem

Three well known Machine Learning algorithms, with different approaches to learning, are applied using the whole set of attributes to predict the survival of cirrhotic patients for the first six months after the setting of the TIPS. The classifiers are selected due to their simplicity and their long tradition in medical diagnose studies.

Naive-Bayes (NB) rule [3] uses the Bayes rule to predict the class for each test instance, assuming that features are independent to each other given the class. The probability for discrete features is estimated from data using maximum likelihood estimation and applying the Laplace correction. A normal distribution is assumed to estimate the class conditional probabilities for continuous attributes. Unknown values in the test instance are skipped.

C4.5 [26] is a popular algorithm that summarises the data in the form of a decision tree. Nodes in a decision tree correspond to features, and, branches to their associated values. The leaves of the tree correspond to the classes. In order to avoid overfitting the data C4.5 employs a simplification pruning mechanism.

CN2 [5] is a well known algorithm that learns a set of independent if-then rules. It tries to construct rules that cover a large amount of examples of a specific class and few examples of the rest of classes.

Costs of medical tests are not considered in the construction of classification models and accuracy maximization and satisfactory human comprehension are the goals of our research. Due to the low number of cases, the *leave-one-out* [16] procedure is used to estimate the accuracy of each classifier. Experiments are run in a SUN-SPARC computer.

The accuracy estimates of three supervised classifiers using the entire set of attributes can be seen in Table 2 under the 'no-FSS' (no Feature Subset Selection) column. At this stage of the study, the obtained accuracy results, specially for the NB classifier, were good enough in our medical staff's opinion. The human interpretability and graphical representation of C4.5 and CN2 classification models were also satisfactory for our medical experts. However, we saw room for improvement using the Feature Subset Selection (FSS) approach.

4   Selecting features: Feature Subset Selection by probabilistic tree structures

It has long been proved that the classification accuracy of supervised classifiers is not monotonic with respect to the addition of features. Irrelevant or redundant features, depending on the specific characteristics of the supervised classifier, may degrade the predictive accuracy of the classification model. FSS objective will be the detection of the features that hurt the performance of the classification algorithm. In addition, thanks to the deletion of features, the obtained classifier probably will be less complex and more understandable by humans and a reduction in the cost of adquisition of the data can be achieved (this is a critical issue in medicine, when the costs of some medical tests are high).

FSS can be viewed as a search problem [20], with each state in the search space specifying a subset of the possible features of the task. Exhaustive evaluation of possible feature subsets is usually unfeasible in practice due to the large amount of computational effort required. In this way, many search heuristics are proposed in the literature.

4.1   Four classic Feature Subset Selection methods

We have used the following well known FSS methods in the experimentation phase:

– Sequential Forward Selection (SFS) is a classic hill-climbing search algorithm [15] which starts from an empty subset of features and sequentially selects features until no improvement is achieved in the evaluation function value;
– Sequential Backward Elimination (SBE) is another classic hill-climbing algorithm [15] which starts from the full set of features and sequentially deletes features until no improvement is achieved in the evaluation function value;
– Genetic Algorithm search with one-point crossover (GA-o);
– Genetic Algorithm search with uniform crossover (GA-u).

Genetic Algorithms (GAs) [13] are one of the best known techniques for solving optimization problems. The GA is a population based search method. First, a population of individuals[1] (in our case feature subsets) is generated, then promising individuals are selected, and finally new individuals which will form the new population are generated using crossover and mutation operators. On the other hand, SFS and SBE, instead of working with a population of solutions, try to optimize a single feature subset.

Although the optimal selection of parameters is still an open problem on GAs [12], for both GA algorithms, guided by the recommendations of Bäck [1], the probability of crossover is set to 1.0 and the mutation probability to $1/d$, being d the number of variables of the domain (these values are so common in the literature). Fitness-proportionate selection is used to select individuals for crossover. The population size is set to 1,000 and the new population is formed by the best members from both old population and offspring[2]. The criterion for halting the genetic search is the following: GA-o and GA-u stop when in a sampled new population of solutions no individual is found with an evaluation function value that improves the best individual found in the previous generation. Thus, the best solution of the previous population is returned as the result of the genetic search. We want to control the risk of overspecialization with this severe criteria.

4.2 FSS-TREE, a new EDA-inspired method to select features

Genetic Algorithms are mainly criticized for three aspects [19]:

– the large number of parameters and their associated refered optimal selection or tunning process;
– the extremely difficult prediction of the movements of the populations in the search space;
– their incapacity to solve the well known deceptive problems [11].

In an attempt to solve the previous problems using an evolutionary and population-based search method, the Estimation of Distribution Algorithm (EDA) [19] [23] appears. In EDA, there are no crossover nor mutation operators: the new population is sampled from a probability distribution which is estimated from the selected individuals. Figure 1 shows the basic structure of the EDA approach.

---

[1] The terms 'individual' and 'solution' are used indistinctly.
[2] As 'offspring' is known the set of newly created solutions.

EDA
    $D_0 \leftarrow$ Generate N individuals (the initial population) randomly.
    Repeat for $l = 1, 2, \ldots$ until a stop criterion is met.
        $D^s_{l-1} \leftarrow$ Select $S \leq N$ individuals from D_{l-1} according to a selection method.
        $p_l(\mathbf{x}) = p(\mathbf{x}|D^s_{l-1}) \leftarrow$ Estimate the joint probability distribution of an individual being among the selected inviduals.
        $D_l \leftarrow$ Sample N individuals (the new population) from $p_l(\mathbf{x})$.

Fig. 1. Main structure of the EDA approach.

The EDA algorithm can be used to solve the FSS problem, representing each individual of the EDA search as a possible feature subset solution. A common notation can be used to represent an individual (or feature subset): for a full d feature problem, there are d bits in each individual, each bit indicating whether a feature is present (1) or absent (0).

The main problem of EDA resides on how the joint d-dimensional probability distribution $p_l(\mathbf{x})$ is estimated. Obviously, the computation of 2^d probabilities (for a domain with d binary variables) is impractical. Bayesian networks [19] could be an attractive paradigm to make the factorization of the probability distribution of best individuals. However, due to the large amount of attributes in our database, a huge number of individuals is needed to induce a reliable Bayesian network [10]. In our study, we have used dependency-trees [4], a simple and well known model to estimate probabilistic distributions.

A dependency tree assumes some kind of dependences among the attributes of the database, restricting $p_l(\mathbf{x})$ to factorizations in which the conditional probability distribution for any one bit depends on the value of at most one other bit. In Bayesian network terms, this means we are restricting our probability models to networks in which each node can have at most one parent. We use the method proposed by Chow and Liu [4] to find the optimal model within these restrictions. The induced tree is optimal in the sense that among all possible trees, its probabilistic structure maximizes the likelihood of selected solutions when they are drawn from any unknown distribution. We call the application to the feature subset selection problem of this search algorithm as FSS-TREE. Figure 2 summarizes the FSS-TREE algorithm.

As GA FSS approaches, FSS-TREE is also a randomized and population-based FSS algorithm. The absence of crossover and mutation operators (implicit to Genetic Algorithms) to evolve the population is one of its biggest attractions. A population size of $1,000$ individuals is set up for FSS-TREE and it uses the same stop criteria as both GA approaches. The new population is also formed by the best members from both old population and sampled offspring.

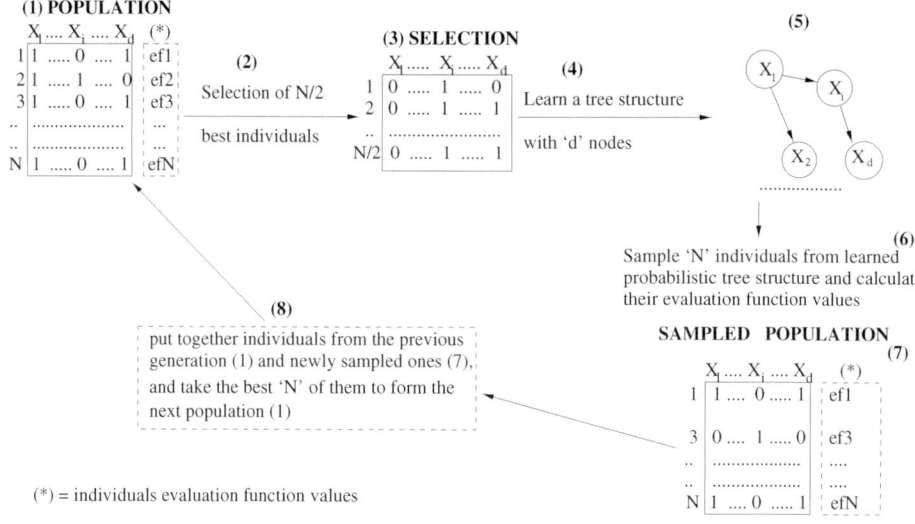

Fig. 2. FSS-TREE algorithm.

4.3   Evaluation function of FSS methods

To assess the goodness of each proposed feature subset for a specific classifier, a *wrapper* [17] approach is applied. In the same way as supervised classifiers when no feature selection is applied, this wrapper approach estimates, by the leave-one-out procedure, the goodness of the specific learning algorithm (NB, C4.5 or CN2) using only the feature subset found by the search algorithm. Thus, the study database is projected maintaining the values of the selected features and the class variable for the whole of 107 patients: over this projected dataset the goodness of the proposed feature subset using the specific classifier is estimated by the leave-one-out estimation technique. By means of the application of the *wrapper* scheme we guarantee the optimality of selected features respect to the specific classifier [17].

5   Experimental results

SFS and SBE are deterministic algorithms which are only run once for each classifier. Due to their randomized nature, GA-o, GA-u and FSS-TREE are run 10 times for each classifier. Coupled with the leave-one-out estimation of the predictive accuracy of three classifiers without feature selection and SFS and SBE selection methods, Table 2 also reflects the leave-one-out accuracy estimation of the best run of each randomized FSS method. Apart from the standard deviation of the leave-one-out estimation, Table 2 reflects the cardinality of the best feature subset for each FSS method and classifier. Note that when no FSS method is applied, CN2 and C4.5 classifiers, on their own, can discard a subset of the features.

Table 2. Estimated accuracy percentage coupled with the standard deviation of the leave-one-out process (first row) and the cardinalities of finally selected feature subsets (second row) for each classifier. For randomized FSS algorithms, the results of the most accurate run are reflected.

	no-FSS	SFS	SBE	GA-o	GA-u	FSS-TREE
NB	75.70 ± 4.17	82.24 ± 3.71	80.37 ± 3.86	85.05 ± 3.46	85.05 ± 3.46	86.92 ± 3.28
	77	3	72	8	9	10
CN2	69.92 ± 4.96	81.15 ± 3.59	79.53 ± 4.27	84.97 ± 2.57	84.16 ± 2.52	85.88 ± 2.85
	32	6	30	5	9	7
C4.5	61.66 ± 4.62	85.19 ± 2.66	80.00 ± 4.37	85.73 ± 4.22	86.11 ± 3.63	87.95 ± 2.63
	6	3	6	3	4	5

As randomized FSS techniques are run 10 times, Table 3 reflects the average accuracy percentages and cardinality of selected subsets of these 10 runs, coupled with the associated standard deviations of these averages.

Table 3. Average accuracy percentages (first row) and cardinalities of finally selected feature subsets (second row) of ten runs for each randomized FSS method and classifier. The standard deviations of accuracy and cardinality averages are also reported.

	GA-o	GA-u	FSS-TREE
NB	84.67 ± 0.51	84.48 ± 0.51	86.28 ± 0.54
	10.2 ± 3.11	9.4 ± 2.88	10.6 ± 0.57
CN2	84.43 ± 0.40	84.12 ± 0.06	85.26 ± 0.54
	9.0 ± 3.46	11.0 ± 3.46	8.3 ± 2.30
C4.5	85.30 ± 0.37	85.30 ± 0.70	86.34 ± 1.38
	4.0 ± 1.73	3.3 ± 0.57	3.7 ± 0.95

Several conclusions can be extracted from the results of Tables 2 and 3:
- with the aid of FSS techniques, all supervised classifiers obtain better accuracy levels than the no-FSS approach using feature subsets that need less than 85% of the attributes of the whole feature set. We suspect that this dimensionality reduction and accuracy improvement is possible due to the large amount of correlations that appear among the features of the study database. 162 pairwise correlations statistically significant at the $\alpha = 0.01$ level and other 168 pairwise correlations at the $\alpha = 0.05$ level by means of the Pearson coefficient are detected among the features of the study database. As a clear example, *Child score* and *Pugh score* variables are a linear combination of other five features of the study. FSS methods are able to mainly detect these groups of correlated features

that hurt the accuracy level of supervised classifiers. Our physicians collected a large number of features they thought they could affect the survival of the patients. However, FSS algorithms are able to discover these correlations and just with a small portion of them, the supervised classifiers are able to acceptably discriminate between both categories of the problem;

• the dimensionality reduction is coupled with significant accuracy improvements with respect to the accuracy of the whole feature set. For all supervised classifiers, when a cross-validated paired t test is applied between the no-FSS approach and each run of any FSS method (except SBE with NB), accuracy differences are always statistically significant at the $\alpha = 0.05$ level;

• due to the low number of patients and the intrinsic high standard deviation, it is not likely to establish statistically significant accuracy differences among the FSS algorithms. Although the non significance of accuracy differences, randomized FSS methods achieve better accuracy levels for all supervised classifiers than SFS and SBE. However, in the case of the C4.5 classifier, the accuracy level achieved by SFS is close to the accuracy of randomized FSS methods. The explanation to these accuracy differences among sequential and population-based FSS methods appears in the works of Vafaie and De Jong [30] and Kudo and Sklansky [18], where they highlight the tendency of greedy-like sequential searches as SFS and SBE to get trapped on local peaks of the search space: thus, they defend the use of population based search methods as more robust search engines in the FSS problem;

• the low standard deviation of the average accuracy of 10 runs for each randomized FSS method must be noted: this gives us an idea about the stability of the models induced by these methods. Among them, FSS-TREE, apart from the single classification models with the best predictive accuracy for three supervised classifiers, achieves the best average accuracy results. Several studies have shown the superiority of the EDA approach respect to the GA approaches in several optimization problems [19] [24]: the reason for this superiority resides in the ability of the EDA approach to capture the underlying structure of the problem. When this happens, the EDA approach can be able to discover better fitted areas of the search space than GA techniques. Thus, we can suppose that this occurs in our problem. In this way, Table 4 presents an intuitive comparison among our randomized methods. As each randomized FSS method is run 10 times, among all randomized methods we have 30 runs: Table 4 shows have many of the best 10 out of these 30 runs belong to each method. Table 4 clearly states the stability in the superior accuracy achieved by the predictive models induced by the features selected by FSS-TREE: for all supervised classifiers, more than half of the best 10 subsets found by randomized FSS methods belong to FSS-TREE;

• we note a high stability degree in the medical findings selected by FSS methods. Although the low standard deviation in the number of findings selected by randomized FSS methods gives us an idea of stability, our objective is to find out which specific attributes are selected by different runs of a randomized FSS method. As FSS-TREE is the method with the best average accuracy for all

Table 4. For each supervised classifier, the amount of the best 10 randomized runs which belong to each FSS method

	GA-o	GA-u	FSS-TREE
NB	0	0	10
CN2	2	1	7
C4.5	2	2	6

classifiers, its behaviour with respect to the stability in the selection of features is analyzed. As FSS-TREE is run 10 times for each classifier, Table 5 reflects the amount of runs in which each medical finding is included in the final models. The attributes that appear in the best subset are also indicated. Table 5 shows a high degree of stability in the attributes selected by the 10 runs of FSS-TREE for each classifier. This stability in the selection of features also occurs for the rest of the randomized FSS methods. As the wrapper approach is used to assure the optimality of selected features with respect to the specific supervised classifier, we analyze each classifier separately:

• NB uses in 10 runs, 16 different features with a mean of 10.6 ± 0.57 features per execution. 6 out of 10 models are minor variations of each other and the rest do not highly vary. The presence of *Parcial thrombin time, PRA* and *Gamma-globulin* findings in all the executions must be noted;

• CN2 uses 21 different features with a mean of 8.3 ± 2.30 features per execution. The 10 models can be divided into 3 groups of near identical rule sets within each group of executions. The presence of the *Previous sclerotherapy* finding is noted in all the executions;

• C4.5 uses 8 different features with a mean of 3.7 ± 0.95 features per execution. All the models are minor variations of each other and 6 runs output the same tree. The *Gamma-globulin* finding appears in all the trees.

When the classification models are presented to the medical staff, they have noted a large improvement in comprehensibility among the models induced with the aid of FSS techniques and those that are constructed without FSS. The dimensionality reduction carried out by the FSS process has reduced the complexity and the amount of variables to be input to the classification models, converting them to paper-based models [7] which can be more easily used in everyday practice. Thus, by this dimensionality reduction, the confidence and acceptance in the models of our medical staff has increased.

Physicians, apart from the high accuracy levels, highlight the transparency and user-executable (ability for mental check) levels [22] of the graphical output produced by decision trees and the set of decision rules. With the reduction in the number of needed measurements, an obvious reduction of the derived economic costs is achieved. We also have a lower amount of possibly troublesome medical test for the future patients.

Table 5. For FSS-TREE, this table lists the amount of runs each that medical finding appears in the models induced by each classifier. An asterisk indicates the findings that appear in the best found feature subset. We do not reflect the attributes that are not never selected by FSS-TREE.

	NB	CN2	C4.5
History finding attributes:			
Gender	6	0	0
Weight	4*	0	0
Etiology of cirrhosis	0	3	0
Indication of TIPS	0	4*	0
Previous sclerotherapy	0	10*	0
Restriction of proteins	0	0	3
Number of hepatic encephalopathies	0	0	3
Dose of furosemide	3	0	0
Spontaneous bacterial peritonitis	6	3	0
Kidney failure	0	0	0
Organic nephropathy	4*	6	0
Laboratory finding attributes:			
Hematocrit	3	0	2*
White blood cell count	4*	0	0
Urine sodium	0	0	0
Serum potassium	7*	0	0
Urine potassium	0	3	0
Plasma osmolarity	0	0	0
Urine osmolarity	0	4*	0
Urea	0	3	0
Creatinine clearance	3	0	0
Fractional sodium excretion	0	0	0
Diuresis	0	5*	0
GOT	0	0	8
GPT	0	3	0
Serum total bilirubin (mg/dl)	0	2	0
Serum conjugated bilirubin (mg/dl)	4*	0	0
Serum albumin (g/dl)	3	0	0
Plateletes	0	3	0
Prothrombin time (%)	0	3	5
Parcial thrombin time	10*	4*	2*
PRA	10*	0	0
Proteins	6	0	0
FNG	0	3	0
Aldosterone	4*	0	0
Epinephrine	0	0	2*
Gamma-globulin	10*	3	10*
CHILD score	0	7*	0
PUGH score	6	6	0
Doppler sonography:			
Portal flow left	0	0	0
Spleen lenght (cm)	3	0	0
Endoscopy:			
Portal gastropathy	0	4*	0
Hemodinamic parameters:			
Free hepatic venous pressure	4*	0	0
Wedged hepatic venous pressure	3	0	0
Hepatic venous pressure gradient (HVPG)	0	3	0
Central venous pressure	0	0	2*
Angiography:			
Portal thrombosis	0	0	0

6   Summary and Future Work

A medical problem, the prediction of the survival of cirrhotic patients treated with TIPS, has been focused from a machine learning perspective, with the aim of obtaining a classification rule for the indication or contraindication of TIPS in cirrhotic patients. With the application of several feature selection techniques the predictive accuracy of applied classifiers is largely improved. Among feature selection techniques, FSS-TREE, a new randomized algorithm inspired on the new EDA (Estimation of Distribution Algorithm) paradigm, has obtained the best accuracy results for all supervised classifiers. Coupled with this improvement, more compact models with fewer attributes have been obtained, which could be easier understood and applied by our medical staff.

In the future, we plan to use a database with near 300 attributes to deal with the problem of survival in cirrhotic patients treated with TIPS, which also collects patients measurements one month after the placement of TIPS. For this work, we plan to apply other probability distribution factorization models, different to dependency trees, to factorize the distribution of selected solutions in the EDA approach.

Acknowledgments

This work was supported by the PI 96/12 grant from Gobierno Vasco - Departamento de Educación, Universidades e Investigación and the grant UPV 140.226-EB131/99 from University of the Basque Country.

References

1. Bäck, T.: Evolutionary Algorithms is Theory and Practice. Oxford University Press (1996)
2. Bornman, P.C., Krige, J.E.J., Terblanche, J.: Management of oesophageal varices. Lancet **343** (1994) 1079-84
3. Cestnik, B.: Estimating Probabilities: a crucial task in Machine Learning. Proceedings ECAI-90 (1990) 147-149
4. Chow, C., Liu, C.: Approximating discrete probability distributions with dependence trees. IEEE Transactions on Information Theory **14** (1968) 462-467
5. Clark, P., Niblett, R.: The CN2 induction algorithm. Machine Learning **3** (1989) 261-284
6. Conn, H.O.: A peek at the Child-Turcotte classification. Hepatology **1** (1981) 1-7
7. Cooper, G.F., Aliferis, C.F., Ambrosino, R., Aronis, J., Buchanan, B.G., Caruana, R., Fine, M.J., Glymour, C., Gordon, G., Hanusa, B.H., Janosky, J.E., Meek, C., Mitchell, T., Richardson, T., Spirtes, P.: An evaluation of machine-learning methods for predicting pneumonia mortality. Artificial Intelligence in Medicine **9** (1997) 107-138
8. D'Amico, G., Pagliaro, L., Bosch, J.: The treatment of portal hypertension: a meta-analytic review. Hepatology **22** (1995) 332-354
9. Draper D., Fouskakis, D.: Stochastic Optimization in Health Policy: Preliminary Results and Problem Formulation. Journal of Global Optimization, in press
10. Friedman, N., Yakhini, Z.: On the Sample Complexity of Learning Bayesian Networks. Proceedings of the Twelveth Conference on Uncertainty in Artificial Intelligence (1996) 274-282
11. Goldberg, D.E.: Genetic algorithms in search, optimization, and machine learning. Addison-Wesley (1989)

12. Grefenstatte, J.J.: Optimization of Control Parameters for Genetic Algorithms. IEEE Transactions on Systems, Man, and Cybernetics **1** (1986) 122-128
13. Holland, J.: Adaptation in Natural and Artificial Systems. University of Michigan Press (1975)
14. Jelonek J., Stefanowski, J.: Feature subset selection for classification of histological images. Artificial Intelligence in Medicine **9** (1997) 227-239
15. Kittler, J.: Feature set search algorithms. Pattern Recognition and Signal Processing. Sithoff and Noordhoff, Alphen aan den Rijn (1978) 41-60
16. Kohavi, R.: A study of cross-validation and bootstrap for accuracy estimation and model selection. Proceedings IJCAI-95 (1995) 1137-1143
17. Kohavi, R., John, G.: Wrappers for feature subset selection. Artificial Intelligence **97** (1994) 273-324
18. Kudo, M., Sklansky, J.: Comparison of algorithms that select features for pattern classifiers. Pattern Recognition **33** (2000) 25-41
19. Larrañaga, P., Etxeberria, R., Lozano, J.A., Peña, J.M.: Optimization by learning and simulation of Bayesian and Gaussian networks. Technical Report EHU-KZAA-IK-4/99. University of the Basque Country, Spain (1999)
20. Liu H., Motoda H.: Feature Selection for Knowledge Discovery and Data Mining. Kluwer Academic Publishers, Norwell MA (1998)
21. Malinchoc, M., Kamath, P.S., Gordon, F.D., Peine, C.J., Rank, J., ter Borg, P.C.J.: A model to Predict Poor Survival in Patients Undergoing Transjugular Intrahepatic Portosystemic Shunts. Hepatology **31** (2000) 864-871
22. Michie, D.: Personal models of rationality. Journal of Statistical Planning Inference **25** (1990) 381-399
23. Müehlenbein, H., Paaß, G.: From recombination of genes to the estimation of distributions. Binary parameters. Lecture Notes in Computer Science 1411: Parallel Problem Solving from Nature – PPSN IV (1996) 178-187
24. Pelikan, M., Goldberg, D.E., Cantú-Paz, E.: Linkage Problem, Distribution Estimation, and Bayesian Networks. IlliGAL Report No. 98013. University of Illinois at Urbana-Champaign (1998)
25. Pugh, R.N.H., Murray-Lion, I.M., Dawson, J.L., Pictioni M.C., Williams, R.: Transection of the esophagus for bleeding oesophageal varices. British Journal of Surgery **60** (1973) 646-649
26. Quinlan, J.R.: C4.5: Programs for Machine Learning. Morgan Kaufmann, San Mateo CA (1993)
27. Róssle, M., Richter, G.M., Nóldge, G., Palmaz, J.C., Wenz, W., Gerok, W.: New operative treatment for variceal haemorrhage. Lancet **2** (1989) 153
28. Róssle, M., Siegerstetter, V., Huber, M., Ochs, A.: The first decade of the transjugular intrahepatic portosystemic shunt (TIPS): state of the art. Liver **18** (1998) 73-89
29. Saunders, J.B., Walters, J.R.F., Davies, P., Paton, A.: A 20-year prospective study of cirrhosis. British Journal of Medicine **282** (1981) 263-266
30. Vafaie, H., De Jong, K.: Robust feature selection algorithms. Proceedings of the Fifth International Conference on Tools with Artificial Intelligence (1993) 356-363

Deconvolution and Credible Intervals using Markov Chain Monte Carlo Method

Roman Hovorka

City University, London EC1V 0HB, UK
r.hovorka@soi.city.ac.uk,
WWW home page: http://www.city.ac.uk/min

Abstract. In certain applications, e.g. during reconstruction of pulsatile hormone secretion, the traditional deterministic deconvolution tec hniques fail primarily due to ill conditioning. To overcome these problems, deconvolution was formulated using a stochastic approach within the Bayesian modelling framework. The stochastic deconvolution with a piece-wise constan t definition of the signal (the input function) cannot be solved analytically but the solution was found by employing Markov chain Monte Carlo method. A computationally efficient sampling algorithm combined with a discrete deconvolution method was employed. An example analysis demonstrated the application of the stochastic deconvolution method to the estimation of hormone (insulin) secretion.

1 Introduction

Novel statistical computational approaches enable solutions to a wide range of problems, which cannot be handled b y traditional methods. In particular, Markov chain Monte Carlo (MCMC) methods [1] ha vebeen applied to characterise multidimensional probability distributions in the areas of, for example, image analysis, population pharmacokinetics, and gene mapping [2, 3].

Deconvolution is a method for signal reconstruction and belongs to the family of model-independent approaches. Deconvolution estimates a large number of parameters as opposed to model-based methods, which use a model structure to reduce dimensionality of the parameter space.

Under certain conditions deconvolution becomes ill conditioned. The combination of *frequent* sampling and a *slow* (in relation to variations in the input function) unit impulse response causes the measurement error to be amplified. The calculated signal (the input function) then displays erratic behaviour and is sensitive to small variations in measurements.

Ill conditioning has been tackled by, for example, a regularisation method [4, 5]. Other methods ha ve also been dev elopedbut all adopt additional assumption(s) about the underlying signal. Often, it is the assumption of *smoothness* of the signal. Smoothing carried out prior to processing (replacing measurements by moving averages) or during processing (introduction of a regularisation component) av oidssuccessfully ill conditioning but also looses information about variability of the signal.

R.W. Brause and E. Hanisch (Eds.): ISMDA 2000, LNCS 1933, pp. 111–121, 2000.

All information could be retained if deconvolution is formulated in probabilistic terms. Deconvolution then calculates the signal but also propagates the measurement error through the deconvolution operation to the signal estimate. This is the objective of stochastic deconvolution.

The present work describes the formulation of stochastic deconvolution and uses an MCMC method to calculate the solution in an example taken from a biomedical field.

2   Methodology

2.1   Discrete Convolution

The general convolution integral has the form

$$c(t) = \int_{-\infty}^{t} u(t - \tau)r(\tau)d\tau + \epsilon(t) \tag{1}$$

where $c(t)$ represents the measurement, $u(t)$ represents the unit impulse response, $r(t)$ represents the input function, and $\epsilon(t)$ represents the measurement error. It will be assumed further in the text that the unit response is described by a sum of exponentials, i.e. $u(t) = \sum_{i=1}^{K} A_i e^{-a_i t}$, as traditional in the biomedical field.

The discrete version of the convolution integral treats the input as a piecewise constant function, which is specified by a time series $\mathbf{r} = \{r_i\}$, $i = 1 \ldots N$. The discrete version of the convolution integral given by Eq. 1 is written as

$$\mathbf{c} = \mathbf{A}\mathbf{r} + \boldsymbol{\epsilon}, \tag{2}$$

where $\mathbf{c} = \{c_j\}$, $j = 1 \ldots M$, is a set of measurements, $\boldsymbol{\epsilon} = \{\epsilon_j\}$, $j = 1 \ldots M$, is a set of measurement errors, and $\mathbf{A}$ is an $M \times N$ convolution matrix[6]. The measurement errors ϵ_j are assumed to be independent and normally distributed with a constant coefficient of variation CV, $\epsilon_j \sim N(0, \left[\frac{CV}{100}c_j\right]^2)$.

Elements a_{ij} of $\mathbf{A}$ are calculated as $a_{ij} = \int_{t_j-1}^{t_j} u(t_i - \tau)d\tau$ assuming that the measurement time grid and the input function time grid coincide (i.e. $N = M$).

2.2   Stochastic Deconvolution

The stochastic formulation of convolution gives stochastic interpretation to the input function $\mathbf{r}$. The Bayesian modelling framework was employed in the formulation.

In the present formulation, components r_i of the input function are treated as random variables, which are assumed to be identically distributed with a non-informative, uniform prior distribution

$$p(r_i) = \begin{cases} const & \text{if } r_{\max} \geq r_i \geq 0 \\ 0 & \text{otherwise,} \end{cases}$$

where $r_{\max}$ is a suitable bound.

In the absence of information about the measurement error, the coefficient of variation CV is assumed to have an improper non-informed prior distribution [7]

$$p(CV) \propto \frac{1}{CV}. \tag{3}$$

The objective of the stochastic deconvolution is to calculate the *posterior* distribution $\pi(\boldsymbol{\theta})$ of the stochastic vector $\boldsymbol{\theta}$, which contains the input function and the measurement error, $\boldsymbol{\theta} = \{\mathbf{r}, CV\}$, employing the Bayesian theorem

$$\pi(\boldsymbol{\theta}) \propto p(\mathbf{c}|\boldsymbol{\theta})p(\boldsymbol{\theta}). \tag{4}$$

The conditional probability $p(\mathbf{c}|\boldsymbol{\theta})$ is calculated according to the standard multivariate normal density with a diagonal covariance matrix,

$$p(\mathbf{c}|\boldsymbol{\theta}) = \prod_{i=1}^{N} \frac{1}{\frac{CV}{100}c'_i\sqrt{2\pi}} \exp\left[-\frac{1}{2}\left(\frac{c_i - c'_i}{\frac{CV}{100}c'_i}\right)^2\right], \tag{5}$$

where c'_i is obtained by discrete convolution, i.e. $\mathbf{c}' = \mathbf{A}\mathbf{r}$.

The posterior distribution $\pi(\boldsymbol{\theta})$ summarises the input function and can be used to calculate, for example, marginal distributions associated with component r_i or can be used to derive other characteristics of the input function, e.g. its spectrum, using fully and coherently the stochastic approach.

2.3   Solution using Markov Chain Monte Carlo Method

A closed-form solution of Eq. 4 does not exist due to, for example, the truncated type of distribution associated with $\mathbf{r}$ and other methods have to be used to characterise/describe the posterior distribution $\pi(\boldsymbol{\theta})$.

MCMC methods enable a sample from the posterior distribution $\pi(\boldsymbol{\theta})$ to be generated. A general MCMC method, the Metropolis-Hastings algorithm [8, 9, 10] starts with an arbitrary initial parameter vector $\boldsymbol{\theta}^{(0)}$, and iteratively generates Markov chain (a sample from $\pi(\boldsymbol{\theta})$) with elements $\boldsymbol{\theta}^{(k)}$.

In the present implementation, the Metropolis-Hastings algorithm generates a new element $\boldsymbol{\theta}^{(k+1)}$ of the Markov chain on a *component-by-component* basis using $N + 1$ transition kernels $q_j(\cdot)$ (similar to Gibbs sampling). During one iteration step, the algorithm considers, in turn, candidate components θ'_j, $j = 1 \ldots N+1$, of a newly generated chain element $\boldsymbol{\theta}'$ and decides on their acceptance using acceptance ratios $\alpha_j(\cdot, \cdot)$, namely

$$\boldsymbol{\theta}' = \boldsymbol{\theta}^{(k)}$$

θ'_1 from $q_1(\theta_1)$;

$\quad$ accept using $\alpha_1((\theta_1^{(k)} \ldots \theta_{N+1}^{(k)}), \boldsymbol{\theta}')$

θ'_2 from $q_2(\theta_2)$;

$$\text{accept using } \alpha_2((\theta_1', \theta_2^{(k)} \ldots \theta_{N+1}^{(k)}), \boldsymbol{\theta}')$$

$$\vdots$$

$$\theta_{N+1}' \text{ from } q_{N+1}(\theta_{N+1});$$

$$\text{accept using } \alpha_{N+1}((\theta_1' \ldots \theta_N', \theta_{N+1}^{(k)}), \boldsymbol{\theta}')$$

$$\boldsymbol{\theta}^{(k+1)} = \boldsymbol{\theta}',$$

where the acceptance ratios are defined as [10]

$$\alpha_j(\boldsymbol{\theta}, \boldsymbol{\theta}') = \min \left\{ 1, \frac{\pi(\boldsymbol{\theta}')q_j(\theta_j)}{\pi(\boldsymbol{\theta})q_j(\theta_j')} \right\}.$$

The transition kernels are function of the newly generated components and are independent of, for example, the previous element on the chain $\boldsymbol{\theta}^{(k)}$. The kernel $q_j(\theta_j)$ in our implementation is an approximation of the conditional density of the j-th component given all other components,

$$q_j(\theta_j) \approx \pi(\theta_j | \boldsymbol{\theta}_{-j}),$$

where $\boldsymbol{\theta}_{-j} = (\theta_i; i \neq j)$. The conditional density $\pi(\theta_j | \boldsymbol{\theta}_{-j})$ is evaluated up to a proportionality constant with the use of Eqs. 4 & 5

$$\pi(\theta_j | \boldsymbol{\theta}_{-j}) \propto \pi(\theta_j, \boldsymbol{\theta}_{-j})$$
$$\propto p(\mathbf{c} | \theta_j, \boldsymbol{\theta}_{-j}) p(\theta_j, \boldsymbol{\theta}_{-j}).$$

The approach described by Gilks *et al* [11] has been adopted to approximate and to sample from the conditional density. This approach employs adaptive rejection sampling [10] and is similar to Gibbs sampling with an addition of a rejection Metropolis step. The approximations of the conditional densities are calculated at each iteration step and involve a limited number (units to maximum tens of units) evaluations of posterior densities.

2.4   FastConvolution

The calculation of the acceptance ratio $\alpha_j(\cdot, \cdot)$ requires the evaluation of the posterior densities $\pi(\theta_j | \boldsymbol{\theta}_{-j})$. In fact, the calculation of the posterior density is computationally the most expensive operation primarily due to the involvement of discrete convolution, see Eq. 2, which is a matrix-vector multiplication. The discrete convolution is carried out when calculating approximations $q_j(\theta_j)$ of the conditional densities $\pi(\theta_j | \boldsymbol{\theta}_{-j})$.

An efficient algorithm was employed, which enables the discrete convolution to be carried out with memory and computational complexity $O(n)$ under the condition that the unit impulse is described by a sum of exponentials [6].

3   Example Analysis

The use of stochastic deconvolution is demonstrated on an example adopted from the field of hormonal secretion. In particular, the rate of appearance of C-peptide is estimated. C-peptide is a protein secreted in a one-to-one molar ratio with the hormone insulin. It is wellestablished that short-term oscillations of insulin secretion with a frequency of one pulse every 10-15 minutes are present in healthy subjects [12] and that impaired glucose tolerance such as that associated with diabetes leads to impaired pulsatility [13]. However, analytical errors and ill conditioning of deconvolution still make the assessment of frequent pulsatility difficult using traditional deterministic deconvolution techniques [14, 15].

In the example, data wereprocessed from a healthy male subject (age 21 years, body-mass-index 24.9 kg m^{-2}) who was studied under fasting conditions after overnight fast. Sixteen replicate plasma C-peptide measurements taken every two minutes over two hours, see Fig. 1, wereemployed to estimate C-peptide secretion as a piece-wise constant function with an equidistant two-minute step. Detailed description of the experiment can be found elsewhere [14].

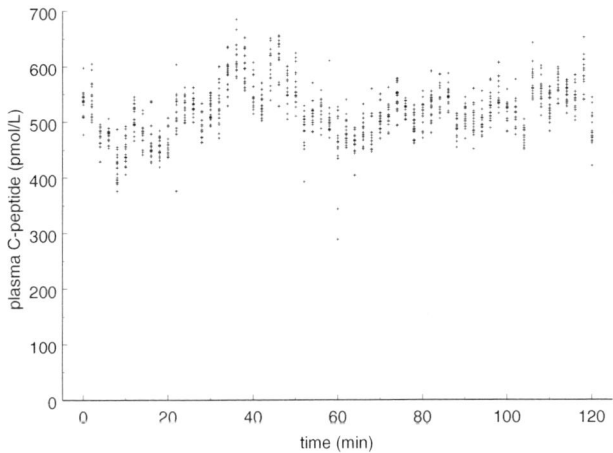

Fig. 1. Plasma C-peptide concentration in a healthy subject during fasting conditions. Samples were taken every two mintes and each sample was subjected to sixteen replicate biochemical analyses.

The unit impulse response (pmol L^{-1} per pmol) was described by a sum of two exponentials, $u(t) = 0.180e^{-0.1400t} + 0.057e^{-0.0216t}$, where t is in minutes. The linear coefficients and exponents wereobtainedusing the well-established population model of C-peptide kinetics [16].

The total number of random variables was 62, i.e. 61 variables representing elements of the input function r_i, $i = 0 \ldots 60$ (r_0 represents an assumed constant secretion prior to the first measurement at time t_0), and a coefficient of variation CV of the measurement error of the C-peptide assay. Although some general information about the intra-assay precision of the C-peptide assay was known, a non-informative prior given by Eq. 3 was employed as the measurement data set was considered to provide sufficient information for the estimation of CV from the data.

A Markov chain with 75,000 elements was generated. The first 25,000 elements were discarded (the burn-in sub-chain). A subsequent analysis employed every 5th element (thinning) from the remaining 50,000 elements to reduce autocorrelation. Formal criteria for the assessment of convergence using the CODA package [1] were employed.

4   Results

The Markov chain representing a sample from a marginal distribution of one component of the input function (r_{37}) is shown in Fig. 2. The plot demonstrates acceptable mixing. The burn-in sub-chain is not shown.

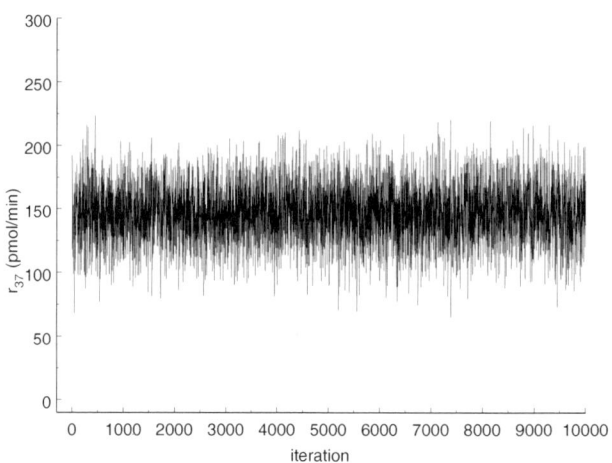

Fig. 2. Markov chain of one component of the input function (r_{37}). Overall, 75,000 elements were generated; 25,000 elements were in the burn-in sub-chain (not shown); every 5th element from the remaining 50,000 elements are shown and were subjected to the analysis.

The secretory profile represented as a piece-wise constant function is shown in Fig. 3. The plot shows 95% credible region (CR) of the secretory profile (marginals of components r_0 to r_{60}) and clearly demonstrates the pulsatile nature of C-peptide secretion. Often, the CR are relatively narrow and overlap betw een adjacent components of the input function. How ev er, surges and, on the other hand, short periods of a nearly complete secretory rests are detectable. No immediately apparent structure was ob vious within the secretory profile, i.e. it w as not clear whether insulin is secreted in repeated, bell-shaped pulses.

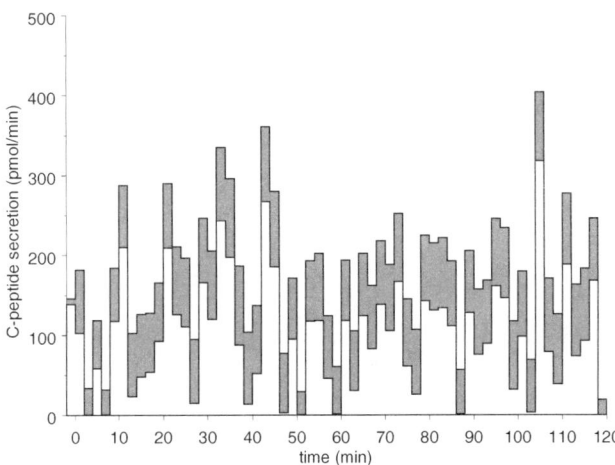

Fig. 3. C-peptide secretion calculated by the discrete stochastic decon volution.The 95% credible regions are giv en for each component of the piece-wise constan tinput function.

The estimates (median and 95% CR) of the measurement error and derived parameters, i.e. number-of-peaks (number of r_j higher than neighbouring values r_{j-1} and r_{j+1}), pulse-mass (the sum of the input function betw een t w o secretion troughs excluding trapezoidal area below the tw o troughs (non-pulsatile secretion)), and interpulse-time (the time difference betw een t w o secretion peaks) are sho wn in T able 1. A tigh 95% CR for number-of-peaks was observed. On the other hand, a wide 95% CR for pulse-mass was present. The measurement error associated with plasma C-peptide measurements w as close to the reported values of CV of the C-peptide assay (4–6%).

The spectral analysis (discrete Fourier transformation of each element of the Markov chain) suggested one major frequency at around 12 minutes per pulse. The normalised spectrum (% of total pow er) is sho wn in Fig. 4 indicating that only this frequency contains more than 10% of the total spectrum (P > 0.05). The median value suggests that this frequency con tributes about 15% to the total spectrum. A t a higher frequency range, a n umber of frequencies suggest its presence in the input function with the culminating frequency of one pulse ev ery 5 minutes. On the opposite side of the spectrum, it is demonstrated that frequencies at the range of one pulse every 14 to 30 minutes do not contribute.

Table 1. Estimates of derived parameters of C-peptide secretion in a healthy subject during fasting conditions.

	median	95% CR
number of peaks (per 120 min)	21	18 – 23
pulse mass (pmol)	359	139 – 1157
pulse mass (% of total)	56	51 – 62
interpulse time (min)	6	4 – 10
measurement error (%)	5.3	5.0 – 5.5

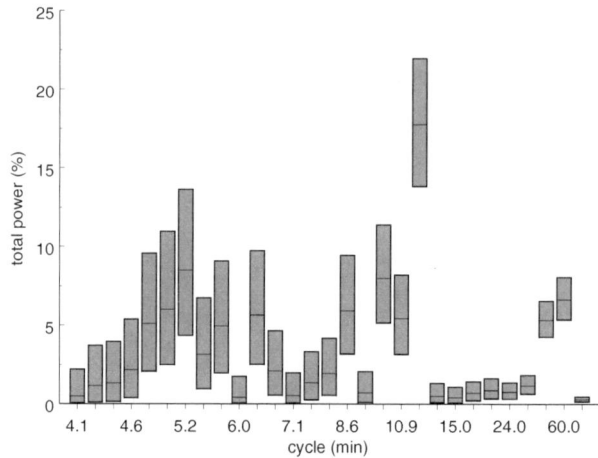

Fig. 4. The spectrum associated with the estimated stochastic profile of C-peptide secretion. The median and 95% credible regions are given.

5   Discussion

Deconvolution (signal reconstruction) is often ill conditioned. This results in the amplification of the measurement error and erratic estimates of the signal (the input function). Existing solutions in biomedical and other fields exploit maximum entropy [18], spline functions [19] polynomials [20], predefined input functions [21], system identification methods [22], reparametrization [23], and regularisation [6]. Most of these methods, e.g. regularisation, are appropriate at situations where the estimated signal is known to be approximately continuous. This does not necessary mean that the "underlying" signal must be also smooth. Consider situation with a highly discontinuous signal but a long sampling (measurement) interval. It follows that infrequent sampling will not allow the discontinuous signal to be reconstructed. Instead, a quantity representing an "average" signal between two adjacent measurements will be obtained. As the sampling interval is prolonged, the "average" values become less discontinuous (due to central limit theorem) and smoothing algorithms become appropriate.

The challenge is to estimate a discontinuous signal. Or at least to estimate its characteristics and to construct confidence intervals of these estimates. The stochastic deconvolution has the potential to facilitate these calculations.

The formal specification of discrete stochastic deconvolution using the Bayesian modelling paradigm is simple. The formalism allows to specify constraints, conditional independence/dependence of input function components r_i, and prior information about both the input function and the measurement error. The constraint in the example is due to non-negativity of the input function. Physiologically, negative secretion rates are not feasible. This constraint is imposed by specifying zero prior probability of the input function for negative secretion values.

Recently, the Gibbs sampler [24] has been employed to solve stochastic deconvolution within the Bayesian framework. However, the approach was limited to the unit impulse response being described by a single exponential, a constraint imposed by the need to express (analytically) full conditionals within the Gibbs formulation. A comprehensive treatment has recently published dealing with Bayesian reconstruction of one-dimensional functions with the use of the regularisation method [25]. The present work differs by focusing on non-regular, i.e. pulsatile functions.

The present example treats adjacent secretion rates conditionally independent and drawn from the same distribution. It is also possible to consider conditional dependence and a more elaborated prior probability. Physiological considerations and experimental results on the cell/organ level should guide these modifications, which are outside the present work. It is however worthwhile to stress that the present approach, i.e. a non-negative uniform prior for the input function with conditional independence between components is the most general, physiologically feasible specification and can serve as a benchmark. Results from these calculations can be instrumental for the formulation of other more elaborated prior distributions. They can also guide construction of suitable candidate models of pulsatile secretion.

The unit impulse response in the present example is obtained from experiments, which involve intravenous dosing with C-peptide and subsequent sampling of central (venous) blood. However, endogenous C-peptide enters hepatic circulation prior to entering the central circulation. Exogenous dosing avoids this first step, which is likely to result in delaying endogenous C-peptide appearance in central circulation. It may therefore be appropriate to use the sum of *three* rather than two exponentials in the description of the unit impulse response to represent the (fast) mixing of C-peptide in the hepatic circulation. If this conjecture is correct, the true pulsatility of C-peptide secretion is even more enhanced than currently thought. The fast mixing cannot be observed during exogenous C-peptide dosing. This additional work is outside the scope of the present paper but suggests how the stochastic framework could be used to explore physiologically relevant details.

The example employed unique, frequently sampled data with a replicate analysis of measurements. These data, at least from the conceptual point of view, are most suitable to address the issue of pulsatility of hormone (insulin) secretion. Traditional deterministic techniques encounter problems [14] due to ill conditioning (amplification of the measurement error). Moving averages and smoothing are the traditional solutions to ill conditioning but reduce the information content of data.

The stochastic formulation of deconvolution is able to incorporate all data in the analysis and fully exploits data to provide confidence intervals (credible regions) of estimated values and derived parameters. Informally, the stochastic deconvolution method estimates the measurement error and *transform* the effect of this error onto values of interest, e.g. the input function. The transformation of the error is not trivial due to the involvement of deconvolution.

The results obtained in the example analysis confirm pulsatility of insulin secretion, e.g. rapid oscillations with one pulse every 12 minutes.

In conclusion, the Markov chain Monte Carlo technique was employed to obtain a solution to the discrete stochastic deconvolution. The solution using the Metropolis-Hastings algorithm is general and allows extensions and modifications of prior distributions.

Acknowledgement

The clinical data were provided by Professor K.S. Polonsky and his colleagues. The work was in part supported by the EC-FP5 project ADICOL (IST-1999-14027).

References

[1] W. R. Gilks, S. Richardson, and D. J. Spiegelhalter, *Markov Chain Monte Carlo in Practice*, Chapman & Hall, London, 1996.

[2] A. F. M. Smith, "Bayesian computational methods", *Phil. Trans. R. Soc. Lond. A*, vol. 337, pp. 369–386, 1991.

[3] A. F. M. Smith and G. O. Roberts, "Bayesian computation via the Gibbs sampler and related Markov-chain Monte-Carlo methods", *J.Roy.Statist.So.B.*, vol. 55, pp. 3–23, 1993.

[4] D. L. Phillips, "A technique for the numerical solution of certain integral equations of the first kind", *J. Assoc. Comput. Mach.*, vol. 9, pp. 97–101, 1962.

[5] S. Twomey, "The application of numerical filtering to the solution of integral equations encountered in indirect sensing measurements", *J. Franklin Inst*, vol. 279, pp. 95–109, 1965.

[6] R. Hovorka, M. J. Chappell, K. R. Godfrey, F. N. Madden, M. K. Rouse, and P. A. Soons, "CODE: A deconvolution program implementing a regularisation method of deconvolution constrained to non-negative values. description and pilot evaluation", *Biopharm. Drug Dispos.*, vol. 19, pp. 39–53, 1998.

[7] A. Jeffreys, *The Theory of Probability*, Cambridge University Press, Cambridge, 1961.

[8] N. Metropolis, A. W. Rosenbluth, M. N. Rosenbluth, A. H. Teller, and E. Teller, "Equation of state calculations by fast computing machine", *J. Chem. Phys.*, vol. 21, pp. 1087–1091, 1953.

[9] W. K. Hastings, "Monte Carlo sampling methods using Markov chains and their applications", *Biometrika*, vol. 57, pp. 97–109, 1970.

[10] S. Chib and E. Greenberg, "Understanding the Metropolis-Hastings algorithm", *A mer. Statist*, vol. 49, pp. 327–335, 1995.

[11] W. R. Gilks, N. G. Best, and K. K. C. T an, "Adaptive rejection Metropolis sampling within Gibbs sampling", *Appl. Statist.*, vol. 44, pp. 455–472, 1995.

[12] D. R. Matthews, D. A. Lang, M. A. Burnett, and R. C. T urner, "Control of pulsatile insulin secretion in man", *Diab etolo gia*, vol. 24, pp. 231–237, 1983.

[13] B. Gumbiner, E. V. V an Cauter, W. F. Beltz, T. M. Ditzler, K. Griver, K. S. P olonsky and R. R. Henry, "Abnormalities of insulin pulsatilit y and glucose oscillations during meals in obese noninsulin-dependent diabetic patients: effects of w eigh t reduction", *J. Clin. Endocrinol. Metab.*, vol. 81, pp. 2061–2068, 1996.

[14] N. M. O'Meara, J. Sturis, J. D. Blackman, D. C. Roland, E. V an Cauter, and K. S. Polonsky , "Analytical problems in detecting rapid insulin secretory pulses in normal humans", *A m. J. Physiol*, vol. 264, pp. E231–E238, 1993.

[15] R. Ho vork aand R. H. Jones, "How to measure insulin secretion", *Diabetes/Metabolism Rev.*, vol. 10, pp. 91–117, 1994.

[16] E. V. V an Cauter, F. Mestrez, J. Sturis, and K. S. P olonsky , "Estimation of insulin-secretion rates from C-peptide levels - comparison of individual and standard kinetic-parameters for C-peptide clearance", *Diab etes*, vol. 41, pp. 368–377, 1992.

[17] N. Best, M. K. Co wles, and S. K. Vines, *CODA: Convergenc e Diagnosis and Output A nalysis Softwar e for Gibbs Sampling Output, V ersion 0.40*, MRC Biostatistics Unit, Cambridge, 1997.

[18] M. K. Charter and S. F. Gull, "Maximum en trop y and its application to the calculation of drug absorption rates", *J. Pharmacokin. Biopharm.*, vol. 15, pp. 645–655, 1987.

[19] D. Verotta, "Two constrained deconv olution methods using spline functions", *J. Pharmacokin. Biopharm.*, vol. 21, pp. 609–636, 1993.

[20] D. J. Cutler, "Numerical deconv olution by least squares: Use of polynomials to represen t the input function", *J. Pharmacokin. Biopharm.*, vol. 6, pp. 243–263, 1978.

[21] D. J. Cutler, "Numerical decon v olution using least squares: Use of prescribed input functions", *J. Pharmacokin. Biopharm.*, vol. 6, pp. 227–241, 1978.

[22] S. V ajda, K. R. Godfrey and P . Valk o, "Numerical deconvolution using system iden tification methods", *J. Pharmacokin. Biopharm.*, vol. 16, pp. 85–107, 1988.

[23] P. Veng-Pedersen and N. B. Modi, "An algorithm for constrained deconv olution based on reparametrization", *J. Pharm. Sci.*, vol. 81, pp. 175–180, 1992.

[24] R. Bellazzi, G. Magni, and G. De Nicolao, "Gibbs sampling for signal reconstruction", in *Pr oceedings of the 3rd IFA C International Symposium Modelling and Control in Biomedical Systems (Including Biolo gical Systems)*, D. A. Linkens and E. R. Carson, Eds., Oxford, 1997, pp. 271–276, Elsevier.

[25] P . Magni, R. Bellazzi, and G. De Nicolao, "Ba yesian function learning using MCMC methods", *IEEE T rans. Pattn. A nal. Mach. Intell.*, vol. 20, pp. 1319–1331, 1999.

Graphical Explanation in Bayesian Networks

Carmen Lacave[1], Roberto Atienza[2], and Francisco J. Díez[2]

[1]Dept. Computer Science
University of Castilla-La Mancha
Paseo Universidad, s/n,
13071 Ciudad Real, Spain
clacave@inf-cr.uclm.es

[2] Dept. Artificial Intelligence
UNED
Senda del Rey, 9
28040 Madrid, Spain
{ratienza,fjdiez}@dia.uned.es

Abstract. Bayesian networks have proved to be an appropriate tool for medical diagnosis, because uncertain reasoning in this field is based on a combination of causal knowledge and statistical data. However, a condition for the acceptance of a medical expert system is the ability to explain the diagnosis. This is a difficult task, because probabilistic inference seems to have little relation with human thinking. The current paper focuses on the graphic interface that constitutes one of the explanation capabilities of Elvira, a software tool for the edition and evaluation of graphical probabilistic models. The method we describe consists in working with different evidence cases and simultaneously displaying the corresponding probabilities.

1 Introduction

Bayesian Networks (BNs) [9, 6] provide a way to build expert systems by using probability as a measure for uncertainty. A Bayesian network consists of an acyclic directed graph (ADG), whose nodes represent random variables, together with a probability distribution over its variables that satisfies the *d-separation* property [9]. This property implies that the joint probability distribution can be factored as the product of the probability of each node conditioned on its parents. The probabilities of a BN can be obtained by human experts' judgment and/or from the literature on the specific domain to be modeled.

A necessary condition for the wide acceptance and use of Bayesian expert systems in medicine is that they are endowed with an explanation facility that shows how the results were obtained, or at least that they are reasonable [12]. However, most users find it difficult to understand the reasoning process involved in probabilistic inference, because these methods seem to have little relation with human reasoning. Therefore, in our opinion a necessary condition for a Bayesian network to be considered an expert system is that it is endowed with an explanation capability.

Explanation in BNs may be verbal or graphical. There are also two levels of explanation, micro and macro [10]; the former tries to justify the variation of the probability of a certain node; in contrast, explanation at the macro level analyses the main lines of reasoning producing the conclusions. Some of the explanation methods proposed in the literature are: micro-level explanations [10], INSITE [11], explanation

R.W. Brause and E. Hanisch (Eds.): ISMDA 2000, LNCS 1933, pp. 122–129, 2000.

in qualitative networks [3, 5], explanation based on scenarios [3, 5], explanation in DIAVAL [1], BANTER [4], and the graphic method developed by Madigan et al. [8]. A detailed review can be found in [7].

There are currently several software packages for the edition and evaluation of Bayesian networks and influence diagrams.[1] However, none of them is able to explain the user the results of evidence propagation. We have tried to overcome this shortcoming in Elvira, a new environment under development as a joint project of several Spanish universities. It is implemented in Java, so that it can run in different platforms. It has a user-friendly graphic interface and algorithms for inference, abduction, learning, and decision making. The current paper focuses on a particular aspect of Elvira's explanation capability, more specifically, on the ability to simultaneously displaying and managing several evidence cases.

2   Graphical Explanation in Elvira

The explanation capability of Elvira is based on a system of windows and menus. It offers verbal and graphic explanations at the micro level, such as information about specific nodes or links. In this paper, due to space restriction, we only describe the possibility of simultaneously displaying several posterior probabilities for each node, corresponding to different evidence cases, and the management of evidence cases through a monitor that permits to create, delete, edit and explain them.

The terminology we use in this paper is as follows. A *finding* is a piece of information that states with certainty the value of a random variable; a finding may be, for example, the assertion that the patient is a male; other findings might be that he is 54 year old, that he presents with fever, that he does not usually have headaches, etc. The set of findings is usually called *evidence*. Each non-contradictory set of findings constitutes an *evidence case*. Probabilistic reasoning consists of computing the posterior probability of the unobserved variables given the findings of a certain case; this process is sometimes called *evidence propagation* and is based on the application of Bayes theorem.

2.1   Graphical Display of Probabilities

Elvira has three main modes: edition (for graphically editing Bayesian networks and influence diagrams), learning (for building a network from a database) and inference (for propagating evidence); when the user selects this latter mode, Elvira compiles the current network and computes the prior probabilities. Figure 1 shows the main window of Elvira in inference mode. In this example, the network contains one diagnostic node, paludism, and four possible findings: blood group, country of origin, fever and the result of an analytical test. We consider four evidence cases: in the first

---

[1] See http://www.dia.uned.es/~fjdiez/bayes/#software for a collection of web pages listing BNs tools.

one, there is no evidence; in the second one, the only finding is „severe fever"; the third case adds a new finding, a positive result in a certain test; the fourth case corresponds to severe fever plus a negative result in the test.

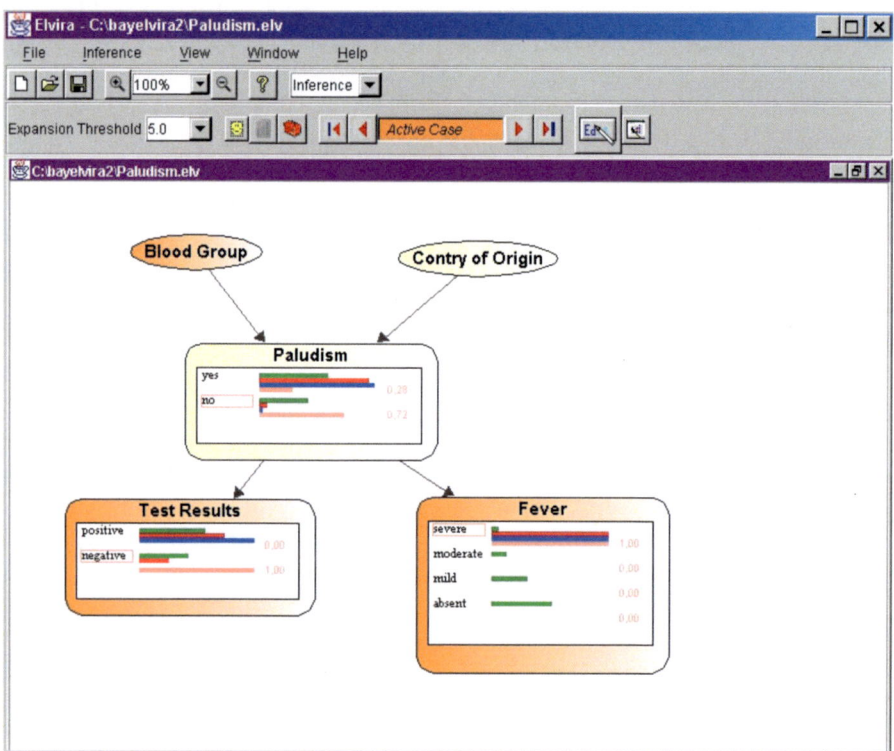

Fig. 1. Elvira main window in inference mode.

In this figure, only three of the five nodes are expanded; they are drawn as rounded rectangles, containing the name of the variable and a line for each value/state, which displays its name, a bar proportional to its probability and the numerical value of its probability. If there are several evidence cases selected in the Editor of Cases (see Sec. 2.2), a different bar is displayed for each case, although only the numerical probability of the current case is displayed. The most probable value for the current case is highlighted by a surrounding rectangle. The color of the bars and the highlighting rectangles are specific of each case.

A finding can be introduced by double-clicking on the corresponding line of the expanded node or by opening the Editor of Cases. This finding is added to the current evidence case and the background color of the window changes, so that the user can easily identify the findings of the current case.

Each node has an *importance factor* assigned by a human expert (its default value is 7.0).[2] When switching to inference mode, the nodes whose importance factor is greater or equal than the *expansion threshold* are automatically expanded. The user can later modify this threshold, or explicitly expand/contract some nodes by selecting them and clicking on the corresponding toolbar buttons or by right-clicking on a node, which opens a contextual menu.

2.2 Management of Cases

In Elvira, the user can assign a name and a comment to each evidence case. A monitor of cases controls how many cases are stored and displayed.

Visualizing Cases. At each moment there is one current evidence case; all the findings introduced by the user are added to this case, until the decides to generate a new case or to select one of the cases previously introduced. Of course, the user can also remove some of the findings of the current case. The first evidence case corresponds to the absence of evidence; the probabilities are then the a priori probabilities. Since this case does not admit any evidence, when switching to *inference mode*, a second case is automatically generated, in order to store the findings entered by the user.

Figure 1 shows that when Elvira is in inference mode, the main window contains an explanation bar. One of the widgets of this bar displays the *expansion threshold*. It also holds buttons for generating a *new case*, *expanding/contracting* the selected nodes and modifying the node *options*. There is also a text field that displays the name and color of the current case, together with buttons for navigating across the set of evidence cases.

Monitor of Cases. If the user wishes to further control which cases are stored and displayed, he/she can open the monitor of cases (Figure 2 shows the monitor for the evidence cases discussed in the previous example). This monitor contains two icons for *creating* and *editing* evidence cases—we describe the case editor below—, a *delete* button for removing cases from memory, and an *options* button for setting the number of stored/displayed cases and other properties. Each stored case correspond to a file in a three-column table: the first cell of the file contains a checkbox for indicating whether the case is displayed or not; the second cell is an editable field for introducing the name of the case; and the third cell allows the user to change the color assigned to that case.

---

[2] This factor is the same as the *relevance factor* used in the expert system DIAVAL for selecting the main diagnoses [1, 2], and is the equivalent of the *importance factor* of each concept in MYCIN [13]. In Elvira we use the original term „importance" in order to avoid confusion with the term „relevance", which has a specific meaning in the context of explanation in Bayesian networks.

Editor of Cases. The editor of cases, not displayed in this paper, allows the user to modify the evidence of an existing case or to introduce evidence to a new one. A pull-down menu gives access to the list of variables in the network, so that the user can enter additional findings. The main utility of this editor is to enter or remove evidence when the number of variables is so high that it becomes impossible or cumbersome to display the whole network on a screen.

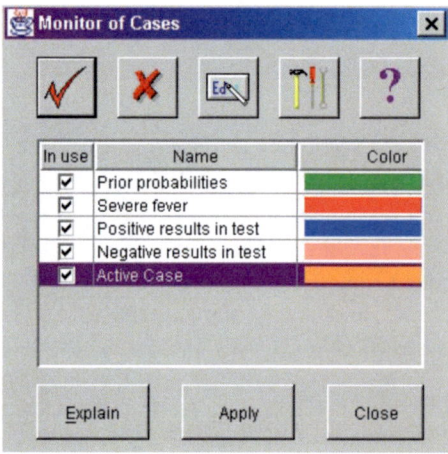

Fig. 2. Monitor of cases.

3 Applications

These facilities permit the user to observe the variations in the probability due to the addition of removal of specific findings. For example, Figures 1 and 2 might correspond to a patient who presents with fever; the doctor using this prototype network can immediately observe how such finding has increased the probability with respect to its prior value (the prevalence in the general population). The doctor then considers the possibility of ordering a analytical test; a criterion for this decision may be whether the result of the test will allow him/her to arrive at a diagnosis with a reasonable certainty. Elvira permits to analyze this question by distinguishing several evidence cases, corresponding to different findings. The comparison of different evidence cases may also be useful for determining which finding or combination of findings has been more influential in the final diagnosis.

   The capability of explanation in Elvira has been applied to PARTIN Bayesian network. It has been designed for helping the user to predict the localization of prostate cancer when it is present with certainty. It is based on the same signs and tests than the Partin Tables, a protocol that gives the user the probability of having the cancer located at a certain place.

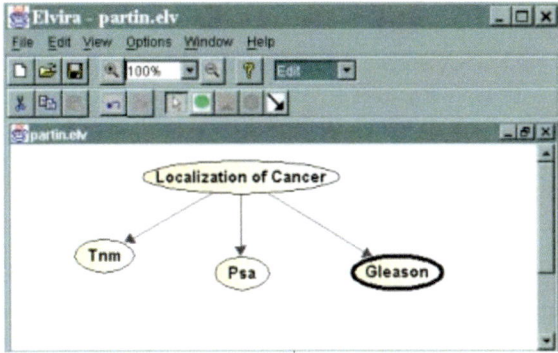

Fig. 3. PARTIN bnet

Another application of the explanation tools of Elvira was to help the user to do differential diagnosis among three infectious diseases — mononucleosis, kalazar and botonose fever— whose symptoms are similar.

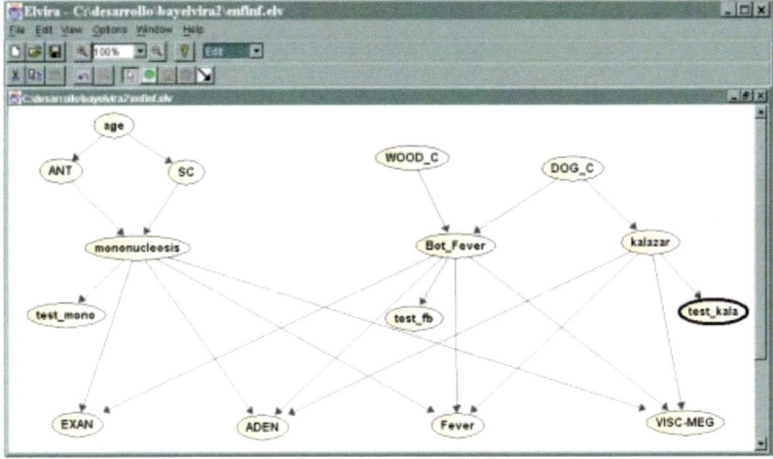

Fig. 4. ENFINF bnet

The explanation tool has also been very useful for the debugging of Elvira's inference algorithms.

4 Conclusions

One of key factors for the acceptance of Bayesian expert systems in real-world domain is their capability to explain their reasoning, in order to justify the results and recommendations they offer, due to the fact that algorithms for probabilistic inference are quite different from intuitive human reasoning, at least apparently. For this reason, Bayesian reasoning is difficult to be understood by untrained users. Although some methods have been proposed, they are still insufficient to generate end-user explanations in BNs.

In this paper we have described one aspect of the explanation capability of Elvira, a software tool for editing and evaluating graphical probabilistic models. It consists of simultaneously displaying the probabilities associated to different evidence cases, supported by a monitor of cases and an editor of cases, which offer the user the possibility of entering evidence and selecting the information he/she wishes to see.

In summary, the contribution of this paper consists in the development of a set of tools for working with several evidence cases and simultaneously displaying the corresponding probabilities. This is one of the explanation tools that will contribute to the application of Bayesian networks in medicine, either as decision support systems or as instructional tools. Naturally, a lot of research is still necessary in this line. Our future efforts will focus on generating macro explanations by using sensitivity analysis, study of reasoning chains in the net, conflict analysis, etc., offering new explanation options, and generating verbal explanations, not only for Bayesian networks, but also for influence diagrams.

References

1. Díez, F. J., *Sistema Experto Bayesiano para Ecocardiografía*. PhD Thesis, Dept. Informática y Automática, UNED, 1994. In Spanish.
2. Díez, F. J., Mira, J., Iturralde, E., and Zubillaga, S., „DIAVAL, a Bayesian expert system for echocardiography", *Artificial Intelligence in Medicine* **10** (1997) 59-73.
3. Druzdzel, M., *Probabilistic Reasoning in Decision Support Systems: From Computation to Common Sense*. PhD Thesis. Department of Engineering and Public Policy, Carnegie Mellon University, Pittsburgh, PA, 1993.
4. Haddawy, P., Jacobson, J., Kahn, C., „BANTER: A Bayesian network tutoring shell", *Artificial Intelligence in Medicine* **10** (1997) 177-200.
5. Henrion, M., Druzdzel, M., „Qualitative propagation and scenario-based approaches to explanation of probabilistic reasoning", *Proceedings of the 6th Conference on Uncertainty in Artificial Intelligence*, July 1990, pp. 17-32.
6. Jensen, F. V., *An Introduction to Bayesian Networks*, UCL Press, London, 1996.
7. Lacave, C., and Díez, F. J., „A review of explanation methods for Bayesian networks", Technical Report IA-00-01, Dept. Inteligencia Artificial, UNED, Madrid, 2000.
8. Madigan, D., Mosurski, K., Almond, R., „Graphical explanations in belief networks", *Journal of Computational and Graphics Statistics* **6**, 2 (1997) 160-181.

9. Pearl, J., *Probabilistic Reasoning in Intelligent Systems: Networks of Plausible Inference*, Morgan Kaufmann, San Francisco, CA, 1988. 2nd printing, 1991.
10. Sember, P., Zukerman, I., „Strategies for generating micro explanations for Bayesian belief networks", *Proceedings of the 5th Conference on Uncertainty in AI*, pp. 295-302.
11. Suermondt, H. J., *Explanation in Bayesian Belief Networks*, PhD Thesis, Dept. Computer Science, Stanford University, 1992.
12. Wallis, J. W., and Shortliffe, E. H., „Customized explanations using causal knowledge", in Buchanan, B. G., and Shortliffe, E. H., *Rule-Based Expert Systems: The MYCIN Experiments of the Stanford Heuristic Programming Project*, Addison-Wesley, Reading, MA, 1984, chapter 20, pp. 371--388.
13. Yu, V. L., Fagan, L. M., et al., „An evaluation of MYCIN's advice", in Buchanan, B. G., and Shortliffe, E.H., *Rule-Based Expert Systems: The MYCIN Experiments of the Stanford Heuristic Programming Project*, Addison-Wesley, Reading, MA, 1984, chapter 31, pp. 589-596.

About the Analysis of Septic Shock Patient Data

Jürgen Paetz[1,2], Fred Hamker[1,2], and Sven Thöne[2]

[1] J.W. Goethe-Universität Frankfurt am Main,
Fachbereich Informatik, AG Adaptive Systemarchitektur
Robert-Mayer-Straße 11-15, D-60054 Frankfurt am Main, Germany
[2] Klinikum der J.W. Goethe-Universität,
Klinik für Allgemein- und Gefäßchirurgie
Theodor-Stern-Kai 7, D-60590 Frankfurt am Main, Germany
paetz@cs.uni-frankfurt.de
http://www.medan.de

Abstract. In intensive care medicine doctors are aware of a high mortality rate of septic shock patients. In this contribution we present the problems and the results of a retrospective, data driven analysis of two studies made in Frankfurt am Main between 1993 and 1997. Our approach includes the necessary steps of data mining, i.e. building up a data base, cleaning and preprocessing the data and finally choosing an adequate analysis for the medical patient data. We chose an architecture mainly based on a supervised neural network. The patient data is classified into two classes (survived and deceased). The importance of this classification for an early warning system is discussed.

1 Introduction – Medical and Data Background

In abdominal intensive care medicine patients are in a very bad condition. Often patients develop a *septic shock*, a phenomenon that is related to mechanisms of the immune system (see [1]) which is still a subject for research. The septic shock is associated with a high mortality rate of about 50%. It is always related to measurements out of the ordinary and often related to multiorgan failure. The exact medical definition for the septic shock and the epidemiology of 656 intensive care unit patients (47 with a septic shock, 25 of them deceased) is elaborated in a study made between November 1995 and December 1997 at the Klinikum der J.W. Goethe-Universität Frankfurt am Main [2]. The data of this study and another study made in the same clinic between November 1993 and November 1995 is the basis of our work. We set up a list of 140 variables, including readings (temperature, blood pressure, ...), drugs (dobutrex, dobutamin, ...) and therapy (diabetes, livercirrhosis, ...). – Our data base consists of 874 patients. 70 patients of all have a septic shock. 24 of the septic shock patients and 69 of all patients are deceased.

2 Preprocessing the Patient Data

Very important for medical data analysis, especially for retrospective evaluations is the preprocessing of the data. In medical data mining, after data-collection and

R.W. Brause and E. Hanisch (Eds.): ISMDA 2000, LNCS 1933, pp. 130–137, 2000.

problem-definition, preprocessing is the third step.[1] Clearly, the quality of the results from data analysis strongly depends on the successful execution of the steps data-collection, problem-definition and preprocessing. The three steps are an interdisciplinary work from data analysts and doctors. The problems and our approaches to them are listed below:

1. We had medical data from two different studies. With the help of doctors we set up a common list of variables. Different units had to be adapted. Some variables are only measured in one of the two studies. It happened that time stamps were not clearly identifiable. Some data entries like see above or zero were not interpretable. So some database entries had to be ignored. The result is one common study with an unified relational database design including input- and output-programs and basic visualization programs.

2. Typing errors were detected by checking principal limit values of the variables. Blood pressure can not be 1200 (a missing decimal point). Typing errors in the date (03.12.96 instead of 30.12.96) were checked with the admission and the discharge day.

3. Naturally our medical data material is very inhomogenous, a fact that has to be emphasized. Each of the patients has a different period of time staying in the intensive care unit. For each patient a different number of variables (readings, drugs, therapies) is documented. So we had to select patients, variables and periods of time. Because different data are measured at different times of day with a different frequency (see table 1), which gave hard to interpretate multivariate time series, we used sampling-methods to get the measurements in regular 24 hours time intervals.

Table 1. Average of sampling rate of four measured variables from all patients without any preprocessing.

variable	days	hours	min
systolic blood pressure	1	12	11
temperature	1	12	31
thrombocytes	1	18	13
lactate	5	0	53

4. A lot of variables showed a high number of missing values (internally coded with -9999) caused by faults or simply by seldom measurements, see table 2 on the next page. The treatment of missing values in the analysis with neural networks is described in more detail in section 3.2.

In conclusion it is almost impossible to get 100% clean data from an enormous amount of different patient records. Nevertheless, we are sure that we have

---

[1] In a *prospective* evaluation the problem-definition phase takes place before the data-collection phase.

Table 2. Available measurements from septic shock patients after 24-hours sampling for six variables.

variable	measurements
systolic blood pressure	83.27 %
temperature	82.69 %
thrombocytes	73.60 %
inspiratorical O2-concentration	65.81 %
lactate	18.38 %
lipase	1.45 %

cleaned the data as good as possible with an enormous amount of time to allow analysis, see chapter 4.

3   The Concept of an Early Warning System

The first of two subsections presents the principal idea of an early warning system. The second subsection describes our neural network approach.

3.1   Principal Idea

The patients often change their conditions quickly. To assist the doctor to protect the patient's life, the main idea concerning the septic shock problem is not to make a prognosis about the survival of the patients, but to build up an early warning system to give individual warnings about the patient's critical condition to the doctor. The principle of such a system is shown in figure 1. In the periods of time U_i patients are uncritical, in K_j they are critical. The aim of an early warning system is to give an alarm as early as possible in the transition phases W_k $(k = 1, 3)$ and of course in K_j.

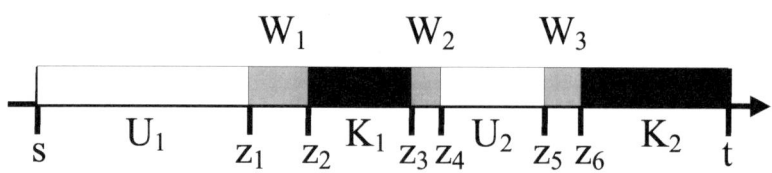

Fig. 1. The concept of an early warning system: s = time of admission, t = time of death, $z_1, \ldots, z_6$ = change of state: begin and end, U_1, U_2 = uncritical period of time, K_1, K_2 = critical period of time and $W_1, \ldots, W_3$ = period of time: change of state.

To achieve knowledge about a patient being in a critical illness condition, we need to classify the vectors $(x_1, ..., x_n)^t$ composed of measurements or drugs x_i, $i = 1, \ldots, n$ with the outcome y_s (survived) resp. y_d (deceased).

Critical illness states are defined as those states which are located in areas of the input space showing a majority of measurements from deceased patients, see [8]. By detecting those states we expect to achieve a reliable warning, which should be as early as possible.

3.2   The Neural Network Approach

In the last years many authors contributed to machine learning, data mining, intelligent data analysis and neural networks in medicine (see [3] and [4]). Concerning our problem supervised neural networks have the following positive aspects: nonlinear classification, fault tolerance, learning from data and generalization ability. The aim of this contribution is not a comparison of statistical with neural network methods (see [5]) but to select an appropriate method that can easily be adapted to our data. Here, our aim is to detect critical illness states with a classification method. Linear classifiers did not seem to be suitable for a classification after having a look at the data. In addition, a nonlinear method surely detects a linear separability.

The neural network chosen for our classification is the supervised growing neural gas (abbr. SGNG, see [6]).[2] Compared to the multilayer perceptron, trained with backpropagation (see [9]), which has reached a wide public, this network achieved similar results on classsification tasks, see [7]. The results are presented in chapter 4.2. Its additional advantage is the ability to insert neurons within the learning process to adapt its structure to the data. The algorithm with its slight modifications and its parameters is noted down in detail in [8]. – It is based on the idea of radial basis functions (abbr. RBF, see [9]). The centers of the radial basis functions are connected through an additional graph that is adapted within the learning process. The graph structure allows to adapt not only the parameters (weights, radii) of the best matching neuron but also those of its neighbours (adjacent neurons).

One feature we additionally integrated into the SGNG algorithm is the toleration of the missing values within the adaptation and activation phase. If $x = (x_1, \ldots, x_n)^t$ is a n-dimensional data vector, you can project the vector x, so that no missing value is in the projected vector $x_p := (x_{i_1}, \ldots, x_{i_m})^t$, $\{x_{i_1}, \ldots, x_{i_m}\} \subset \{1, \ldots, n\}$, $m \leq n$, $x_{i_1}, \ldots, x_{i_m}$ are not missing values. Due to the fact that the SGNG is based only on distance calculations between vectors, it is possible to apply this standard projection argument to the adaptation and activation calculations of the SGNG, so that all calculations are done with the

---

[2] Logistic regression is a statistical alternative to supervised neural networks.

projected vectors x_p. Preliminary experiments showed that it is not appropriate to project to less than the half of the variables; sample vectors with more than 50% missing values are omitted. This procedure causes a statistical bias, but we believe that it is not high because the most part of the data is missing randomly.

4   Results

We give an impression of our results achieved up to now. We are aware of the problem that data from only 70 patients with a septic shock, including missing values in some variables, are not sufficient for excellent results but we are able to give some hints and first results in the right direction with the data available at the moment.

4.1   Basic Statistical Analysis

We calculated some statistical standard measures for each of the variables (mean, standard deviation etc.) including all patients or only the septic shock patients combined with all days or comprising only the last day of their stay in the intensive care unit. We detected some distinctions but they are usually not significant. Q-Q-plots show that the distributions are usually normal with an overlap of values from deceased and survived patients. A correlation analysis of the data shows high absolute values for the correlations between medicaments and variables, so surely the medicaments complicate the data analysis. Correlations between variables and {survived, deceased} are not high or not significant.

More interesting are the correlations COR between variables X, Z, calculated one time with the sets X_d, Z_d of samples from deceased and one time with the sets X_s, Z_s of samples from survived patients and the corresponding differences taken from all patients and all days, listed in the table 3 on the next page. The significance level was calculated with SPSS 9.0. The correlations with significance level 0.01 are marked with an asterisk.

Both correlation values for the pairs urea, creatinin and arterial pO2, potassium are significant (level 0.01), so that the difference could be an indicator for survived or deceased patients. Therefore, these variables have to be measured very often to calculate the correlation in a time window during the patients actual stay at hospital. - In addition to the results in the section 4.2 an idea is to train a neural network with the correlation values to find out the exact threshold for a warning based on correlation values or combinations or modifications of such values (for first results see [8]). This seems to be reasonable because doctors reported that the interdependence of variables, measured from critical illness patients, could be disturbed.

Table 3. Correlations between two variables (all patients, all days of hospital stay) with the highest correlation differences ≥ 0.3 betweeen survived and deceased patients and frequency of measurement of each variable $\geq 20\%$. Significant correlations (level 0.01) are marked with an asterisk. GGT is the abbreviation of gammaglutamyltransferase.

variable X	variable Z	$COR(X_s, Z_s)$	$COR(X_d, Z_d)$	difference
inspir. O2-concentration	pH	-0.03	-0.39*	0.36
leukocytes	GGT	0.00	0.32*	0.32
iron (Fe)	GGT	0.31*	0.01	0.30
(total) bilirubin	urea	0.26*	-0.07	0.33
urea	creatinin	0.14*	0.57*	0.43
fibrinogen	creatinin in urine	0.05	-0.31*	0.36
arterial pO2	potassium (K)	-0.13*	0.18*	0.31
thromboplastintime	chloride	0.24*	-0.07	0.31

4.2   Classification of Septic Shock Patient Data

In this section we use the neural network architecture described in section 3.2. The doctors gave a recommendation which variables are the most important ones for a classification. The chosen variable set V is composed of: pO2 (arterial), pCO2 (arterial), pH, leukocytes, thromboplastintime, thrombocytes, lactate, creatinin, heart frequency, volume of urine, systolic blood pressure, frequency of artificial respiratory, inspiratorical O2-concentration, antithrombine III, dopamine and dobutrex. The variables are normalized (mean 0, standard deviation 1) for analysis. The classiﬁcation is based on 2068 measurement vectors (16-dimensional samples) from variable set V taken from 70 septic shock patients. 348 are deleted because of too many missing values in the sample. With 75% of the 1720 remaining samples the SGNG was trained and with 25 % samples from completely other patients than in the training set it was tested.

Table 4. Correct classifications, sensitivity, specifity with standard deviation, minimum and maximum in % from three repetitions.

measure	mean value	standard deviation	minimum	maximum
correct classification	67.84	6.96	61.17	75.05
sensitivity	24.94	4.85	19.38	28.30
specifity	91.61	2.53	89.74	94.49

The network chosen was the one with the lowest error on the smoothed test error function. Three repetitions of the complete learning process with different, randomly selected divisions of the data were made. The results are presented in table 4. To achieve a generally applicable result ten repetitions would be better but here it is already clear that with the low number of data samples the results can only have a prototypical character, even with more cleverly thought-out benchmark strategies. Some additional results are reported in [8]. On average

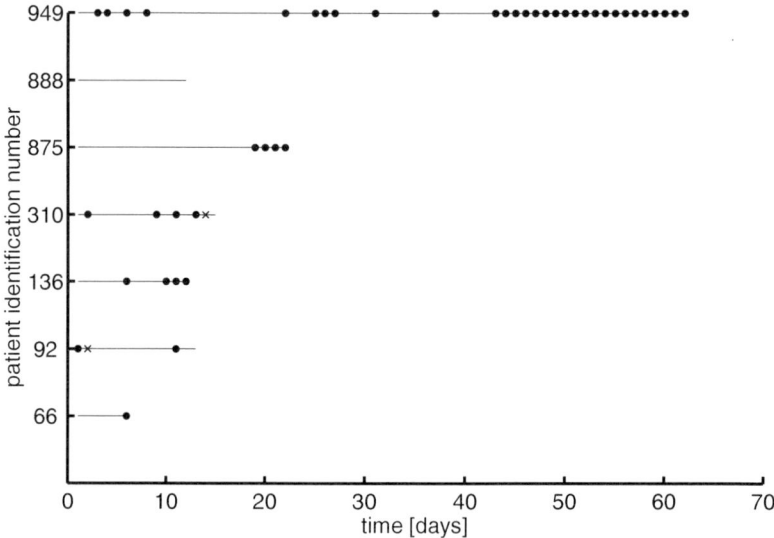

Fig. 2. Deceased septic shock patients during their hospital stay with warnings (filled circles). A too high number of missing values causes some missing states (crosses). If there is no marking then no warning is given.

we have an alarm rate ($= 1-$ specifity) of 8.39 % for survived patients showing also a critical state and a detection of about 1 out of 4 critical illness states. For such a complex problem it is a not too bad but clearly no excellent result. An explanation for this result are the different, individual measurements of each patient. In figure 2 the resulting warnings from classification are shown for 7 out of 24 deceased patients with a septic shock (to give an impression of the warnings over time). Not for each deceased patient exists a warning (patient with number 888) and some warnings are given too late (patient with number 66), i.e. the doctors knew already that the patient had become critical. So the ideal time to warn the doctor has not yet been found for all patients and it remains as future work.

5   Conclusion

We have presented a data analysis approach for the important medical problem septic shock. The results are basically encouraging for the doctors to achieve an early warning system for septic shock patients but the results are not final.

In spite of some severe restrictions of the data we succeeded in achieving some results by using several preprocessing steps. In the near future it is desirable to improve the performance of the results.

Further work will be a comparison of the achieved results with scores, that are known to have limitations in classifying individual patients (see [10]). Some results from cluster analysis are presented in [8]. To improve the results we are collecting data from septic shock patients from 166 clinics in Germany to evaluate our algorithms on this larger amount of patient data. Another approach is adaptive rule generation to explain the class boundaries in the data and at the same time to find out the necessary variables for the early warning system.

Acknowledgement: The work was done within the DFG-project MEDAN (Medical Data Analysis with Neural Networks). The authors like to thank all the participants of the MEDAN working group especially Prof. Hanisch and Dr. Brause and all other persons involved in the MEDAN project for supporting our work.

References

1. Fein, A.M. et al. (eds.): Sepsis and Multiorgan Failure, Williams & Wilkins Baltimore (1997)
2. Wade, S., Büssow, M., Hanisch, E.: Epidemiologie von SIRS, Sepsis und septischem Schock bei chirurgischen Intensivpatienten. Der Chirurg **69** (1998) 648–655
3. Lavrač: Machine Learning for Data Mining in Medicine. In: Horn, W. et al (eds.): AIMDM'99. LNAI 1620. Springer-Verlag Berlin Heidelberg (1999) 47-62
4. Brause, R.: Revolutionieren Neuronale Netze unsere Vorhersagefähigkeiten? Zentralblatt für Chirurgie **124** (1999) 692–698
5. Schumacher, M., Roßner, R., Vach, W.: Neural Networks and Logistic Regression: Part I. Computational Statistics & Data Analysis **21** (1996) 661–682
6. Fritzke, B.: Fast Learning with Incremental RBF Networks. Neural Processing Letters **1**(1) (1994) 2–5
7. Heinke, D., Hamker, F.: Comparing Neural Networks: A Benchmark on Growing Neural Gas, Growing Cell Structures, and Fuzzy ARTMAP. IEEE Transactions on Neural Networks **9**(6) (1998) 1279–1291
8. Hamker, F., Paetz, J., Thöne, S.: Detektion von kritischen Zuständen von Patienten mit der Diagnose "Septischer Schock" mit einem RBF-Netz. Interner Bericht, Fachbereich Informatik, J.W. Goethe-Universität Frankfurt am Main (2000)
9. Haykin, S.: Neural Networks: A Comprehensive Foundation. Prentice Hall (1999) 2nd edition
10. Neugebauer, E., Lefering, R.: Scoresysteme und Datenbanken in der Intensivmedizin - Notwendigkeit und Grenzen. Intensivmedizin **33** (1996) 445–447

Data Mining and Knowledge Discovery in Medical Applications Using Self-Organizing Maps

Thomas Villmann[+]*, Wieland Hermann[++] and Michael Geyer[+]
[+]Clinic for Psychotherapy, University Leipzig
04109 Leipzig, K.-Tauchnitz-Str. 25, Germany
[++]Clinic of Neurology, University Leipzig
04103 Leipzig, Liebigstr. 22a, Germany

Abstract

In the contribution the authors discuss the application of *Self-Organizing Maps* (SOMs) for data mining and knowledge discovery in medicine. Thereby, the usually assumed but not verified topology preservation is in the main focus. Extensions of the usual SOM are offered to obtain correct results. The authors give examples for applications such as visualization and clustering.

1 Introduction

Self-organizing maps (SOM) as a special type of artificial neural networks play in increasing role in the area of data analysis, data mining and knowledge discovery in medical applications which are inspired by neural representation of sensoric signals in the cortex in the brain [10].In technical context SOMs project data from some (high-dimensional) input space $V \subseteq \Re^{D_V}$ (D_V - dimensionality of input space) onto a position in some output space A such that a continuous change of a parameter of the input data should lead to a continuous change of the position of a localized excitation in the neural map. The latter property is called *topology preservation*. In this way the SOM determines a *non-linear principal component analysis* (PCA) of the data. Using the topology preservation of the map one can now project high-dimensional data adequately into a lower-dimensional (discrete) parameter space model represented by the neuron lattice. However, a major disadvantage of the usual SOM is that the topology preservation can not be assumed all the way. It is dependent on the lattice topology , i.e. the structure of the output space A which has at least approximately to match the shape of the (usual) unknown shape of the data space. Usually, A

---

*corresponding author, email: villmann@informatik.uni-leipzig.de

R.W. Brause and E. Hanisch (Eds.): ISMDA 2000, LNCS 1933, pp. 138–151, 2000.

is chosen to be rectangular (or it high-dimensional derivatives) which implies a correct choice of the dimensionality of $\mathcal{A}$ and adequate length ratios of the edges. Finally, for a trained network one has to proof the topology preservation or to include structure adaptation to obtain accurate results.

To obtain a proper representation advanced methods for SOM learning are necessary. In the present paper we highlight some of them and show applications in data visualization and data mining. Especially we emphasize the faithful learning of the map which includes structure adaptation to obtain topology preserving mapping as well as magnification control for optimization of the information transfer.

2   The SOM and Extensions for Suitable Data Modelling

As usual, we assume the output space $\mathcal{A}$ is to be a $D_{\mathcal{A}}$-dimensional hypercube such that the neurons are situated on positions $\mathbf{r} = (r_1, r_2, r_3, ..., r_{D_{\mathcal{A}}})$, $1 < r_j < n_j$ with $N = n_1 \times n_2 \times ... \times n_{D_{\mathcal{A}}}$ as the overall number of neurons.[1] Associated to each neuron $\mathbf{r} \in \mathcal{A}$, is a weight vector $\mathbf{w_r} \in \mathcal{V}$. The map $\Psi_{\mathcal{V} \to \mathcal{A}}$ is realized by a winner take all rule

$$\Psi_{\mathcal{V} \to \mathcal{A}} : \mathbf{v} \mapsto \mathbf{s} = \operatorname*{argmin}_{\mathbf{r} \in \mathcal{A}} \|\mathbf{v} - \mathbf{w_r}\| \tag{2.1}$$

whereas the back mapping is defined as $\Psi_{\mathcal{A} \to \mathcal{V}} : \mathbf{r} \mapsto \mathbf{w_r}$. Both functions determine the map $\mathcal{M} = (\Psi_{\mathcal{V} \to \mathcal{A}}, \Psi_{\mathcal{A} \to \mathcal{V}})$ realized by the network. All data points $\mathbf{v} \in \mathcal{V}$ which are mapped onto the neuron $\mathbf{r}$ perform its (masked) receptive field $\Omega_{\mathbf{r}}$. To achieve the map $\mathcal{M}$, SOMs adapt the pointer positions with respect to a presented sequence of data points $\mathbf{v} \in \mathcal{V}$ selected according to the data distribution $\mathcal{P}(\mathcal{V})$:

$$\triangle \mathbf{w_r} = \epsilon h_{\mathbf{rs}} (\mathbf{v} - \mathbf{w_r}) . \tag{2.2}$$

$h_{\mathbf{rs}}$ is the neighborhood function depending on the best matching neuron according to (2.1), usually chosen to be of Gaussian shape: $h_{\mathbf{rs}} = \exp\left(-\frac{\|\mathbf{r} - \mathbf{s}\|^2}{2\sigma^2}\right)$.

Thereby, topology preservation in SOMs is understood as preserving of the continuity of the mapping from the input space onto the output space, exactly spoken: it is equivalent to the *continuity* of $\mathcal{M}$ between the *topological spaces* with properly chosen metrices in both $\mathcal{M}$ and $\mathcal{V}$. Because of the lack of space we refer to [17] for a detailed consideration. This property of *neighborhood preservation* depends on an important feature of the SOM: the *a priori* defined output space topology. If the topology of $\mathcal{A}$ does not match that of the data shape, neighborhood violations are inevitable [17] (see Fig. 1). On the other hand, a higher degree of topology preservation, in general, improves the accuracy

---

[1] Yet other arrangements are also admissible which can be described by a connectivity matrix. Here we only consider hypercubes.

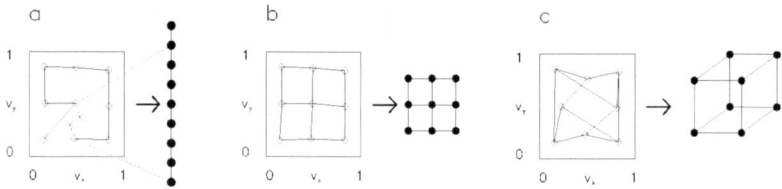

Figure 1: A map learning algorithm can achieve an optimal neighborhood preservation only, if the output space topology roughly matches the effective structure of the data in the input space.

of the map [3]. Yet, many SOM application only use the two-dimensional lattice of the standard SOM which is in contrast to the demanded feature of topology preserving projection. Hence, the interpretation of the map may fail. Therefore, in real applications the topology preservation of the map has to be proofed and, if necessary, a structure adaptation of the lattice has to be added manually or by advanced algorithms as presented below.

Several approaches were developed to judge the degree of topology preservation for a given map [2]. A robust tool is the topographic product P [3] which comprise the information about violations of the topology preservation in a single value. P can take positive and negative values indicating that the dimensionality of the grid $\mathcal{A}$ is too low dimensional or too high, respectively, for representation of the given data. If one obtains P approximately zero the shape of the lattice matches the data distribution. For a detailed introduction and analysis of the properties we refer to [3] and [17].

To overcome the problem of prior specified lattices one can adapt also the shape of the grid in addition to the usual weight vector dynamic. One approach is the now *Growing* SOM (GSOM) [4] which realizes an data driven structure adaptation, however, always remaining a hypercube structure of the grid which allows a simple post-processing. During the learning scheme both the lattice dimension and the edge length ratios are adapted (in addition to the weight vectors), i.e. we allow a variable overall dimensionality and variable dimensions along the individual directions in the hypercube. It can be taken as a non-linear principle component analysis.

The GSOM starts from an initial 2-neuron chain, learns like a regular SOM, adds neurons to the output space with respect to a certain criterion to be described below, learns again, adds again, etc., until a prespecified maximum number $N_{\max}$ of neurons is distributed but always remaining the output space topology to be of the form $n_1 \times n_2 \times ...$, with $n_j = 1$ for $j > D_A$, where D_A is the current dimensionality of $\mathcal{A}$.[2] Hence, the initial configuration is $2 \times 1 \times 1 \times ...$, $D_A = 1$. From there it can grow either by adding nodes in one of the directions which are already spanned by the output space,

---

[2] Hence, the initial configuration is $2 \times 1 \times 1 \times ...$, $D_A = 1$.

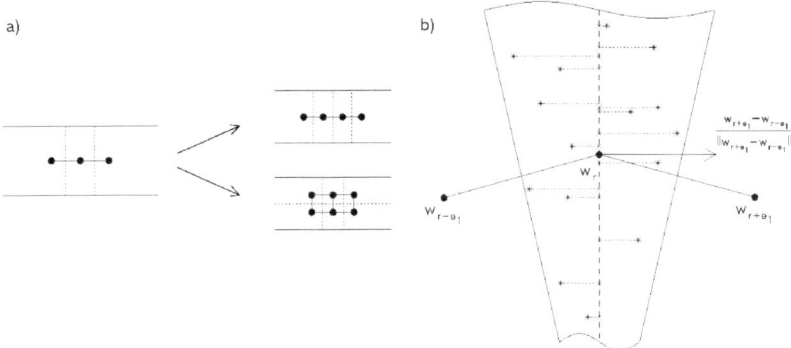

Figure 2: a) (left) Illustration of the basic decision to be made during the growth procedure: an output space lattice can either grow in an existing direction or it can extend into a new direction. b) (right) Illustration of the criterion for determining the correct growth direction. Consider the center neuron with receptive field center position $\mathbf{w_r}$ in a hypothetical one-dimensional chain of neurons. From the receptive-field-center positions $\mathbf{w_{r+e_1}}$ and $\mathbf{w_{r-e_1}}$ of its output space neighbors the local input space direction $\frac{\mathbf{w_{r+e_1}} - \mathbf{w_{r-e_1}}}{\|\mathbf{w_{r+e_1}} - \mathbf{w_{r-e_1}}\|}$ can be estimated (large arrow) which corresponds to output space direction $\mathbf{e_1}$. The stimuli (stars) within the Voronoi cell of neuron $\mathbf{r}$ can now be decomposed into a parallel and a perpendicular part relative to this local direction. The average of the relative size of the resp. decomposition amplitudes then determines whether the output space is extended along $\mathbf{e_1}$ or whether a new dimension is added.

i.e. by having $n_i \rightarrow n_i + 1$, $i \leq D_A$, or by adding a new dimension, i.e. $(n_{D_A+1} = 1) \rightarrow (n_{D_A+1} = 2)$, $D_A \rightarrow D_A + 1$ (see Fig 2a)). This decision is made on the basis of the receptive fields $\Omega_\mathbf{r}$. When reconstructing $\mathbf{v} \in \mathcal{V}$ from neuron $\mathbf{r}$, an error $\theta = \mathbf{v} - \mathbf{w_r}$ remains decomposed along the different directions, which result from projecting back the output space grid into the input space $\mathcal{A}$:

$$\theta = \mathbf{v} - \mathbf{w_r} = \sum_{i=1}^{D_A} a_i(\mathbf{v}) \frac{\mathbf{w_{r+e_i}} - \mathbf{w_{r-e_i}}}{\|\mathbf{w_{r+e_i}} - \mathbf{w_{r-e_i}}\|} + \mathbf{v}' \tag{2.3}$$

Thereby, $\mathbf{e_i}$ denotes the unit vector in direction i of $\mathcal{A}$.[3] and Considering a receptive field $\Omega_\mathbf{r}$ and determining its first principle components $\boldsymbol{\omega}_{PCA}$ allows a further decomposition of $\mathbf{v}'$. Projection of $\mathbf{v}'$ onto the direction of $\boldsymbol{\omega}_{PCA}$ then yields

$$a_{D_A+1}(\mathbf{v}) : \mathbf{v}' = a_{D_A+1}(\mathbf{v}) \frac{\boldsymbol{\omega}_{PCA}}{\|\boldsymbol{\omega}_{PCA}\|} + \mathbf{v}''. \tag{2.4}$$

---

[3] At the border of the output space grid, where not two, but just one neighboring neuron is available, we use $\frac{\mathbf{w_r} - \mathbf{w_{r-e_i}}}{\|\mathbf{w_r} - \mathbf{w_{r-e_i}}\|}$ or $\frac{\mathbf{w_{r+e_i}} - \mathbf{w_r}}{\|\mathbf{w_{r-e_i}} - \mathbf{w_r}\|}$ to compute the backprojection of the output space direction $\mathbf{e_i}$ into the input space.

The *criterion for the growing* now is to add nodes in that direction which has on average the largest error (normalized) expected amplitudes $\tilde{a}_i$:

$$\tilde{a}_i = \sqrt{\frac{n_i}{n_i + 1}} \sum_{\mathbf{v}} \frac{\mid a_i(\mathbf{v}) \mid}{\sqrt{\sum_{j=1}^{D_A+1} a_j^2(\mathbf{v})}}, i = 1, ..., D_A + 1 \qquad (2.5)$$

After each growth step, a new learning phase has to take place, in order to readjust the map. For a detailed study of the algorithm we refer to [4] or [16].

A further extension of the basic SOM concerns the so-called magnification : the usual SOM distributes the pointers $\mathbf{W} = \{\mathbf{w_r}\}$ according to the input distribution: $P(\mathcal{V}) \sim P(\mathbf{W})^\alpha$ with the magnification factor $\alpha = \frac{2}{3}$ [12].[4] The first approach to influence the magnification of a learning vector quantizer was proposed in [5]. The algorithm converge such that the winning probabilities of all neurons are equalized which is related to a maximization of the entropy and, hence, the resulted magnification is equal to the unit. However, a arbitrary magnification can not be achieved. BAUER ET AL. in [1] introduced a local learning parameter $\epsilon_\mathbf{r}$ with $\langle \epsilon_\mathbf{r} \rangle \propto P(\mathcal{V})^m$ in (2.2) which now reads as

$$\triangle \mathbf{w_r} = \epsilon_s h_{\mathbf{rs}} (\mathbf{v} - \mathbf{w_r}) . \qquad (2.6)$$

This local learning rule leads to a relation $P(\mathcal{V}) \sim P(\mathbf{W})^{\alpha'}$ with $\alpha' = \alpha(m + 1)$ and, hence, allows a magnification control. Especially, one can achieve a resolution $\alpha' = 1$ which maximizes the mutual information (corresponding to a maximization of the entropy) [11], [15].

The most common method for visualization of SOMs is to project the weight vectors in the first dimension of the space spanned by the principle components of the data and connecting these units the respective nodes in the lattice are neighbored [9]. However, assuming the shape of the SOM lattice to be hyper-cubically there exist several approaches to visualize the properties of the map. Here we are concentrating only on a few approaches which are of interest in the below given applications, whereas a expansive overview can be found in [14].

One interesting evaluation is the so-called **U**-matrix introduced by ULTSCH ET AL. [13] the elements $U_{\mathbf{rr'}}$ of which are the distance between the respective weight vectors $\mathbf{w_r}$ and $\mathbf{w_{r'}}$ whereby $\mathbf{r}$ and $\mathbf{r'}$ are neighbored in $\mathcal{A}$

$$\mathbf{U_{rr'}} = \|\mathbf{w_r} - \mathbf{w_{r'}}\| \qquad (2.7)$$

U can be used to determine clusters within the weight vector set and, hence, within the data space. Supposing, the map $\mathcal{M}$ is approximately topology preserving large values refer to cluster borders. If the lattice is a two-dimensional array the respective matrix **U** can easily be viewed and gives a powerful tool for cluster analysis.

Another visualization technique can be used if the lattice $\mathcal{A}$ is three-dimensional. Then we can identify the neurons $\mathbf{r}$ as locations in the color

---

[4]This result is valid for the one-dimensional case and higher dimenional ones which separate.

space $\mathcal{C}$ defined by the intensities of the colors *red, green* and *blue*. In this way we are able to assign to each data point a color via (2.1) which can be utilized for data analysis [18].

3   Visualization applications in medicine

3.1   Analysis of the psychotherapy process

The therapeutical process in psychotherapy usually is organized in a sequence of single therapy sessions. During the therapy the emotional feeling can vary in dependence on the actual situation (emotional excitements, as the result of the therapeutical discussion) which can be observed by individual asses by the therapist. Beside these individual observations there exist a large pool of instruments to judge the emotional situation of both the patient and the therapist which consist in a spectrum of several questionnaires [21]. On the other hand, it is generally known that emotions influence physiological parameters as for instance heart rate, respiration rate, muscle tension and electrodermal conductivity (skin conductance)and vice versa. Hence, the *parallel* observation of them during therapy sessions together with a psychological analysis should lead to a better understanding of the psycho-physiological processes. However, this consideration was never tried before in usual therapy sessions or complete therapies. Thereby, the most difficult thing is that the set of physiological parameters is correlated but have to be considered in a parallel way by a therapist to detect relevant changes [8]. For this purpose a suitable tool is needed for an easy parallel assessment. In the present investigation the therapy of one patient was considered containing $t_{\max} = 37$ single sessions. Each of them usually takes approximately 45 Min.. During the several sessions for both the patient and, additionally, for the therapist the following parameters were simultaneously obtained: *heart rate, muscle tension (by surface electromyogram), skin conductance level (SCL), skin conduction reaction (SCR)*. The value are determined as averages over time intervals of $30s$. In the above outlined approach we are interested in the variation of the parameters. Hence, we investigate only the difference of the parameter for a certain time point in comparison to the previous one. In this way we are independent on the basic level of data in each session which can be influenced by climatic conditions, nourishment, etc.. Yet, only the actual development is considered. In this way we obtain 3105 data vectors for both the patient and the therapist resulting in $n_{\max} = 6210$ data vectors for SOM learning. Subsequently, the data were normalized such that for the resulted vectors $\mathbf{v} \in \mathcal{V} \subseteq \Re^4$ we have for all components j: $\sum_{i=1}^{n_{\max}} v_j = 1$, i.e., all measured parameters are assumed to be of the same importance.

The GSOM was applied to the above described data set. We result a $7 \times 5 \times 7$–lattice as the final shape for the grid $\mathcal{A}$. Thereby, the magnification control scheme (2.6) was inserted to obtain a maximal mutual information, i.e. the control parameter m was chosen as $m = \frac{1}{2}$. We have judged the degree of topology preservation using a special kind of the topographic product which

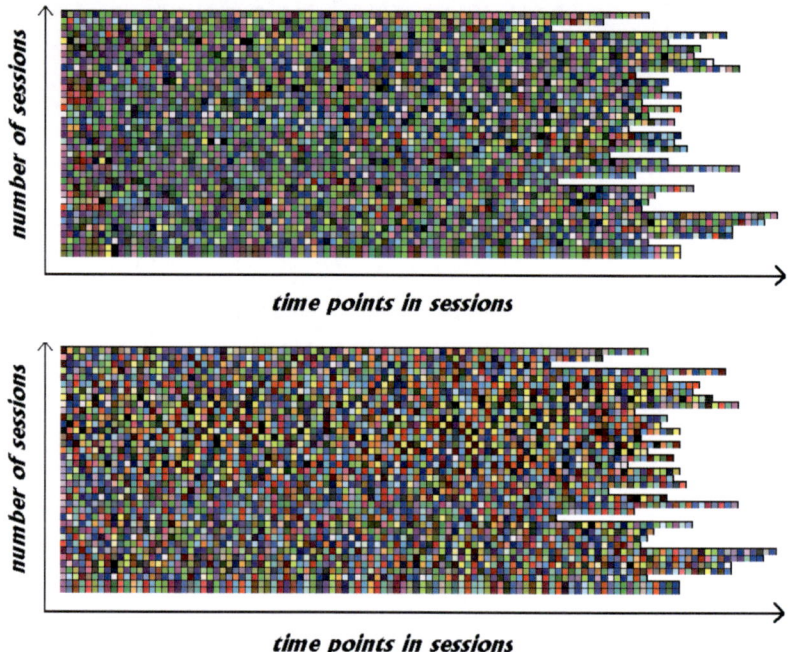

Figure 3: Color description of the variation of the physiological parameters for the patient (above) and the therapist (below) for the complete therapy for each single session. Each colored pixel code a characteristic pattern of change. Global color texture changes within the pictures correspond to variations in the therapy (see text for details). Single colors can be related to charteristic patterns. The color representation is resulted from a GSOM generated $7 \times 5 \times 7$ SOM.

takes the receptive fields of the neurons into account [20] and obtain a value $P = 0.007$ referring to a good topology preservation. The magnification control scheme have lead to a improvement of the entropy: without control the entropy was 94.8% of the maximal possible entropy value [19] in comparison to 96.4% using the control scheme.

Hence, following the above idea of color coding we now are able to give a visualization of the development of the neurophysiological parameters during the therapy which then allow an easy interpretation by the therapists.

In Fig. 3 we plotted for each time point in all sessions the mapped original data according to the above outlined color coding. We observe, for example, a clear change in the distribution of colors after the 20th. session: for the therapist picture the occurrence yellow typed colors is increasing, in the patient picture in the same area the frequency of blue colored pixels is increased. This rough observation can be visualized more detail. In Fig.4 the probability distribution of colors with respect to the session number is depicted. Now, the following in-

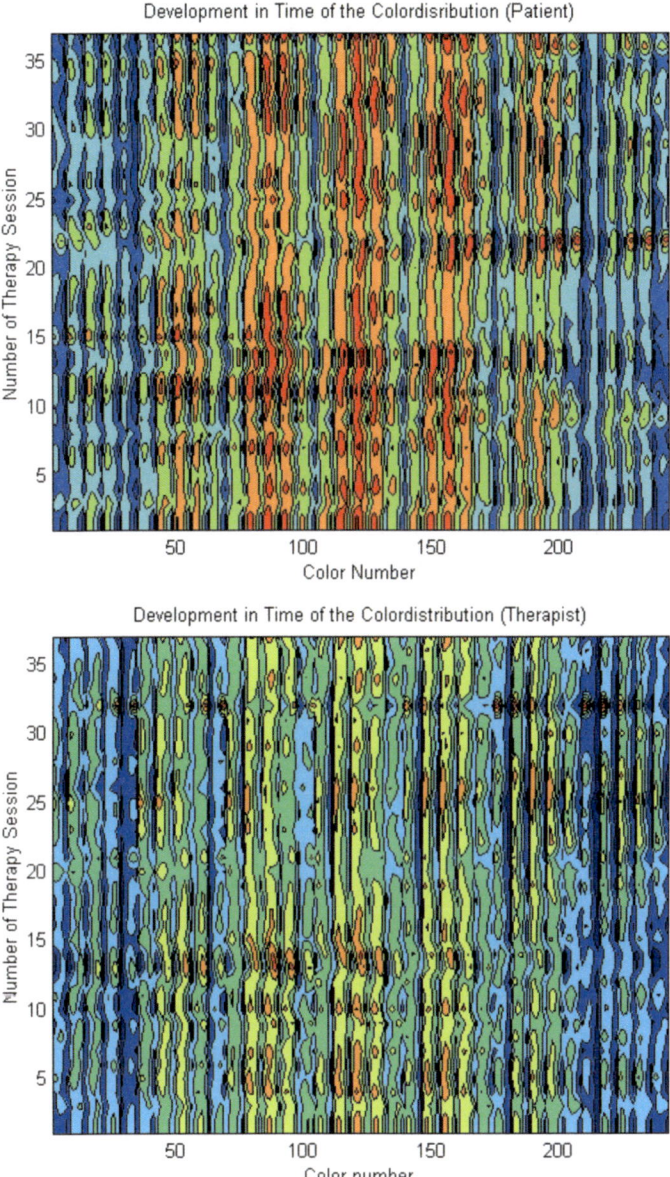

Figure 4: Time development of the probability distribution of the colors according to number of therapy sessions for the patient (above) and the therapist (below).

terpretation (in the sense of psychotherapy research) can be done: this change in the color distribution *is related to a change in the treatment concept regarding the therapeutical interactions*. An second alteration in the color distribution of the therapist picture can be recognized for the last 5 sessions which are indicated by the detachment of the patient from the therapist [7] which plays an important role in the psychotherapy process. This phase is indicated by a drastic change of the patient-therapist-relation. On the other hand, investigating the initial phases of therapy sessions we observe that the frequency of blue-green colors for the patient decreases. We have found that these colors correspond to a decreasing heart rate. This is in agreement to the assessment by therapist where is stated that in the first sessions there was a big emotional pressure and expectation from the patient in the beginning phase which is lost during the following ones. The several phases of the therapy also can be seen in the time development of the color distribution considered in each session (Fig.4). Moreover, it is possible to assign characteristic pattern of parameter changes to specific colors by a deeper analysis. For instance, as mentioned above we found that green-blue colors are related to an decreasing heart rate whereas red indicates an increase. Yellow-green colors symbolize increasing muscle tensions. The rise of electrodermal conductivity is coded by magenta-like colors. However, for a detailed consideration and interpretation further investigations are necessary.

3.2   Determination of fine motoric disturbances to detect patients suffering from Wilson's disease using the U-matrix

The second exemplary application is to determine for probands whether they have a Wilson's disease or not. For this purpose an extensive *test set* was created to examine the fine motoric disturbances of probands containing passive and active motoric control tasks as resting and holding tremor control, forefinger tapping, spiral painting and target tapping. From this set 11 values are derived characterizing the motoric disturbance of the patient [6]. As it was shown in [6] the separated single consideration of each variable does not lead to a clear classification. Moreover, traditional approaches of classical multivariate statistics also have failed. Therefore, we tried an analysis using SOM. Because of the small data set (only 56 probands - 32 patients and 24 random selected probands) we generated additional data for SOM-learning by adding small noise to each original data vector. Thereby, the noise was in the range of less then 10% of the variance of the respective component. Using this extended data set the GSOM results in a two-dimensional (16×13) lattice. Again, we included the magnification control scheme to obtain an optimal information transfer which achieves a value of 93.7% of the maximal possible entropy value (in comparison to 87.2% without control). The topology preservation judged by the topographic product gives $P = 0.012$ referring to an approximate match. After SOM training the matrix $\mathbf{U}$ was computed according to (2.7) and the clusters are determined

Clusters (no shading) - vscopewilson_som_ges_best.som

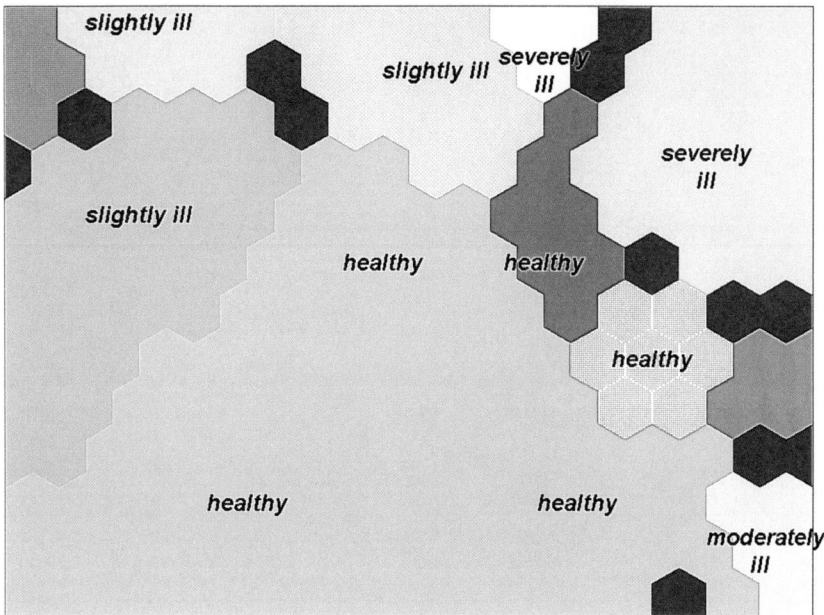

Figure 5: Cluster partition resulted from the GSOM. The vertical direction describes the passive control wheras the horizontal axis correspond to active control. The shadowing is according to the **U**-matrix and gives the clasification of severity of the neurological symptoms. The label of strength of illnes represent the distribution of the strength of the extrapyramidal symptoms in the map. (More details - see text)

by analyzing its structure (Fig. 5).

From a clinical point of view a clear distinction between healthy and ill probands can be made using the resulted cluster partition. Moreover, we can differentiate neurologic and non-neurologic variants of the Wilson's disease on basis of their fine motoric values. Furthermore, one can divide the neurologic variants of Wilson's disease into three subclasses regarding to *clinical symptoms* [6]. However, this subclassification can not be found in the determined cluster partition of motoric disturbances. The SOM based cluster partition corresponds to the severity of neurologic symptoms. This fact is not surprising because of neurological different kinds of Wilson's disease may view similar effects in motoric disturbances. However, the two founded *GSOM lattice dimensions can be assigned to the strength of disturbances for passive and active motoric tasks* by analysis of the respective component planes (Fig.6–Fig.8). We can see that in all parameter planes the topological order is established.

Moreover, the SOM analysis shows that the used test set for fine motoric

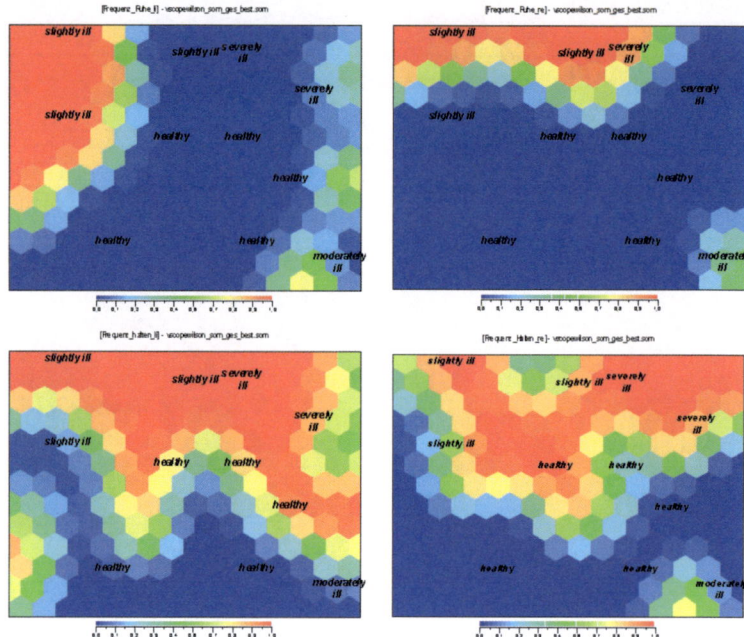

Figure 6: Distribution of the values within the component planes describing passive control abilities: detection of resting tremor - left hand (above left) / right hand (above right), detection of holding tremor - left hand (below left) / right hand (below right).

disturbance detection can be successfully applied to detect and to differentiate probands with extrapyramidal motoric disorders. Thereby, the SOM visualization gives an easy tool for expert assessment.

4   Conclusion

In the present paper we reviewed some advanced approaches to improve the capabilities of the SOM for non-linear PCA, clustering and visualization which are structure adaptation and magnification control. Both extensions together with faithful learning and control of the topology preservation leads to successful applications results. Particularly, the visualization methods (color representation and **U**-matrix consideration) for easy assessment make essential use of the proper data representation by the SOM. We demonstrated the techniques for real world examples both are in medicine which is a innovative area for advanced visualization methods.

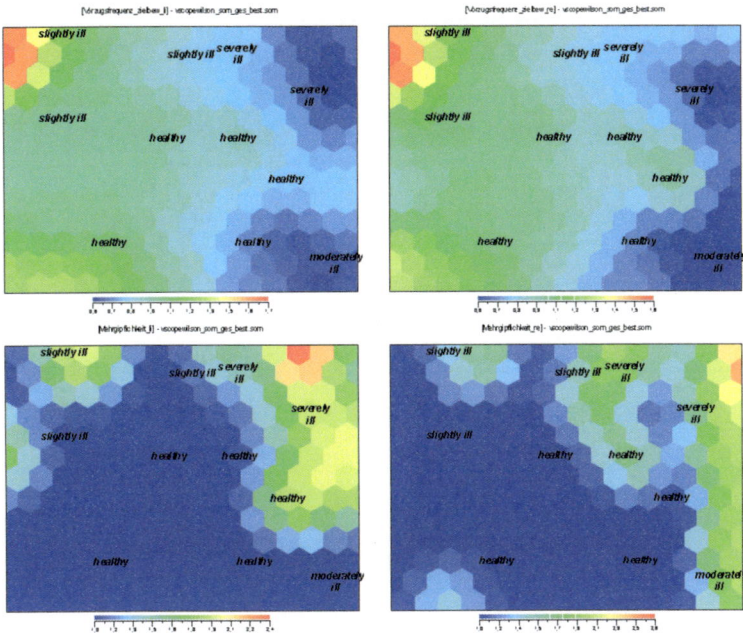

Figure 7: Distribution of the values within the component planes describing active control in case of target tapping: main frequency - left hand (above left), main frequency - right hand (above right), occurence of additional frequencies - left hand (below left) and right hand (below right).

References

[1] H.-U. Bauer, R. Der, and M. Herrmann. Controlling the magnification factor of self–organizing feature maps. *Neural Computation*, 8(4):757–771, 1996.

[2] H.-U. Bauer, M. Herrmann, and T. Villmann. Neural maps and topographic vector quantization. *Neural Networks*, 12(4–5):659–676, 1999.

[3] H.-U. Bauer and K. R. Pawelzik. Quantifying the neighborhood preservation of Self-Organizing Feature Maps. *IEEE Trans. on Neural Networks*, 3(4):570–579, 1992.

[4] H.-U. Bauer and T. Villmann. Growing a Hypercubical Output Space in a Self–Organizing Feature Map. *IEEE Transactions on Neural Networks*, 8(2):218–226, 1997.

[5] D. DeSieno. Adding a conscience to competitive learning. In *Proc. ICNN'88, Int. Conf. on Neural Networks*, pages 117–124, Piscataway, NJ, 1988. IEEE Service Center.

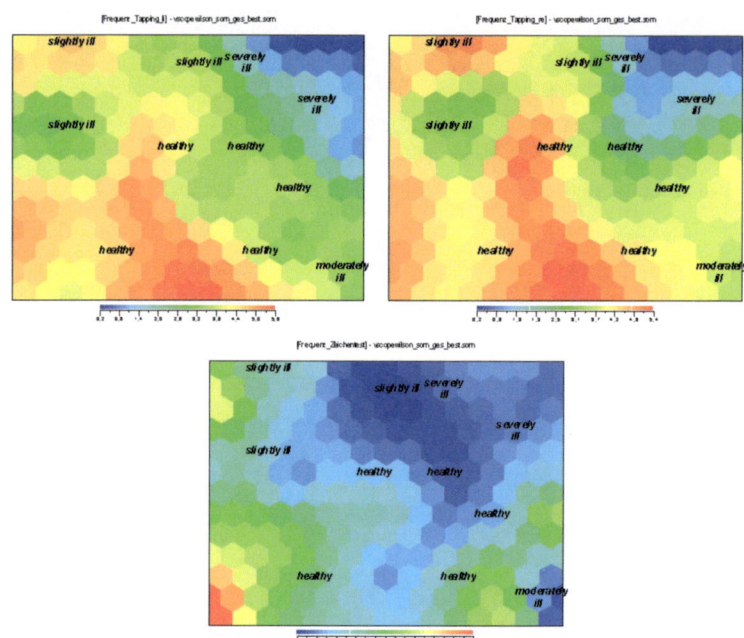

Figure 8: Distribution of the values within the component planes describing active control: forefinger tapping frequency - left hand (above left), forefinger tapping frequency - right hand (above right), spiral drawing frequency (below).

[6] W. Hermann, T. Villmann, M. de Groot, F. Grahmann, and A. Wagner. Kinesiologische Diagnostik bei Morbus Wilson. *Klinische Neurophysiologie - Zeitschrift für Funktionsdiagnostik des Nervensystems*, 2:94–100, 2000.

[7] H. Hess. *Untersuchungen Zur Abbildung Des Prozeßgeschehens und der Effektivität in der Intendiert-Dynamischen Gruppenpsychotherapie.* PhD thesis, Humbold University Berlin (Germany), 1986.

[8] W. Hubert and R. de Jong-Meyer. Psychophysiological response patterns to positive and negative film stimuli. *Biological Psychology*, 31(1):79–93, 1991.

[9] S. Kaski, J. Nikkilä, and T. Kohonen. Methods for interpreting a self-organized map in data analysis. In *Proc. Of European Symposium on Artificial Neural Networks (ESANN'98)*, pages 185–190, Brussels, Belgium, 1998. D facto publications.

[10] T. Kohonen. *Self-Organizing Maps.* Springer, Berlin, Heidelberg, 1995. (Second Extended Edition 1997).

[11] R. Linsker. How to generate maps by maximizing the mutual information between input and output signals. *Neural Computation*, 1:402–411, 1989.

[12] H. Ritter and K. Schulten. On the stationary state of Kohonen's self-organizing sensory mapping. *Biol. Cyb.*, 54:99–106, 1986.

[13] A. Ultsch. Self organized feature maps for monitoring and knowledge aquisition of a chemical process. In S. Gielen and B. Kappen, editors, *Proc. ICANN'93, Int. Conf. on Artificial Neural Networks*, pages 864–867, London, UK, 1993. Springer.

[14] J. Vesanto. SOM-based data visualization methods. *Intelligent Data Analysis*, 3(7):123–456, 1999.

[15] T. Villmann. Controling strategies for the magnification factor in the neural gas network. *Neural Network World*, 10(4):739–750, 2000.

[16] T. Villmann and H.-U. Bauer. Applications of the growing self-organizing map. *Neurocomputing*, 21(1-3):91–100, 1998.

[17] T. Villmann, R. Der, M. Herrmann, and T. Martinetz. Topology Preservation in Self–Organizing Feature Maps: Exact Definition and Measurement. *IEEE Transactions on Neural Networks*, 8(2):256–266, 1997.

[18] T. Villmann, W. Hermann, and M. Geyer. Variants of self-organizing maps for data mining and data visualization in medicine. *Neural Network World*, 10(4):751–762, 2000.

[19] T. Villmann and M. Herrmann. Magnification control in neural maps. In *Proc. Of European Symposium on Artificial Neural Networks (ESANN'98)*, pages 191–196, Brussels, Belgium, 1998. D facto publications.

[20] T. Villmann and A. Hessel. Analyzing psychotherapy process time series using neural maps. In D. Wilshaw, editor, *Proceedings of the International Conference on Artificial Neural Networks (ICANN'99)*, pages 767–772. IEE Press, 1999.

[21] G. Westhoff. *Handbuch Psychosozialer Meßinstrumente*. Hogrefe-Verlag, Göttingen, 1993.

Analysis of Nonlinear Differential Equations: Parameter Estimation and Model Selection

Werner Horbelt[1], Thorsten Müller[1], Jens Timmer[1],
Werner Melzer[2], and Karl Winkler[3]

[1] Freiburger Zentrum für Datenanalyse und Modellbildung,
Eckerstr. 1, D–79104 Freiburg, Germany
{horbelt, jeti}@fdm.uni-freiburg.de
http://www.fdm.uni-freiburg.de
[2] Institut für Angewandte Physiologie, Universität Ulm, 89069 Ulm, Germany
[3] Universitätsklinik Freiburg

Abstract. We have implemented a method for estimating parameters in systems of nonlinear differential equations which is superior to conventional approaches with respect to reliability and effectiveness. The method is based on the multiple shooting approach introduced by Bock (1983). Different models are compared with respect to their adequacy by means of likelihood ratio tests. We demonstrate the advantages of the algorithm with simulated data and present applications from calcium dynamics in skeletal muscle cells and the human lipoprotein metabolism.

1 Introduction

Many problems in medical data analysis require the modeling of dynamical data with a set of nonlinear differential equations. Mostly the model comprises system states and parameters not accessible by direct measurements. The goal is to estimate the unknown parameters and the hidden components from time series of a single observable and to investigate the compatibility of a model with measurements.

A widely used approach is to approximate the model with a linear set of equations. These can be solved analytically and a least squares fit between the model trajectories and the measurements can be implemented easily. However, the linear approximation might introduce systematic errors and there is no way to detect the limits of the simplified model.

Thus it is preferable to calculate the solutions of the nonlinear model numerically and to fit it iteratively to the measured data. The objective function that is to be minimized, is highly nonlinear and has numerous local minima apart from the global one that corresponds to the best choice of the parameters. This problem is adressed by a multiple shooting algorithm introduced in [1,2].

After defining the class of problems considered, we demonstrate the performance of the method in Section 3. Then we show applications from two different research areas.

R.W. Brause and E. Hanisch (Eds.): ISMDA 2000, LNCS 1933, pp. 152–159, 2000.

2   Methods

2.1   Definition of the Problem

Consider a time-continuous, dynamical process described by a set of m nonlinear ordinary differential equations (ODE)

$$\dot{\mathbf{x}} = \mathbf{f}(t, \mathbf{x}, \mathbf{p}), \quad \mathbf{x} \in \mathbf{R}^m, \quad t \in [t_0, t_1], \tag{1}$$

with a set of unknown parameters $\mathbf{p} \in \mathbf{R}^p$. The initial values $\mathbf{x}_0 = \mathbf{x}(t_0)$ are treated as additional parameters and are included in $\mathbf{p}$.

The scalar time series $\{y_i\}$ represents a measurement of the system state $\mathbf{x}(t_i)$ at discrete times t_i via the observation function g:

$$y_i = g(\mathbf{x}(t_i, \mathbf{p}), \mathbf{p}) + \eta_i, \quad i = 1..N. \tag{2}$$

Here, η_i denotes independent normally distributed random numbers with zero mean and variance σ_i^2, accounting for measurement noise. We aim at identifying the set of parameters $\hat{\mathbf{p}}$, for which the solution $\mathbf{x}(t, \hat{\mathbf{p}})$ of (1) is closest to the observed dynamics y_i. To this end, the objective function $\chi^2(\mathbf{p})$ is defined as the sum of squared residues between the data and the model, weighted with the inverse variances of the data:

$$\chi^2(\mathbf{p}) = \sum_{i=1}^{N} \left(\frac{y_i - g(\mathbf{x}(t_i, \mathbf{p}), \mathbf{p})}{\sigma_i} \right)^2 \tag{3}$$

The parameters $\hat{\mathbf{p}}$ are identified as the ones minimizing $\chi^2(\mathbf{p})$.

2.2   The Initial Value Approach

If the problem of parameter identification in ODE systems is treated in the same way as other problems of non-linear regression, one is led to the so-called initial value approach: Starting from some initial guess of the parameter vector, the model equations are solved over the whole fitting interval $[0, T]$. Then a steepest descent method, a generalized Gauss-Newton method or a sequential quadratic programming method is used to minimize $\chi^2(\mathbf{p})$. [3,4]. The Gauss-Newton method and its descendants are well suited to least squares minimization because they exploit the structure of χ^2 as a sum of squared residues, resulting in a second order approximation of χ^2 though only first order derivatives must be supplied.

Compared with regression, where an explicit function is used as a model, this task is more difficult because the ODE trajectory $\mathbf{x}(t, \mathbf{p})$ is very sensitive to the parameters, especially in the case of complex dynamical systems. Badly chosen initial estimates can preclude most routines from yielding any solution at all because the trial trajectory might diverge. Since $\chi^2(\mathbf{p})$ shows a highly non-linear dependence on the parameters $\mathbf{p}$, it will usually have several local minima apart from the global one that corresponds to the true parameters [5]. Noise on the data destabilizes the fit further.

2.3   Multiple Shooting

The multiple shooting method for estimating parameters was established by Bock (1981, 1983). The motivation is that the initial value effectively neglects information on the dynamics of the system present in the measurements. Even though the time course of at least one component, the observation, is known rather accurately, the initial value approach does not take advantage of any but the very first observation in the fitting interval. If the parameters are far off from the correct ones, the trial trajectory soon loses contact to the measurements.

With Bock's elegant approach, one partitions the fitting interval into many subintervals, each having its own initial values. While the ordinary parameters $\mathbf{p}$ are unique over the full interval, the local initial values are optimized separately during the iteration. The measurements are used to get initial guesses for them.

This approach leads to an initially discontinuous trajectory, which is, however, close to the measurements. The final trajectory must of course be continuous, i.e. constraints must be imposed that force the computed solution at the end of one subinterval to be equal to the local initial values of the next subinterval. This leads to a *nonlinear programming problem*:

$$\text{Minimize } \chi^2(\mathbf{p}) \text{ subject to the continuity constraints.} \tag{4}$$

When the Gauss-Newton method is used to solve this problem, the continuity constraints can be treated very efficiently due to their special structure. The additional variables introduced by the subintervals do not increase the computation time excessively.

Furthermore, the constraints are considered only in a linearized form. Thus the iterative process is allowed to proceed to the final continuous solution through "forbidden ground": the iterates will generally be discontinuous trajectories. This freedom allows the method to stay close to the observed data, prevents divergence of the numerical solution and reduces the problem of local minima. Details of the mathematical and implementational aspects of the method are given in Bock (1983).

2.4   Other Features

At the convergence point, the variance-/covariance matrix of the estimated parameters is computed. When the model is overparameterized, the algorithm signals rank deficiency. Additional constraints on the parameters or trajectories, e.g., boundaries for parameters and state variables, can easily be implemented in (4). Furthermore, our algorithm is able to take into account multiple data sets simultaneously (multiexperiment case). Each parameter can be varied independently, forced to be the same for all data sets or fixed to a given value.

3   Demonstration

To illustrate the behavior of the multiple shooting algorithm we examined the restricted Lotka-Volterra system

$$\dot{x} = k_1\, x - k_2\, xy \qquad (5)$$
$$\dot{y} = k_2\, xy - k_3\, y \qquad (6)$$

with parameters $k_1 = 1.0$, $k_2 = 1.5$ and $k_3 = 2.0$ and initial values $x_0 = 0.3$ and $y_0 = 0.8$. The simulated curves were sampled with $\Delta t = 0.2$. Observational noise with a standard deviation of 0.1 was added to the signal. Only the first components of the data were taken as observations. The starting guesses for the parameters were half the true values.

When trying to estimate the parameters with the initial value approach, the algorithm ran into a local minimum (s. left column of Fig. 1). On the other hand, the multiple shooting algorithm converged to the global minimum (right column). The true trajectory is perfectly reproduced. The estimated parameters deviate from the true values by less than 1%. Even under much worse conditions, the parameters could be estimated reliably.

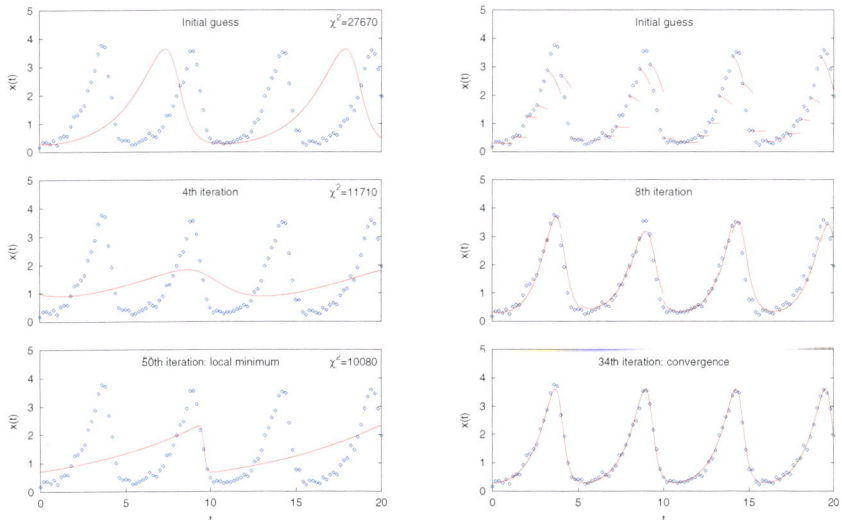

Fig. 1. Fit of the Lotka-Volterra system with the initial value approach and the multiple shooting approach. Three stages of the iterative process are shown in each case. It can be seen clearly that in the multiple shooting case the trajectory is discontinuous initially and becomes continuous at the end

4   Applications

In this Section we show two applications of the algorithm to problems from physiology and medicine. Fig. 2 shows schematically the two compartment models.

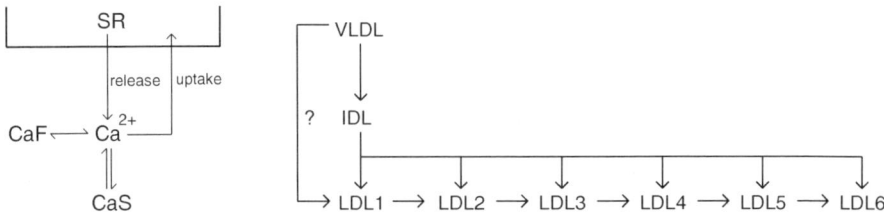

Fig. 2. Schemes for the two applications. Left: compartment model of the Ca^{2+} dynamics in skeletal muscle cells. Right: compartment model of human lipoprotein metabolism

4.1   Analysis of Ca^{2+} Release in Skeletal Muscle Cells

In skeletal muscle cells, Ca^{2+} ions are stored in the sarcoplasmic reticulum (SR). They are released from the SR into the cell plasma, binding to various compounds. The concentration of free Ca^{2+} is observed experimentally by optical measurements [7]. The goal is to determine the release rate time course.

A simple compartment model of the Ca^{2+} distribution is shown in the left

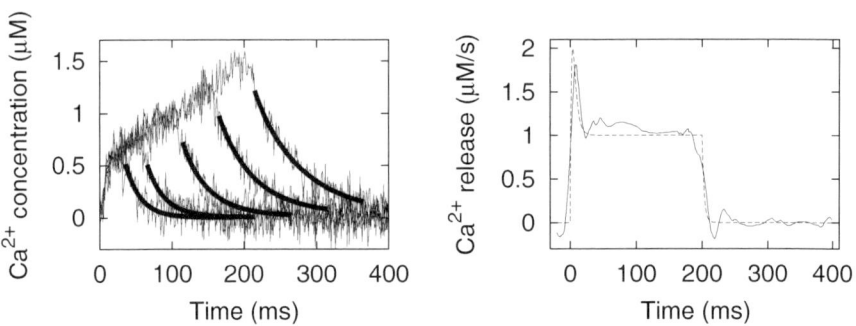

Fig. 3. Left: Simultaneous fit of model trajectories (thick lines) to five different simulated noisy Ca^{2+} transients (thin lines). Of each transient only that part was used for the fit, in which the release was known to be zero. Right: Simulated Ca^{2+} release used to generate one of the transients (dashed line) and release curve calculated from that transient with the parameters estimated in the fit

part of Fig. 2. It contains an instantaneously equilibrating non-saturating compartment CaF whose occupancy is a multiple of the free calcium concentration

Ca^{2+}, a saturable slow compartment CaS, described by two rate constants and the total concentration of binding sites, and a slow non-saturable uptake with one associated rate constant.

Using simulated calcium transients with known underlying release rates we tested the ability of our algorithm to determine the time course of the release under different conditions. The determination of the release rate involves two steps.

At first the dynamical system under study is characterized, i.e. the unknown parameters are determined by analyzing the Ca^{2+} transients in a time interval in which the release is known to vanish. In a second step, the release curve is calculated using the measurements and the fully specified model. The result is shown in Fig. 3. The analysis reproduced in a satisfactory way the characteristics of the input release rate. For details and technicalities, see [6].

4.2   Human Lipoprotein Metabolism

Lipoproteins mediate the transport of cholesterol and triglyceride through the plasma. All contain the Apolipoprotein B-100 (ApoB) and can be subdivided into very low (VLDL), intermediate (IDL) and low (LDL) lipoproteins with help

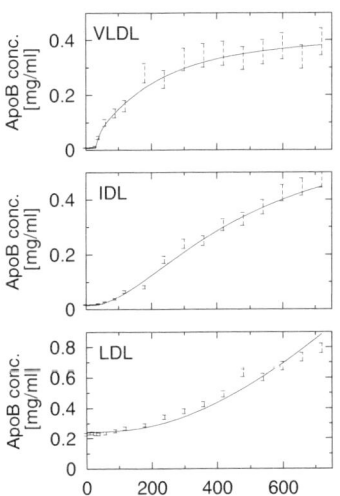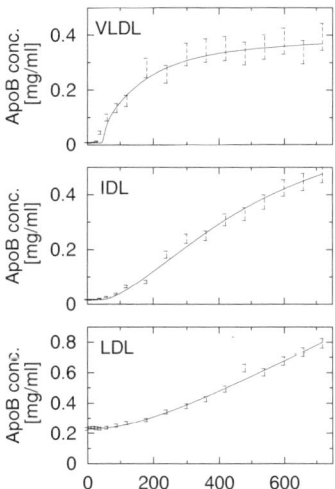

Fig. 4. Fit with the smaller model (*left*) and the larger model including a pathway between the VLDL compartment and the first LDL compartment (*right*). Five multiple shooting intervals were used for each trajectory

of their density. Modelling the dynamics of the transfer of ApoB from VLDL to LDL through a delipidation chain can be done with help of a compartmental model (see Fig. 2) [8].

It is still unclear if there exists a metabolism mechanism other than the delipidation chain. Especially the direct pathway from VLDL to LDL through cell membrane receptors might be possible.

Or mathematically: Is the larger compartment model with a pathway between VLDL and LDL superior to the smaller model?

Minimizing the objective function $\chi^2(\mathbf{p})$ with a data set leads to a minimum χ^2-value of 103.8 for the smaller model and a minimum χ^2-value of 55.0 for the larger model (see Fig. 4). The theoretical distribution of the test statistic is a mixture of $\chi^2(\mathbf{p})$-distributions with the 95% level at 2.7. Calculating the test statistic with the data set (i.e. the minimum χ^2-values) reveals a value of 48.3; the null hypothesis has to be rejected, the larger model has to be preferred.

5   Summary

The strategy of multiple shooting is a powerful tool for estimating parameters in systems of ordinary differential equations. We demonstrated its applicability to three different systems. For the Lotka-Volterra model we showed that it is possible to get reliable estimates of the parameters under conditions for which the initial value approach failed. The procedure was successfully applied to the analysis of Ca^{2+} release in skeletal muscle cells and to measurements of the human lipoprotein metabolism. Likelihood ratio tests were used to choose among different models.

References

1. H. G. Bock, in *Modelling of Chemical Reaction Systems*, edited by K. Ebert, P. Deuflhard, and W. Jäger (Springer, Heidelberg and New York, 1981), pp. 102–125.
2. H. G. Bock, in *Numerical Treatment of Inverse Problems in Differential and Integral Equations*, edited by P. Deuflhard and E. Hairer (Birkhäuser, Basel, 1983), pp. 95–121.
3. L. Edsberg and P. Wedin, Optim. Methods Softw. **6**, 193 (1995).
4. K. Schittkowski, in *Recent Trends in Optimization Theory and Applications*, edited by R. Agarwal (World Scientific, Singapore, 1995), pp. 353–370.
5. O. Richter, P. Nörtersheuser, and W. Pestemer, Science Total Env. **123/124**, 435 (1992).
6. J. Timmer, T. Müller, and W. Melzer, Biophys. J. **74**, 1694 (1998).
7. A. Struk, G. Szücs, H. Kemmer, and W. Melzer, Cell Calcium **23**, 23 (1998).
8. K. Winkler *et al.*, Atherosclerosis **144**, 167 (1999).
9. J. Timmer, H. Rust, W. Horbelt, and H. Voss, PLA, submitted (2000).

Medical Expert Evaluation of Machine Learning Results for a Coronary Heart Disease Database

Dragan Gamberger[1], Goran Krstačić[2], and Tomislav Šmuc[1]

[1] Rudjer Bošković Institute, Bijenička 54,10000 Zagreb, Croatia
E-mail: dragan.gamberger@irb.hr
[2] Institute for Prevention of Cardiovascular Disease and Rehabilitation,
Dra škovićeva 13, 10000 Zagreb, Croatia

Abstract. A set of machine learning experiments w as performed on the atherosclerotic coronary heart disease data collected in the regular medical practice, with intention to evaluate established medical diagnostic practice, in vestigate the relations bet ween the results of less important diagnostic tests, and detect novel regularities in patients' data. The results of these experiments were evaluated by the medical expert for their soundness with respect to the existing kno wledge in the domain, and potential for the generation of new and useful medical knowledge. The performed experiments generally verify the existing medical practice in non-invasive diagnosis of atherosclerotic coronary heart disease, but also demonstrate how the synergy of medical and machine learning expertise helps in the inference of a new knowledge and potentially could increase efficiency and reliability of the medical diagnostic process.

1 Introduction

Improv ement and rationalization of diagnostic procedures and treatment of atherosclerotic coronary heart disease (ACHD), one of the world's most frequent causes of mortality, are important problems of medical practice. The usual procedure in ACHD diagnosis consists of several diagnostic levels and the amount of available information for a patient at the end is large [12]. The goal of rational diagnostic procedures is to establish the conclusive diagnosis of A CHD and to plan the most appropriate management of the disease using only the necessary diagnostic steps. This can be achieved by evaluating all the information collected by different diagnostic methods according to their importance and diagnostic value [4].

Non-inv asiv e medical diagnostic practice today uses a series of anamnestic information, laboratory testing, and diagnostic measurements. T ypically diagnosis is based on a few important and v erified diagnostic tests including ST segment depression in exercise testing [1], long term ECG recording [3], and echocardiography measurements. Although significance of other av ailable information is known and prov ed in medical theory, it is mainly used as qualitative confirmation of the diagnosis based on the main factors.

R.W. Brause and E. Hanisch (Eds.): ISMDA 2000, LNCS 1933, pp. 159–168, 2000.

The importance of the ACHD diagnosis has stimulated different statistical analyses of patients' data [5, 8]. The results have been interesting, but mostly of scientific and less of practical importance. Recent applications of intelligent data analysis methods can be divided into several closely related categories like decision support tools [11], educational systems [2], and detection systems [6]. The core of these applications are different machine learning algorithms whose main objective is to construct highly accurate classifiers, sometimes with special properties that might be useful for diagnostic practice [9, 10].

The goal of this work is to broaden the scope of the application of intelligent data analyses methods by testing how iterative and interactive methodology involving both machine learning and medical expertise can help in improvement of regular medical practice. The idea is based on the assumption that machine learning methods are capable of objective interpretation of available information contained in collected patient database. The topics of this research are: a) evaluation of established medical diagnostic practice, b) evaluation of diagnostic tests and anamnestic data generally treated as less reliable diagnostic predictors in everyday medical practice, and c) detection of novel regularities in patient data applicable in diagnostic practice. The last two items have their motivation especially for situations in which important diagnostic parameters are not reliable or not available.

The methodology described in this work is specific in two ways: 1) the patient classification in the database is done by medical expert, and therefore is not necessarily exact 2) the aim of the supervised learning algorithm was not induction of the most accurate classification rules, but extraction of useful information hidden in the available database. Thus, common use of supervised learning tools for building classifiers is extended by performing a set of inductive learning experiments using different subsets of diagnostic results(descriptors), all under supervision and evaluation of medical expert. The results obtained through applying this methodology are manifold, and can be transformed into improved quality of the database, a new knowledge about the specific cases, and possibly new knowledge about the disease itself.

In the following section we describe the data set available for the inductive learner. In Section 3 the information extracted from the data set by different machine learning experiments is presented while Section 4 summarizes medical expert evaluation of the obtained results especially in the sense of their usefulness in medical practice.

2   Data Set

For this work, a database representing typical medical practice in ACHD diagnosis has been prepared. The data describe patients who entered the Institute for Prevention of Cardiovascular Disease and Rehabilitation, Zagreb Croatia, during a period of few months. The set of descriptors represents all potentially interesting and typically available information about patients. The descriptor set includes 10 anamnestic items like age, body mass index (BMI), family anamnesis

(F.A.), stress, diabetes mellitus (D.M.), 6 items with laboratory test results like cholesterol, uric acid, and fibrinogen (FIB), the resting ECG data (5 items), the exercise test data (5 items), echocardiogram results (2 items), vectorcardiogram results (2 items), and long term continuous ECG recording data (HOL) in 3 items. It makes all together 33 data items. Only patients with complete data have been included into the data set, resulting in the data set with 150 patients. The descriptors are cited in Tables 1 and 2.

descriptor	abbr. name	characteristics
anamnestic data		
sex	SEX	1-man 2-woman
age	AGE	continuous (years)
height	H	continuous (m)
weight	W	continuous (kg)
body mass index	BMI	continuous ($kg\ m^{-2}$)
family anamnesis	F.A.	1-negative 2-positive
present smoking	P.S.	1-negative 2-positive 3-very positive
diabetes mellitus	D.M.	1-negative 2-pos. medicament therapy 3-pos. insulin therapy
hypertension	HYP	1-negative 2-positive 3-very positive
stress	STR	1-negative 2-positive 3-very positive
laboratory tests		
total cholesterol	T.CH.	continuous ($mmol\ L^{-1}$)
trygliceride	TR	continuous ($mmol\ L^{-1}$)
high density lipoprotein	HDL/CH	continuous ($mmol\ L^{-1}$)
low density lipoprotein	LDL/CH	continuous ($mmol\ L^{-1}$)
uric acid	U.A.	continuous ($\mu mol\ L^{-1}$)
fibrinogen	FIB	continuous ($g\ L^{-1}$)

Table 1. The names and the characteristics of 16 descriptors verified by anamnesis and laboratory testing.

The classification of the patients was performed by the cardiologist and it reflects generally accepted medical knowledge. The classification is mostly based on the results of the most important tests like ST segment depression during exercise testing, but also the NYHA classification [12] and clinically significant metabolic equivalents (METs) are used. Similar parameters can be found in long term ECG recording, except MET and NYHA classification. Dyastolic internal diameter of left ventricular with parasternal short axis view and left ventricular ejection fraction (according to Simpson) are determined from the echocardiogram.

For this research the cardiologist classified patients into 5 groups:

descriptor	abbr. name	characteristics
resting ECG		
heart rate	HR	continuous (beats min^{-1})
ST segment depression	ECGst	1-negative 2-positive 1mm 3-positive $\geq$ 2mm
serious arrhythmias	ECGrhyt	1-negative 2-positive
conduction disorders	ECGcd	1-negative 2-positive
left ventricular hypertrophy	ECGhlv	1-negative 2-positive
exercise ECG		
ST segment depression	ExECGst	1-negative 2-positive 1mm 3-positive $\geq$ 2mm
serious arrhythmias	ExECGrhyt	1-negative 2-positive
conduction disorders	ExECGcd	1-negative 2-positive
hypertensive reaction	ExECGhyp	1-negative 2-positive
New York Heart Ass. functional class	ExECGNYHA	class I - IV
echocardiography		
left ventr. internal diameter	EchoLVID$_d$	continuous (mm)
left ventr. ejection fraction according to Simpson	EchoLVEF	continuous (%)
vectorcardiography Q		
transmural MI	VCGQ	1-negative 2-positive
left ventricular hypertrophy	VCGhlv	1-negative 2-positive
long term continuous ECG		
serious arrhythmias	HOLrhyt	1-negative 2-positive
conduction disorders	HOLcd	1-negative 2-positive
ST segment depression	HOLst	1-negative 2-positive 1mm 3-positive $\geq$ 2mm

Table 2. The names and the characteristics of 17 descriptors verified with non-invasive diagnostic procedures.

Group I Healthy patients without verified A CHD but with possible present cardiovascular risk factors.

Group II-V These are patients with previous myocardial infarction. They were classified by the results of non-invasiv e cardiovascular tests and their condition after some coronary angioplastic or cardiosurgery treatment. They are all under medicament treatment.

> **Group II** P atien ts with normal results of exercise testing, long term recording and echocardiogram.
>
> **Group III** Patients with ST segment depression 1.00 mm in exercise testing and during long term ECG recording, left ven tricular ejection fraction higher than 55%, METs 10.
>
> **Group IV** P atien ts with ST segmentdepression equal or higher than 2.00 mm in exercise testing and during long term ECG recording, left ventricular ejection fraction less than 55% (40-54%), left ventricular internal diameter more than 6.0 cm, NYHA II-III, METs 5–10.
>
> **Group V** P atien ts ha ving ST segmentelevation or depression > 3.00mm, left ven tricularejection fraction less or equal to 30%, left ven tricular inner diameter greater than 6.5 cm, NYHA III-IV, METs<5.

3   Machine learning results

Experimental results presented in this section are obtained from the database presented in Section 2 by the inductive learning system ILLM [7]. ILLM (Inductive Learning by Logic Minimization) is a minimization based, tw o class, propositional, rule generating inductive system. In contrast to other popular inductive systems it is not statistically or probability based. ILLM starts from a set of implicitly defined literals that are automatically generated from the example set for the given set of descriptors. Rule complexity is measured by the number of different literals used in it. The rule is built of necessary and sufficient conditions in the form of a mixed disjunctive-conjunctive logical expression. The aim of the work was not to compare results of different systems but to explore the possibilities of applying machine induction to generate useful medical knowledge. F or this purpose the application of a deterministic, minimization based system like ILLM, seemed a good choice.

The purpose of the experiments w asto extract as much as possible of the useful kno wledgefrom the av ailable data. Since ILLM system performs rule induction for one target class at a time, for each experiment it was necessary to join groups formed by medical expert into tw o distinctie classes (positive and negative). During the preparation phase of machine learning experiments it w as detected that potentially in teresting differences may be betw een groups II - III and groups III - IV. In majority of experiments the default positive class were patients in groups III - V while groups I and II represented the negative class. In this case the positive class contained about 40% of the total number of patients.

The machine learning experiment settings included: 1) different grouping of patients into 2 classes (positive and negative) with the intention to investigate

Descriptor set	P ositiv e class	Negative class
full	exECGst $\geq 1mm$ **or** (HOLst $\geq 1mm$ **and** ECHOlvef < 62.5) %	exECG $< 1mm$ **and** HOLst $< 1mm$
reduced	ECHOlvef < 63.5 %, age $> 57years$, F.A. = pos. heigh t$< 173cm$, FIB $< 3.65gL^{-1}$, stress = pos. choles. $> 5.59mmolL^{-1}$, weight $> 85kg$	
significantly reduced	F.A. = pos. · D.M. = pos. · age $> 55years$ · heigh t$< 173cm$	age $< 58years$ · trygl < 1.78 · BMI $< 28.02kgm^{-2}$
	F.A. = pos. · BMI $> 26.82kgm^{-2}$ · heigh t$< 173cm$ · choles. $> 6.03mmolL^{-1}$	F.A. = neg. · hypert. = neg. · heigh t$> 168cm$

Table 3. Induction results for different descriptor sets computed for **a)** positive class patients in groups III - V and **b)** negativ e class patients in groups I and II. For the full and the significantly reduced descriptor set, induced rules are presented while in the row for the reduced descriptor set is only the list of 8 most important conditions used in the induced rules for the positive class.

borders between groups formed b y the cardiologist; 2) different subsets of de-scriptors used in rule induction with intention to inv estigate significance and limits for less important descriptors; 3) different values of the acceptable noise level parameter; 4) different covering properties of the induced rules. Selection of the appropriate noise level parameter was the main factor which determined the complexity of the induced rules. The course of the experimen ts was influenced b y the results of previous experiments and their preliminary medical expert eval-uation. The results presented in this section represent only the most significant ones from the machine learning point of view.

In the preprocessing phase ILLM uses saturation based noise detection filter. In the case with the default definition of the positiv eclass and all a vailable descriptors, the noise detection process undoubtedly pointed out three patients. The detection process practically did not depend on the possible changes in the selectable noise acceptance level.

After eliminating the detected three noisy cases from the training set, it was possible to induce a very simple rule for the default positiv eclass. The rule states that a patient is in groups III - V either if his exercise ECG ST segment depression is positive (equal or greater than 1.00 mm) or if both long term ECG ST segment depression is positive and his echocardiography ejection fraction is equal or smaller than 62.5 %. The rule is correct for all positiv epatients and not true for any of the negative patients in the reduced set of 147 cases. The reliable rule for the detection of negative cases is that both exercise ECG and long term ECG ST segment depressions must be less than 1 *mm*. None of the positiv e cases satisfies this rule while it is satisfied by 94 % of the negative cases in the data set. The rules are presented in the first row of Table 3.

The rules generated for the complete descriptor domain show ed absolute importance of the ECG ST segment changes for the A CHD disease diagnosis. This has confirmed that medical expert classification was based almost solely on three main descriptors. Therefore, to induce more information and potentially new kno wledge about the patient population, it w as reasonable to remove the most important descriptors from the dataset in the subsequent learning exper- iments. Induction w as, as expected, more difficult and the induced rules more complex than in the original domain. Because of the rule complexity, second row of Table 3 presents only the list of 8 most important conditions used in the induced rules for the positive class.

The last set of experiments was concentrated on the reliability of predicting A CHD in a non-specialist medical practice. The experiments w ere performed excluding those data which might be unavailable in some basic medical insti- tution. This includes the following list of descriptors: exercise ECG data, long term recording ECG, echocardiography, vectorcardiography data, as well as some laboratory testing like fibrinogen, glucose tolerance test, and lipid profile. The resting ECG data and basic laboratory tests remained included. It was possible to induce four interesting and relative reliable rules that can confirm the posi- tive target class (groups III - V). Each of them cov ers about 20% of the positive cases. For the negative target class four confirmation rules with mean prediction correctness about 25% for negative cases have been constructed. Only tw o rules for the positive class and tw o rules for the negative clas are presented in third row of T able 3. F or illustration, the first rule for the positiv e class states that a patient is ill if it has positiv e family anamnesis , positiv e diabetes mellitus, age over 55 years and height under 173 *cm*. The first confirmation rule for the negative class shows that a patient is in groups I-II if he/she has age under 58 y ears, trygliceride less than $1.78\,mmol\,L^{-1}$, and body mass index less than 28.02 $kg m^{-2}$.

4   Medical expert evaluation of the results

The results present potentially in teresting in terpretation of a vailable patients' data, which is significantly different from the statistical analysis. Noise elimina- tion is important for maintaining data qualit y, although it does not represent new medical kno wledge. The detection of three noisy examples is very illus- trative. Two of them are typical medical outliers representing v ery seriously ill patients who, due to the previous or current medical treatment (cardiological or cardiosurgical procedure, medicament therapy), have at the moment good car- dio vascular condition and heart function. Because of their medical history and present therapy, medical experts have put them into the group III. Detection and elimination of these patients from further machine learning experiments is completely justified but presents no significant information for medical doctors. This is not the case with the third patient. Its inclusion into the noisy set represented a real surprise. The surprise was even greater when it was detected that in this case a mistake occurred, which under different circumstances, could have had dangerous consequences. It was found out that there are two patients with the same name, and that the diagnostic data of the healthy one were by mistake, used in the decision process for the other patient. It can be expected that the mistake would be detected later, during the further patient treatment, but the fact is, that a potentially dangerous mistake have been detected by performed machine learning analysis. This perhaps opens a completely new field for machine learning algorithm applications as a data inconsistency detection supervisor.

In the sense of knowledge, generated rules are much more interesting. At a first glance, the rule that the patient is in groups III-V if he has either positive ST segment depression in exercise ECG or positive ST segment depression in long term ECG recording combined with echocardiogram ejection fraction of left ventricular less than or equal to 62.5 %, only reformulates the known expert knowledge. But the second part of the rule, combination of the long term ECG and echocardiogram results is interesting for two reasons. The first is that this condition successfully detects about 65% of ill patients (groups III - V) while it is false for all 91 patients in groups I and II. From these results it may be concluded that the condition is a reliable way to detect ACHD although it is known that neither ST depression in long term ECG nor echocardiography ejection fraction are reliable symptoms by themselves. In this sense the simultaneous detection of both symptoms represents a reliable sign of the disease which might be interesting for medical practice. At the moment it can represent only a hypothesis that must be verified on a significantly greater number of patients. The second interesting fact about the rule is that the selected echocardiography ejection fraction limit of 62.5% is different from the established medical practice in which positive diagnosis for the impaired heart function is below 56% with normal value 65% +/- 9%. There have been 7% of ill patients in the database, with ejection fraction values between 56% and 62% who have ST depression during long term ECG but no ST depression in exercise ECG. It means that these ill patients could not be detected neither by exercise ECG results nor by echocardiography ejection fraction values if standard limit of 56% is used. Their present diagnosis have been determined by medical doctors based on other auxiliary symptoms, for example increased left ventricular internal diameter. Setting a new, higher patological limit for the echocardiography ejection fraction values, at least in conjunction with long term ECG ST depression, might be a useful correction of the existing medical practice.

The list of induced descriptors and their limits for the reduced descriptor domain contains most of the known facts about the importance of factors like family anamnesis, age, stress, and cholesterol. The induced limits are reasonable.

F or descriptor age, for example the selected limit is 57 years; for fibrinogen the induced limit is 3.65 while most laboratories use 3.80 gL^{-1}; selected limit for total cholesterol is higher than typically used (5.59 instead of 5.00 $mmolL^{-1}$) while for uric acid it is slightly below the standard values.

In some experiments with reduced descriptor domain literals like *present smoking negative* and *tryglic eride under* 2.18 have been detected as properties of the positive class patients. This is in contrast with the existing medical experience that smoking and trygliceride are well known cardiovascular risk factors and these conditions have not been included into T able 3. Detection of these contradictory conditions might be the consequence of a too small number of available data. But their inclusion stimulated additional medical evaluation. It w as detected that most of chronical ACHD patients, which represent the majority in this database, have medicamental therapy for reducing the level of lipids. The consequence is that many chronical ACHD patients actually have low trygliceride lev el. Similarly, it was detected that among chronical ACHD patients there are unproportionally many non-smokers. It is actually not a surprise because doctors suggest non-smoking to all patients and many of them stop smoking after acute coronary syndrome. But it does not mean that present non-smokers ha ve not smoked before which might have influenced the disease. The lesson learned from these unexpected literals is that the present smoking status descriptor of the patient is not appropriate for the estimation of potential risk factors. This suggests refining of this descriptor through addition of patients smoking history to the existing set of descriptors.

The generated confirmation rules for ACHD patients, presented in the last row of T able 3, are interesting because they present an effort in reliable detection of A CHD from relatively simple or easily obtainable data. But it seems even more significant to construct reliable rules for non-ACHD patients with the aim of reducing the number of patients entering specialized cardiovascular institutions. Although the induced rules seem completely reasonable, their broad acceptance b y general medical practitioners, even after thorough medical validation, is not expected. The main reason is the relatively small number of target cases covered b y any of the presented rules. On the other side, the set of rules aimed at detecting ACHD patients points out some significant regularities. In the first place it is the combination of positive family anamnesis with diabetes mellitus as well as the combination of positive family anamnesis with increased body mass index. Information contained in confirmation rules for ACHD patients might be useful for early detection of ACHD by defining the risk population groups which should undertake coronary diagnostic procedures before first disease symptoms.

Conclusion

Medical expert evaluation demonstrated that some of the machine induction results are very in teresting, like the detection of outliers and errors or like the detection of problems in the quality of collected data. Induced descriptor limits in the rules, according to the expert's opinion, could represent new medical

kno wledge. Especially importan in this respect are the results obtained for differen t target patient classes, which either confirmed existing medical practice
or suggest its more or less significant modification. The results are in teresting
for medical practitioners, because they reveal connection betw een known theory
and their everyday experience and detect potentially diagnostically important
combinations of different descriptors.

References

1. A CP/ACC/AHA Task force on Exercise Testing (1990). *Journal of Americ an College Car diolo gy* **16**: 1061-1065.
2. Carrault, G., Cordier, M.O., Quiniou, R., Garreau, M., Bellanger, J.J., Bardou, A.
   (1999) A Model-Based Approach for Learning to Iden tify Cardiac Arrhythmias.
   In *Proc. of Joint Europ ean Conferenc e on Artificial Intelligence in Medicine and
   Medical Decision Making (AIMDM'99)*, 165–174. Springer, Berlin.
3. Detrano, R. et all.(1989) Exercise-induced ST segment depression in the diagnosis of multivessel coronary disease: a meta analysis. *Journal of A meric anColl.
   Car diolo gy* 14:1501–1508.
4. Diamond, G.A.,& F orester, J.S. (1979). Analysis of probability as an aid in the
   clinical diagnosis of coronary artery disease. *New England Journal of Medicine*
   300:1350.
5. Diamond, G.A., Staniloff, H.M., & Forester, J.S. (1983). Computer-assisted diagnosis in the non-invasive evaluation of patients with suspected coronary artery
   disease. *Journal of American Cardiology* **1**:444.
6. F ernandez, E.A., Presedo, J., Barro, S.(1999) An ECG Ischaemic Detection System Based on Self-Organizing Maps and a Sigmoid Function Pre-processing Stage.
   In *Pr oc. of Joint Euop ean Conference on Artificial Intelligence in Medicine and
   Medical Decision Making (AIMDM'99)*, 207–216. Springer, Berlin.
7. Gamberger, D. (1995). A minimization approach to propositional inductive learning. In *Proc. of the 8th European Conferenc e on Machine L earning* 151–160.
   Springer, Berlin.
8. Gerson, C.M. (1987). Test accuracy , test selection and test result interpretation in
   chronic coronary artery disease. In Gerson, C.M. (ed.) *Car diac Nuclar Medicine*,
   pp. 309–347. McGraw Hill.
9. Grošelj, C., Kukar, M., Fetich, J. & Kononenko, I. (1997). Machine learning improves the accuracy of coronary artery disease diagnostic methods. *Computers in
   Car diolgy* **24**: 57–60.
10. Kong, D.F., Del Carlo, C.H., Eisenstein, E.L. (1999). Predicting survival in coro-
    nary disease: machine-learning computer models versus expert clinicians. *Europ an
    He art Journal Abstract Supplement* **20**: 312.
11. T orchio, M.,Battista,S., Bar, F., Pollet, C., Marzuoli, M., Bucchi, M.C., Pagni,
    R., Molino, G.(1999) A Decision Support System for the Identification, Staging,
    and F unctional Evaluation of Liv er Diseases (HEPASCORE). In *Pr oc. of Joint
    European Conference on Artificial Intelligence in Medicine and Medical De cision
    Making (AIMDM'99)*, 158–164. Springer, Berlin.
12. Wayne A.R., Schlan t R.C., Fuster V., In HURST'S: The Heart, Arteries and Veins.
    McGraw c Hill, NY, 1127-1263.

Combining Methodical Procedures from Knowledge Discovery in Databases and Individual-Oriented Simulation
Data Mining in Time Series

Frank Köster[1], Roland Radtke[2], Bernd Westphal[1], and Michael Sonnenschein[1]

[1] Oldenburger Forschungs- und Entwicklungsinstitut
für Informatik-Werkzeuge und -Systeme (OFFIS)
· Escherweg 2 · D-26121 Oldenburg · Germany
[2] Microsoft Corporation · Redmond · United States (WA)
Email: Frank.Koester@Offis.de

Abstract. Systems analysis and the exploration of data are important tasks during the course of environmental epidemiological studies. We examine knowledge discovery in databases combined with individual-oriented modeling and simulation to support the detection of hypotheses about cause-and-effect relationships within environmental systems. An individual-oriented model and detected hypotheses can uncover possible explanations for the current state of health of a study population. Such a model can support future planning and decision making for health-care management. The main goal of attempting to use these methods in epidemiological research is to reduce expenditures in costs and time for a study as well as to improve the analysis and interpretation of available data.

1 Introduction

Systems analysis and the extensive exploration of (sometimes heterogeneous and incomplete) data are important tasks during the process of environmental epidemiological studies. This paper describes an approach to the application of techniques from knowledge discovery in databases (KDD) [22,5] combined with individual-oriented modeling and simulation [4,10] to support the creation of hypotheses about cause-and-effect relationships within populations of individuals interacting with (or being affected by) their environment. These hypotheses can help epidemiologists to gain deeper insights into the occurrence of specific diseases and illnesses [13,15].

Our approach uses individual-oriented modeling and simulation techniques to create a structurally equivalent model of the investigated environmental system and the population of individuals [14]. A special data mining technique is applied to analyze the dynamic and possibly 'emergent' [4] behavior of the simulated model by processing time series which are derived from simulations [13, 15]. Combining these techniques enables us to gain detailed knowledge about

R.W. Brause and E. Hanisch (Eds.): ISMDA 2000, LNCS 1933, pp. 169–182, 2000.

interactions (i.e. cause-and-effect relationships) within the individual-oriented model and the real system. This knowledge can also be helpful, when using individual-oriented modeling and simulation techniques to predict future evolution of a system or structural modified variants of it for different (environmental or individual) situations. In particular, while changing parameters of the model the observed (variant) interactions can be used to describe the shifting of characteristical relationships between components of the modeled system [15].

In the process of modeling it is an important advantage of the individual-oriented approach to be easily applicable to integrate heterogeneous databases (e.g. containing information on the distribution of different agents or geographical data) and knowledge-bases (e.g. containing information on the individual behavior or possible exposure-paths) with respect to each single modeled component in a formal and structured manner [14]. Moreover, these models can be used to estimate missing data within the databases during simulation. For instance, during a simulation the exposure of every single individual to a selected agent can be estimated [15,14]—usually an important but difficult task within environmental epidemiological studies (cf. [21], pages 74–129).

In the past we carried out some technical case-studies [13,15] and developed a set of user-friendly software tools to put this concept into practice. In particular, we developed a special individual-oriented modeling language, a user-friendly tool to control individual-oriented simulations, and a powerful tool for data mining in time series. This set of software tools is intended to help epidemiologists to reduce expenditures in costs and time for an environmental epidemiological study as well as to improve the extensive analysis and interpretation of (heterogeneous and incomplete) available data. Furthermore, the individual-oriented models and detected hypotheses—the gained 'knowledge'—can be used to discover 'new' or previously unknown existing cause-and-effect relationships and support future planning and decision making for health-care management.

Following, Section 2 gives a short introduction to the foundations of our work. In Section 2.1 we give a coarse overview of the process of KDD. Section 2.2 introduces our approach to data mining in time series which is used to analyze individual-oriented simulations discussed in Section 2.3. Section 3 describes the process of KDD combined with individual-oriented modeling and simulation. In Section 4 we give an overview of the software tools we developed which are essential to put our concept into practice. The application of these tools is discussed in Section 5. Finally, Section 6 contains a short summary.

2   Foundations

2.1   KDD and Data Mining

KDD is an interactive and multistage process for the exploration of large databases. In the common literature we usually find characterizations of this process comparable to the following definition suggested by Fayyad et al.:

'KDD is the nontrivial process of identifying valid, novel, potentially useful, and ultimately understandable patterns in data.' ([5], pages 40–41)

During this process we usually distinguish five phases: *Selection, Pre-processing, Transformation, Data Mining,* and *Interpretation* (cf. Fig. 1) [5].

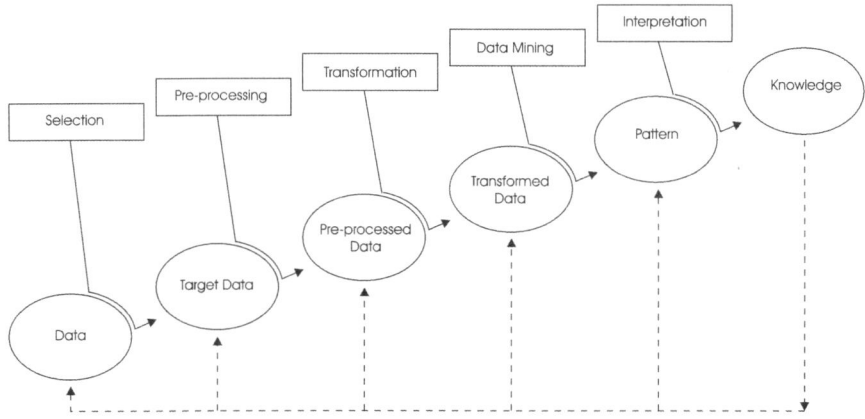

Fig. 1. The process of KDD

Within the first three phases an initial database is created to process in the 4th phase (data mining). The identified patterns (cf. Fig. 1) are interpreted with respect to the area of application and carefully checked for plausibility in the final phase of KDD[1].

In the data mining phase 'intelligent' algorithms (e.g. see the report by Holsheimer and Siebes [12] for an overview) are applied to rummage through the transformed data in order to detect significant patterns. A more concise definition of data mining is given by Woods and Kyral:

'[Data mining is] the automated analysis of large or complex data sets in order to discover significant patterns or trends that would otherwise go unrecognised.' ([22], page 6)

2.2 Application of Evolutionary Algorithms to Data Mining in Time Series

The way our data mining technique works is related to the theory of natural evolution introduced by the naturalist Charles R. Darwin [3]—an evolutionary algorithm. This superclass of algorithms consists of several more or less

---

[1] For further information on this topic we refer the reader to publications by Fayyad et al. (e.g. [5]) or to the book by Woods and Kyral [22].

sharply separated specializations. These are for instance the class of genetic algorithms [11] or approaches to evolutionary and genetic programming [7,16]—to name only some 'main streams' in this area of work. In more detail, the basic principle of our approach to data mining in time series can be assigned to the last-mentioned two classes [13].

Principle: A population of so-called γ-individuals[2] performs an evolution driven forward by the survival (and selection) of the 'fittest'. The γ-individuals are composed of a set of different metrics and functions (e.g. based on descriptive statistics, differential equations, wavelets (e.g. see [18]), or fuzzy graphs (e.g. see [1], pages 282–292)) which are presently arranged in a special tree-based classifier. Within the current implementation of our data mining-tool these γ-individuals are interpretable hypotheses on possible cause-and-effect relationships contained in the data (the individuals' history derived from simulation and coded in time series). A γ-individual is called 'fit', if it separates—using only the given data on the individuals' history—the study population corresponding to additional information on the state of health of the individuals. The fitness is computed by a so-called quality function which defines the goal of the evolution (optimization). To allow γ-individuals to increase their fitness, the two genetic operators *crossover* (recombination) and *mutation* (alteration) are used to create and modify γ-individuals.

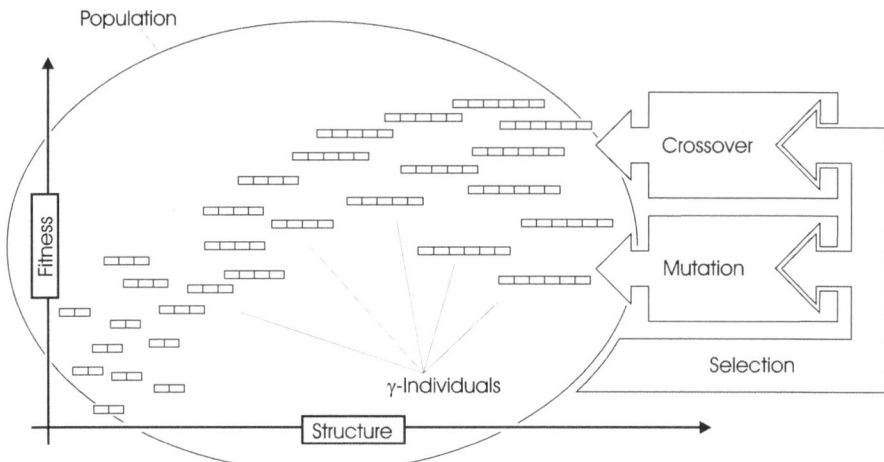

Fig. 2. Scheme of an evolutionary algorithm

---

[2] To distinguish the individuals of the study population from those within the evolutionary algorithm, we name the entities within the evolutionary algorithm γ-individuals.

The fitness of γ-individuals grows with the evolution of generations within the evolutionary algorithm (i.e. the quality of the hypotheses about cause-and-effect relationship grows in the same way).

Figure 2 shows the general structure of an evolutionary algorithm: This figure shows a population of γ-individuals (in this special case) all containing a unique tree-based classifier. In general γ-individuals contain different structures. Furthermore, these γ-individuals all have different fitness values which influence their chance to be selected as the basis for the next generation of γ-individuals generated by the application of operations crossover or mutation.

Goals: For the application to data mining in sets of time series our evolutionary algorithm 'works on' the following tasks to increase the γ-individuals' fitness:

- select the most significant time series from the processed database (e.g. name the most important agents which could be responsible for the occurrence of the examined diseases and illnesses),
- find the most important characteristics within the time series (e.g. describe significant courses of individual exposition to the selected agents which could be responsible for the occurrence of the examined diseases and illnesses),
- explore the most important coherences within the processed database (e.g. describe significant coherences in courses of individual exposition to different agents which could be responsible for the occurrence of the examined diseases and illnesses),
- indicate if the last-mentioned most important characteristics and coherences 'act' protective or not (e.g. indicate the case that a special individual behavior acts possibly protective against the outbreak of the examined diseases and illnesses), and
- present the γ-individuals (i.e. the hypotheses about cause-and-effect relationships) in a comprehensible resp. interpretable way (e.g. reduce their size by simplification of the tree-based classifiers).

2.3   Individual-Oriented Modeling and Simulation

Modeling and simulation techniques which are relevant within the context of this work must be suitable for a detailed description of the behavior of individuals within a heterogeneous and variable environment over time. Furthermore, the approach of combining modeling and simulation and KDD requires to extend or simplify a current version of the model and the ability to easily merge different kind of data and systems knowledge into simulation.

Individual-oriented modeling and simulation offers an approach fulfilling these requirements. These detailed models are created by paying attention to single components of the real system. The components within individual-oriented models are labeled with attributes and rules which specify their current state (e.g. their current position or state of health) and dynamical behavior during the simulation. Usually, the selection and evaluation of the active rules depends on the state of the modeled components. The components can modify their own state or affect other components by processing selected rules. Within individual-oriented models there is no global instance deciding how the modeled components interact while a simulation runs. The behavior of the entire system is a conjunction of the interacting single components (e.g. individuals, environmental polluters etc.). Existing (complex) cause-and-effect relationships on a global level of these models are hidden within the (static) specification of the interaction of their components. So individual-oriented models and simulations can show a kind of unexpected or previously unknown global (dynamic) behavior—'emergence'— which can often be found in the modeled system as well. [3]

The application of individual-oriented techniques for exploratory systems analysis offers some important advantages:

- individual-oriented modeling is a very intuitive approach to the modeling of environmental systems,
- the user does not neccessarily need prior knowledge of global cause-and-effect relationships within the system,
- the complexity of individual-oriented models (e.g. the number of considered components) can be gradually extended or reduced, and
- the (local) dynamics of each modeled component can be investigated with respect to the (local) behavior of all other modeled components within simulation runs.

The analysis of the output of individual-oriented simulations (basically time series containing the individuals' state over time) to find new/unexpected cause-and-effect relationships on a global level is an exciting but difficult task.

3   Combining KDD and Individual-Oriented Techniques

We use individual-oriented modeling and simulation techniques to merge data from different databases and knowledge from the area of application into one homogeneous destination database (transformed data—cf. Fig. 1). This approach offers the benefit of integrating data of different qualities into one model of the real system. Problems arising from differently scaled data can be solved locally within each single component. During the simulation, the output time series (e.g. emission rates of polluters or the individual exposure) can be synchronized to make the analysis of the destination database easier and to avoid missing values.

As an example, consider an individual-oriented model using data from a survey to define rules for each individual which determine its (changing) position within the environment. Such basic behavior can be extended by adding rules to determine the physical activity, which influences the amount of possibly polluted air inhaled by each considered individual. To integrate environmental

---

[3] For further information on individual-oriented modeling and simulation we refer to the book edited by DeAngelis and Gross [4] or publications by Hogeweg and Hesper (e.g. [10]).

data describing the pollution of air, we use a geographic information system (GIS) and data from long term observations of possible polluters, enabling us to approximate the amount of environmental pollution at the current position of each individual.

Figure 3 shows an interactive and multistage process of (individual-oriented) modeling and simulation (derived from a book by Paul A. Fishwick [6]) integrated with the process of KDD. Fig. 3 describes the idea of using individual-oriented modeling and simulation as a powerful tool within the first three phases of KDD. In summary, *Modeling* 'replaces' the phases *Selection* and *Pre-processing*, and *Simulation* 'replaces' the phase of *Transformation* in KDD. The time series derived from simulations can be analyzed by applying the data mining technique mentioned in Sect. 2.2.

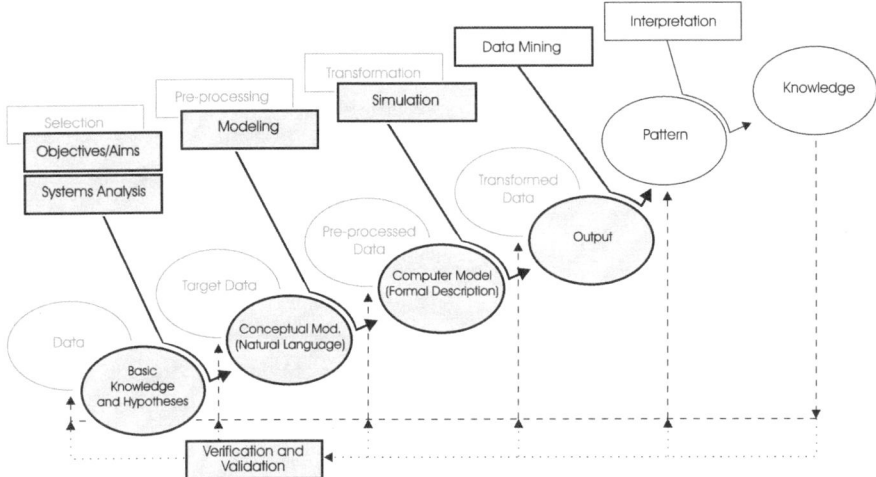

Fig. 3. Combining KDD and individual-oriented modeling and simulation (cf. [13])

Figure 3 also illustrates the well-known fact that we need to examine the question of validity of models and results, whenever we want to use modeling and simulation techniques to solve or understand real-world problems. Fortunately, individual-oriented techniques in conjunction with KDD (in particular data mining) offer a strong approach to qualitative validation [13,15].

4   Tools

In the past we carried out some small and technical case-studies to apply and test the approach mentioned above [13,15]. Since the beginning of this year we are working on a larger 'real' case-study in the context of the *International Study of Asthma and Allergies in Childhood* (ISAAC) [20]. During this case-study we want to prove the ability of our concept and to extend the existing software tools with respect to the special needs of environmental epidemiological research.

The current set of software tools includes different computer programs which are designed to support the entire integrated process of KDD combined with individual-oriented modeling and simulation (cf. Fig. 3). Each of these tools is intended to support different aspects within this process. In the following, we distinguish the aspects *Modeling, Simulation Execution, Simulation Control, Data Mining,* and *Interpretation* resp. *Evaluation* of gained results.

4.1   Modeling

We developed a high-level modeling language called i·EpiSim²-ML (= i·Epi-Sim²-Modeling-Language) to describe individual-oriented models and experiments on these models[4]. Consequently, this modeling language is subdivided into two parts: a model description language called i·EpiSim²-MDL (= i·Epi-Sim²-Modeling-Description-Language) and an experiment description language called i·EpiSim²-EDL (= i·EpiSim²-Experiment-Description-Language).

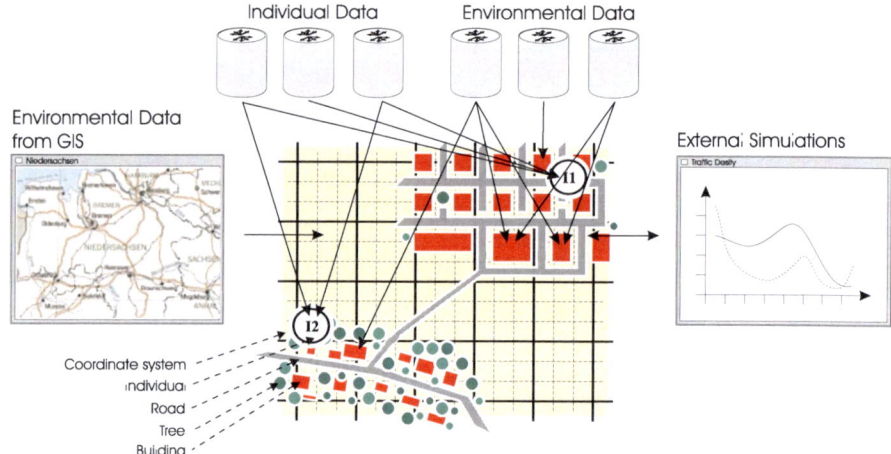

Fig. 4. An individual-oriented model described with i·EpiSim²-ML (scheme)

i·EpiSim²-MDL is used to describe the general environmental structure and abstract components of an individual-oriented model (e.g. types of individuals and their attributes). Regarding this description i·EpiSim²-EDL must be used to specify concrete instances of the environmental structures and components within a simulation (e.g. to define initial values for attributes of concrete simulated individuals).

i·EpiSim²-ML supports the integration of different types of prior systems knowledge, different databases (of observed values), GIS, and other external

---

[4] i·EpiSim² is the name of the software tool described in Sect. 4.3. This name should express the use of individual-oriented techniques (i), different databases, and simulations (²) as a set of (simulation) tools for environmental epidemiology (EpiSim).

models (e.g. for pollution diffusion). Figure 4 shows a scheme of a small model described with i·EpiSim²-ML, different databases, and one external model.

The modeling language is available for Windows-9⋆/Nt-4.0/2000 computer systems and is intended to be used in the phases 1–3 of the integrated process.

4.2 Simulation Execution

To process i·EpiSim²-ML we developed a simulation engine. This simulation engine provides different interfaces to databases by using Open Database Connectivity (Odbc) [19], a special Gis accessed via the internet [8], and external simulations presently by using the High Level Architecture (Hla) [2].

Furthermore, the simulation engine enables other software tools (see Sect. 4.3 for an example) to gain information on the current state of a simulation and to exchange information to control a running simulation by a special data exchange protocol. This protocol can be handled via a socket connection. Thus, it is possible to receive data from a running simulation via the internet and to operate the simulation progress by remote control.

The kernel of this simulation engine is based on an extended version of the class-library EcoSim [17] which is adapted to our needs (especially by the different interfaces mentioned above).

The simulation engine is available for Windows-9⋆/Nt-4.0/2000 computer systems and is intended to be used in phases 1–3 of the integrated process.

4.3 Simulation Control

i·EpiSim² is an interactive software tool to control (individual-oriented) simulations and to provide simple online analysis of simulation data (e.g. aggregation of time series). i·EpiSim² can be used to derive data from simulations and operate the simulation progress via a socket connection (cf. Sect. 4.2). Figure 5 shows a screenshot of a part of the tool's graphical user interface.

Before i·EpiSim² can access a simulation the simulation engine is asked to initialize i·EpiSim² properly: During this step the general structure of the processed model and every single component of the simulation (e.g. the individuals of a study population) must be registered to enable i·EpiSim² to access all relevant information. The already mentioned data exchange protocol (cf. Sect. 4.2) is designed to support this special function.

i·EpiSim² is developed for Windows-9⋆/Nt-4.0/2000 computer systems and is intended to be used in phases 1–3 of the integrated process.

4.4 Data Mining

We developed a non-interactive software tool for data mining in sets of time series called Ea-Mole, and some utilities for the transformation of databases processed with Ea-Mole. The tool is based on an evolutionary algorithm (cf.

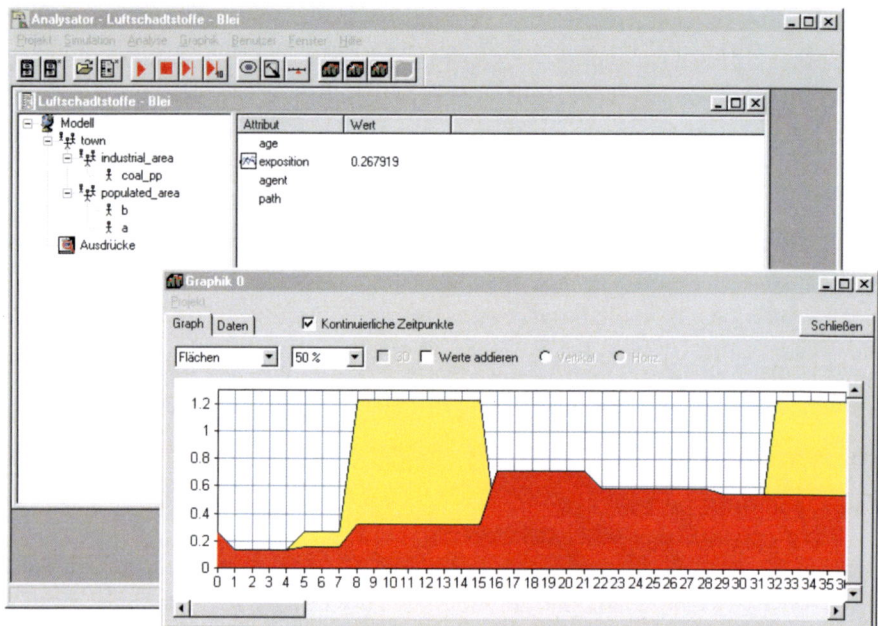

Fig. 5. A tool to control simulations and online analysis of simulation data

Sect. 2.2) and runs on different single- and multiprocessor computer systems
(UNIX, LINUX, and UNICOS/mk). The efficient parallel implementation reduces
the run-time of the evolutionary algorithm (cf. [9]) and enables us to process
very large databases.

To mention a few features of the current implementation of EA-MOLE:

→ The software design of EA-MOLE and the utilities allows the easy integration
  of available domain knowledge.
→ The application of integrated domain knowledge and the analysis process
  itself can be adjusted by different parameters which are organized in a parameter file.
→ EA-MOLE enables the user to access selected status information via the
  internet by sending defined messages to the running program.
→ The tool generates electronic mails to inform a user about the current state
  of the data mining system, the current anaysis progress, and current 'worst'
  and 'best' results.
→ It is possible to continue a previously interrupted data mining process.

EA-MOLE has been implemented on different computer systems mentioned
above and is intended to be used in phase 4 of the integrated process.

4.5   Interpretation resp. Evaluation

To process the γ-individuals produced by EA-MOLE and to support their interpretation and evaluation an interactive software tool has been developed. Figure

6 shows a screenshot of a part of the graphical user interface of this tool named EA-MOLE-VIS.

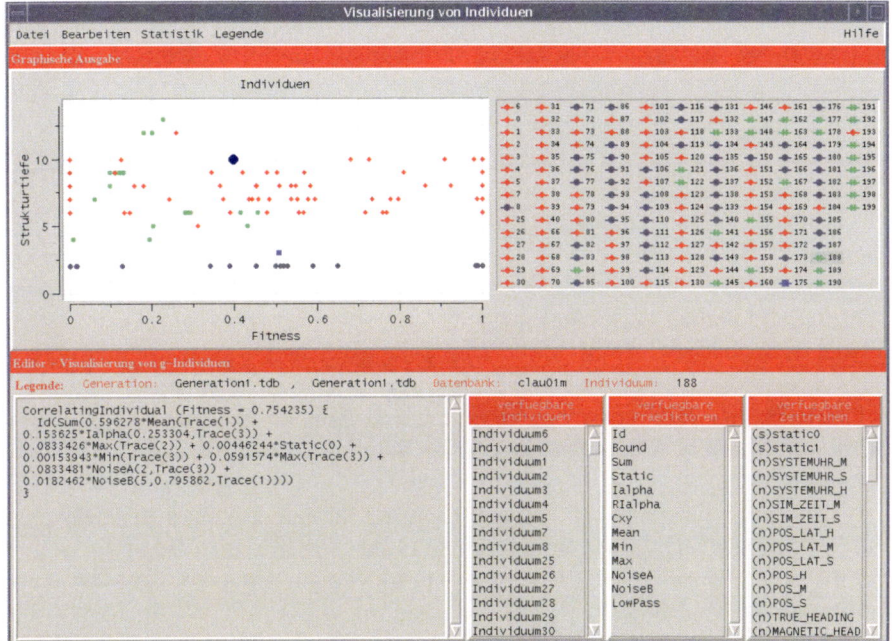

Fig. 6. An interactive tool for interpration resp. evaluation of γ-individuals

Within EA-MOLE-VIS it is possible to filter, simplify, and edit the γ-individuals manually. Thus, this tool enables users with detailed domain knowledge to manually create their hypotheses about cause-and-effect relationships. These hypotheses can be compared with those automatically generated during the data mining process. Furthermore, the manually created hypotheses can be optimized within EA-MOLE (cf. Sect. 4.4).

EA-MOLE-VIS runs on UNIX and LINUX computer systems and is intended to be used in the 'final' phase of the integrated process.

5   Application of the Integrated Process

Our approach uses individual-oriented modeling methods to create a structurally equivalent model of the investigated environmental system as well as the population of individuals (cf. Sect. 2.3, 4.1, 4.2, and 4.3). The advantages of individual-oriented modeling (cf. Sect. 2.3) enables a user to 'play' with the (modeled) system within a computer simulation. The variation of the model's structure resp. of its components can be the key to gain deeper insights into system's dynamics on a detailed or global level.

For instance, during a simulation the exposure of each single individual to selected agents can be estimated over time—usually a difficult task within environmental epidemiological studies ('Personal Sampling'—cf. [21], pages 102–103). In an individual-oriented simulation it is easily possible to estimate the individual exposure depending on its dynamic bahavior (e.g. favorite individual transportations or whereabouts) and on the dynamics of the environment (e.g. variation in local pollution over time). Changing the behavior of single components (e.g. the emission rates of a industrial plant) may lead to a different exposure for the entire population of simulated individuals and, therefore, to different health conditions of the simulated study population.

KDD (in particular data mining—cf. Sect. 2.2, 4.4, and 4.5) can be useful to support the analysis of the environmental system. The gained knowledge can be helpful to uncover responsible agents and the course of exposure over time which are possible causes for the outbreak of an observed disease or cases of illness—explaining the state of health of the investigated study population.

As mentioned before, these insights into system's dynamics can be helpful when using individual-oriented modeling and simulation techniques to predict future evolution of a changed system for different (environmental or individual) situations.

The currently developed software tools are intended to support environmental epidemiological studies and planning in the scope of health-care management. Moreover, simulation of individual-oriented models is offered as a powerful technique to develop and assess procedures aiming at the improvement of environmental conditions to reduce or prevent the occurence of diseases and illnesses.

6   Conclusion and Related Work

In our approach we combine KDD with methods for individual-oriented modeling and simulation. The individual-oriented models and the gained 'knowledge' can be used to discover 'new' or previously unknown existing cause-and-effect relationships and support future decision making and planning for health-care management.

The integration of the methods discussed in this paper seems symbiotic: The application of data mining techniques helps to overcome problems concerning the validity of individual-oriented models resp. simulations [13,15], while individual-oriented modelling and simulation supports the creation of homogeneous and complete databases (transformed data) to be analyzed by data mining techniques. The developed software tools are designed to support the entire process of KDD. In particular, we developed a special individual-oriented modeling language and a powerful tool for data mining in time series which is based on evolutionary algorithms.

The tools EA-MOLE and EA-MOLE-VIS (cf. Sect. 4.4 and 4.5) are in principal not restricted to applications in environmental epidemiology. Merely the components the hypotheses consist of have to be changed to use this general approach within a different area of application. For instance, these tools were applied by the first author for the analysis of data from the field of flight simulation.

Currently we are working on a large case-study (ISAAC [20]) to prove the ability of our concept and to extend the existing software tools with regards to the special needs of environmental epidemiological research. Furthermore, we are planning a software tool which supports the formulation of individual-oriented models on the basis of collected data from environmental epidemiological studies.

References

1. Berthold, M. and Hand, D.J. (eds.): Intelligent Data Analysis: An Introduction. Springer-Verlag (1999).
2. Dahmann, J.S., Kuhl, F., and Wetherly R.: Standards for Simulation: As Simple as Possible But Not Simpler – The High Level Architecture for Simulation. Simulation (Special Issue: High-Level-Architecture) 71:6, 7 378–387 (1998).
3. Darwin, C.R.: The Origin of Species: By Means of Natural Selection or The Preservation of Favoured Races in the Struggle for Life. Oxford Univ. Press – London, a repr. of the 6th ed. (1968).
4. DeAngelis, D.L. and Gross, L.J. (eds.): Individual-based Models and Approaches in Ecology. Chapman Hall (1992).
5. Fayyad, U., Piatetsky-Shapiro, G., and Smyth, P.: From data mining to knowledge discovery in databases. AI Magazine, 17:37–54 (1996).
6. Fishwick, P.A.: Simulation Model Design and Execution – Building Digital Worlds. Prentice-Hall (1995).
7. Fogel, D.B.: Evolutionary Computation: Towards a New Philosophy of Machine Intelligence. IEEE Press, Piscataway, NY (1995).
8. Friebe, J.: Softwarekomponenten für GIS im Internet. In: Hypermedia im Umweltschutz und Betriebliche Umweltinformationssysteme. Metropolis-Verlag (1999).
9. Hoffmeister, F.: Scalable Parallelism by Evolutionary Algorithms. In Grauer, M. and Pressmar, D.B. (eds.), Parallel Computing and Mathematical Opimization, Springer-Verlag, pages 177–198 (1991).
10. Hogeweg, P. and Hesper B.: Individual-Oriented Modeling in Ecology. Mathl. Comput. Modeling, Vol. 13/6, pages 83–90 (1990).
11. Holland, J.H.: Adaption in Natural and Artificial Systems. Univerity of Michigan Press, Ann Arbor (1975).
12. Holsheimer, M. and Siebes, A.P.J.M.: Data Mining: The Search for Knowledge in Databases. Centrum voor Wiskunde en Informatica (CWI), P.O. BOX 94079, 1090 GB Amsterdam, The Netherlands, Report CS-R9406 (1994).
13. Köster, F.: Techniken des Knowledge Discovery in Databases zur Analyse von Simulationen am Beispiel individuenorientierter Simulationsmodelle der Umweltepidemiologie. Bericht zum Workschop der Fachgruppe 4.5 – Modellbildung und Simulation in Umweltanwendungen. 12.-14. März 2000 in Hamburg – im Druck.
14. Köster, F. and Sonnenschein, M.: Individual-Oriented Modeling and Simulation – An Approach to Support Epidemiological Research. In: Anderson, J.G., Katzper, M. (eds.): 1998 Medical Science Simulation Conference. SCS, pages 73–78 (1998).

15. Köster, F. and Sonnenschein, M.: An Approach to the Creation and Validation of Hypotheses about Cause-and-Effect Relationships in Individual-Oriented Models by Knowledge Discovery in Databases. In: Anderson, J.G., Katzper, M. (eds.): 1999 Medical Science Simulation Conference. Scs, pages 139–144 (1999).
16. Koza, J.R.: Genetic Programming: On the Programming of Computers by Means of Natural Selection, Complex Adaptive Systems. Mit Press, Cambridge, Ma (1992).
17. Lorek, H. and Sonnenschein, M.: Object-oriented support for modelling and simulation of individual-oriented ecological models. Ecological Modelling 108, pages 77–96 (1998).
18. Louis, A.K., Maaß, P., and Rieder, A.: Wavelets – Theorie und Anwendungen. Teubner Verlag (1998).
19. Sanders, R.E.: Odbc 3.5 Developer's Guide, McGraw-Hill Series on Data Warehousing and Data Management (1998).
20. Weiland, S.K., von Mutius, E., and Keil, U. (for the Isaac Steering Committee): Die International Study of Asthma and Allergies in Childhood (Isaac): Forschungsstrategie, Methoden und Ausblick. In Allergologie 22:275-82 (1999).
21. World Health Organization (Who): Guidelines on Studies in Environmental Epidemiology. International Program on Chemical Safety, Who – Geneva (1983).
22. Woods, E. and Kyral, E.: Ovum Evaluates: Data Mining. Ovum Evaluates, Ovum Ltd. (1997).

Incosistency Tests for Patient Records
in a Coronary Heart Disease Database

Dragan Gamberger[1], Nada Lavrač[2], Goran Krstačić[3], Tomislav Šmuc[1]

[1] Rudjer Bošković Institute, Bijenička 54, 10000 Zagreb, Croatia
[2] Jožef Stefan Institute, Jamova 39, 1000 Ljubljana, Slovenia
[3] Institute for Prevention of Cardiovascular Disease and Rehabilitation, Draškovićeva 13, 10000 Zagreb, Croatia

Abstract. The work presents the results of inconsistency detection experiments on the data records of an atherosclerotic coronary heart disease database collected in the regular medical practice. Medical expert evaluation of some preliminary inductive learning results have demonstrated that explicit detection of outliers can be useful for maintaining the data qualit y of medical records and that it migh be a key for the improvement of medical decisions and their reliability in the regular medical practice. With the intention of on-line detection of possible data inconsistences, sets of confirmation rules have been developed for the database and their test results are reported in this work.

1 Introduction

The motivation for the research presented in this work stems from the fact that modern medical decision processes are generally based on patient data from many different sources which are typically collected and archiv ed by a multiterminal or distributed computer systems. Such organization enables prompt and high quality decisions by medical doctors, supported by abundance of available data [3,4], but it also enables that errors of different sources, caused by the w ork of many different people and/or instrumentation can directly enter patient records. Detcction of data inconsistencies at the global level of every patient record can help in tracing systematic as well as spurious errors in the data acquisition process and in this way it can be an important part for insuring high quality and reliability of data used for medical decision making. On the other side, the existence of data inconsistencies do not need to be the sign of data errors but may bethe consequence of some un typical medical case. Attracting attention of medical doctors to such patient records may be interesting both from the point of view of medical science as well as for av oiding routine medical errors.

Our interest for inconsistency testing is the result of many inductive learning experiments performed on a database of atherosclerotic coronary heart disease (ACHD) patients [7] prepared at the Institute for Preven tion of Cardiovascular Disease and Rehabilitation, Zagreb Croatia. In the data preparation phase, the saturation filter [6] was used to detect and eliminate outliers from the database.

R.W. Brause and E. Hanisch (Eds.): ISMDA 2000, LNCS 1933, pp. 183–189, 2000.

This is a necessary step in the knowledge discovery process which enables the induction of globally relevan t rules. But medical expert evaluation has demonstrated that the detection of outliers is a very interesting result by itself, which suggested the idea of using noise detection algorithms developed for data preprocessing in inductive machine learning as a tool for data cleaning of patient records. In this w ork t w o differen approaches to the problem of inconsistency testing are presented in Section 2. This is follo w ed b y the presentation of the medical domain used in experiments and the results of the experiments in Sections 3 and 4, respectively. The algorithms used for outlier detection and rule construction are out of the scope of this work since their description can be found in [5, 6].

2   Inconsistency tests

Machine learning approach to inconsistency testing in patient records can be either based on outlier (noise) detection algorithms or on a set of rules that are supposed to be true for the data in patient records. The later approach can be used also for on-line inconsistency testing but it requires the construction of rules with specific propertie in both   cases, testing is based on supervised machine learning algorithms which require that patient records are grouped in tw o or more classes. The classes can be defined either by domain experts or by values of one or more descriptors av ailable in the patient record. Correlation betw een defined classes and data contained in patient records is the main mechanism used in inconsistency detection. Requirement of an appropriate class assignment for all patient records is one of the main restrictions of machine learning approaches to inconsistency testing and it is specially analyzed in Section 4.

Explicit outlier detection The first approach, in the work called *explicit outlier detection* can be without changes used on very different patient records. It is actually a noise detection algorithm for data of tw o classes, described in detail in [6], used in the data preprocessing phase (data cleaning) of inductive learning algorithms. It w orks on the set of records, trying to iden tify significant differences among positively and negatively classified records. Those records which are difficult for correct classification are detected as outliers. The approach is appropriate for off-line data analysis. Its main drawback is its time complexity as well as the fact that for multiclass problems the algorithm must be repeated for every reasonable definition of class positive and class negative records.

Rule-based outlier detection The second approach, called *rule-b ased outlier dete ction* is more appropriate for on-line inconsistency testing. It works with data of one patient record only and the consequence is its simplicity and high execution speed. The approach is actually a set of logical tests that must be satisfied b y every patient record. If one or more of the tests is not satisfied, the record is detected as an outlier. The logical tests are defined b y the set of rules that hold for the patient records in the domain. The main dra wback of the approach is that the set of rules must be developed specially for the tested type of records. Moreover, the used rules must be highly reliable rules with a very small number of mispredictions, leading to false outlier alarms. Such rules can be constructed by domain experts but also by inductive learning algorithms. Because of the required rule reliability, the concept of *confirmation rules* seems appropriate for this task [5]. In this concept, separate rules are constructed for the positive and negative class cases. The confirmation rules for the positive class must be true for many positive cases and for no negative case. If a negative case is detected true for any confirmation rule developed for the positive class, it is a reliable sign that the case is an outlier. In the same way, confirmation rules constructed for the negative class can be used for outlier detection of positive patient records. An additional advantage of the approach is that the user can have the information about the rule which caused the alarm what can be useful in the error detection process. An systematic approach to outlier detection based on different classification algorithms, together with many experimental results demonstrating its usefulness, is presented in [2].

3   Data Set

For this work, a database representing typical medical practice in atherosclerotic coronary heart disease ACHD diagnosis has been prepared. The data describe patients who entered the Institute for Prevention Cardiovascular Disease and Rehabilitation, Zagreb Croatia, in few months period. The set of descriptors represents all potentially interesting and typically available information about patients. The descriptor set includes anamnestic data (10 items), laboratory test results (6), the resting ECG data (5), the exercise test data (5), echocardiogram results (2), vectorcardiogram results (2), and long term continuous ECG recording data (3). It makes altogether 33 descriptors. The complete list of used descriptors can be found in [7], but the used data are not the same in both experiments. The main differences are that in this work ST segment depression descriptors in exercise and long term ECG recording data have real measured continuous values (in contrast to classes negative, positive 1mm, and positive $\geq 2mm$ used in previous experiments), that hypertension descriptor has continuous values, and that some detected errors in the dataset have been accepted by the domain expert and corrected for this work.

The classification in five groups (I-V) for all patients was performed by the cardiologists and it reflects generally accepted medical knowledge. The classification is mostly based on the results of the most important tests. These are: exercise testing, long term ECG recording and echocardiography. In exercise testing ST segment depression or elevation, serious cardiac arrhythmias, and conducting disturbances are the important parameters. Additionally, the NYHA classification and clinically significant metabolic equivalents (METs) are used [1]. Group I are healthy patients without verified ACHD while groups II - V are ill patients with different levels of previous myocardial infarction. Details of the group definitions can be also found in [7].

4   Experimental results and medical evaluation

The domain of 238 patient records practically consists of two sets: the dataset
of 150 patients collected earlier, has been used for preliminary experiments and
rule development, while the set of remaining 88 records collected later, has been
used for test purposes only. The first set will be in the rest of the paper called
the main set and the second one the control set.

Explicit outlier detection results The set of experiments started with
explicit outlier detection for the main set and for the positive and negative classes
as defined in Section 3 by medical doctors. There have been only two detected
outliers (patient records number 28 and 52) and both of them are very interesting
cases. The first one is actually an older patient after a serious cardiosurgical
treatment who was in spite of non-optimal laboratory tests intentionally put into
Group II (patients with normal results of exercise testing, long term recording
and echocardiogram). The second patient was also in Group II but after its
detection as an outlier, medical doctor agreed that Group III would be much
more appropriate for the patient. In the analysis it was detected that the main
reason for its inclusion Group II were good exercise testing results. But
results were misleading because patient t was so weak that he could sustain
only 2 minutes (instead of 7 - 9 minutes) of exercise. It means that an actually
important outlier have been detected, that its detection helped in finding more
appropriate diagnostic group for the patient, and that the medical doctor has
found out that exercise testing results are reliable data only if the tests could be
and have been performed completely and correctly.

T arget set	Detected outliers	
	In main set	In control set
main	28 52	- - -
control	- - -	174 214 227 230
main + control	1 28 43 52 98	174 214 227 230

T able 1. Results of explicit outlier detection for different sets of target patient records.

The same explicit approach to outlier detection was also applied on the control set which resulted in the detection of patient records 174, 214, 227, and
230. The experiment was later repeated for the whole dataset. The result of this
experiment was the detection of the same four detected records from the control
set and in total five records from the main set. Besides examples 28 and 52,
that were detected also in the first experiment, the set of detected records from
the main set included also cases number 1, 43, and 98. Table 1 summarizes the
results of the first three experiments with explicit outlier detection. The results
show weakness of the explicit approach to noise detection demonstrated by the
fact that different outliers have been detected for the main set depending on the
target set.

Medical evaluation showed that cases 1 and 43, patients from Group III, are
not expert recognized outliers. These cases can be accepted as false alarms of the

explicit outlier detection approach. Completely different situation is the patient number 98 from Group III, classified as a serious case but with practically normal results of laboratory tests. Medical doctor accepted the patient as a special case and was satisfied that machine learning methods recognized it as an outlier. Two out of four cases detected in the control set are border line cases (cases number 174 and 227) and the remaining tw o are real medical outliers: one is a difficult coronary patient from Group V with diagnosed cardiopathia dilatativa therefore, not an ACHD patient (number 214), while the other one is an atypical ACHD patient whose disease could be detected only by echocardiography (number 230).

Rule-based outlier detection results With the inten tion to show the application of a rule-based outlier detection approach, the main set was used to induce confirmation rules, explained in Section 2.2, for both classes. The rules for the positive class were $ExECGst > 0.45mm$ and $HOLst > 0.65mm$. Each of these tw orules holds for about 95% of the positiv eclass cases in the main set and none (except explicitly detected outliers) negative class cases in this set. The rules detected the following negative class outliers in the control set: 165, 174, 185, and 227. There was only one confirmation rule for the negative class consisting of tw oconditions $ExECGst \leq 0.45mm \wedge HOLst \leq 0.65mm$. The rule holds for about 98% of negative class cases and for all positive class cases in the main set. The rule detected as outliers positive patient records 214 and 230 in the control set. The results are presented in the first row of Table 2. Comparing results obtained by explicit and rule-based outlier detection it can be noted that the later approach selected the same records as the former approach but that it also detected tw o more records: 165 and 185. The method is interesting because its application is muc h simpler for all other future patient records. Medical ev aluation of the cases 165 and 185 show ed that they are actually not false alarms. One of them is a border line case (case number 185) while in the other case the medical doctor accepted the suggestion and he has changed the patient group classification (case 165).

Classes defined by	Outlier detection	
	Explicit	Rule-based
medical doctors	174 214 227 230	165 174 185 214 227 230
$ExECGst > 0.45mm$	165 174 185 195 197 199 202 227 232 237	165 174 185 195 197 199 202 227 232 237
$HOLst > 0.65mm$	165 185 195 197 199 202 214 230 232 237	165 185 195 197 232

Table 2. Comparison of the outliers detected by explicit and rule-based detection approaches for differently defined patient record classes.

Results obtained by descriptor-based classifiers In all previous experiments inconsistency testing w asbased on classes defined by medical doctors.

Existence of such classification assumes that there exists a dependency between the determined class and record data what practically ensures the quality of the inconsistency tests. In a general case, when there is no expert classification, one or more descriptors from the patient record should be used as a classification parameter. In this situation it is essential to select classifiers for which it can be assumed that their dependency with other data in the record exists. Table 2 in its second and third row includes results obtained for positive classes defined by conditions $ExECGst > 0.45mm$ and $HOLst > 0.65mm$ respectively. In the left column are records detected as outliers in the control set by explicit approach while in the right tone are detected by the rule-based method. In the explicit approach, the target sets included both the main and the control sets. Rules for the rule-based detection have been constructed always from the main set so that its own outliers have been previously excluded from it. The method resulted in successful detection of the most outliers detected based on expert classification. It can be noticed that among outliers occur also some completely new cases, like numbers 195, 197, 232, and 237. Their medical evaluation demonstrated that in three out of four cases the problem was that the patient exercise testing was incomplete and the obtained results were misleading. In the fourth case (number 195) the patient had an asymptomatic (silent) ischaemic heart disease known by its differences between exercise and long term continuous measurements. It must be noted that detection of these four outliers was medically completely justified. Analysis of medical classifications in all four cases showed that medical expert reasoning also successfully detected the problems and that all cases were in appropriate groups in spite of data inconsistencies.

5   Conclusions

This paper introduces two approaches to outlier (inconsistency) detection in medical datasets: explicit outlier detection and rule-based outlier detection. Explicit outlier detection is applicable offline analysis since it operates on the dataset level and involves data cleaning algorithms usually used in machine learning preprocessing. Rule-based outlier detection relies on rules induced upon previously collected data in the same dataset. It is applicable for on-line detection of inconsistencies in future records. We have applied both approaches on the ACHD patient dataset. Experiments were performed with expert classified records as well as with different descriptor-based classifications. The results indicated the sensitivity of both approaches for inconsistency detection. Although detected outliers differed from one experiment to another, most outliers were confirmed as special cases by subsequent medical expert evaluation. In order to detect possible inconsistencies in less important descriptors, experiments with different descriptor subgroups have been performed. Medical evaluation in some of these experiments recognized outliers with similar characteristics representing interesting domain subconcepts. The results could be important both with respect to everyday medical practice as well as for future medical research.

References

1. ACP/ACC/AHA Task force on Exercise Testing (1990). *Journal of Americ an College Car diolo gy* **16**: 1061-1065.
2. Brodley, C.E. & Friedl, M.A. (1999). Identifying mislabeled training data. *Journal of Artificial Intelligence Research,* **11**:131–167.
3. Diamond, G.A.,& F orester, J.S. (1979). Analysis of probability as an aid in the clinical diagnosis of coronary artery disease. *New England Journal of Medicine* **300**:1350.
4. Dorffner, G., Leitgeb, E., & Koller, H. (1999) A comparison of linear and nonlinear classifiers for the detection of coronary artery disease in stress-ECG. In *Proc. of Joint Europ ean Conference on A rtificial Intelligenc e in Medicine and Medical De cision Making (AIMDM'99)* 227–231. Springer, Berlin.
5. Gamberger, D., Lavrač, N., & Grošelj C. (1999) Diagnostic rules of increased reliablit y for critical medical applications. In *Proc. of Joint Europ ean Conferenc e on Artificial Intelligence in Medicine and Medical De cision Making (AIMDM'99)* pp.361–365.
6. Gamberger, D., Lavra č, N., & Grošelj C. (1999) Experiments with noise filtering in a medical domain. In *Proc. of International Conferenc e of Machine L earning (ICML'99)*, pp. 143–151.
7. Gamberger, D., Krstačić, G., & Šmuc, T. (2000) Medical expert evaluation of machine learning results for a coronary heart disease database. In this proceedings.

A MATLAB-Based Software Tool for Changepoint Detection and Nonlinear Regression in Dose-Response Relationships

Stefan Wagenpfeil[1], Uwe Treiber[2], and Antonie Lehmer[2]

[1] Institut für Medizinische Statistik und Epidemiologie der Technischen Universität München, Klinikum rechts der Isar, Ismaninger Str. 22, D-81675 München, Germany
`stefan.wagenpfeil@imse.med.tu-muenchen.de`
`http://www.imse.med.tu-muenchen.de/persons/wagenpfeil/index.html`
[2] Urologische Klinik und Poliklinik der Technischen Universität München, Klinikum rechts der Isar, Ismaninger Str. 22, D-81675 München, Germany

Abstract. Resulting from a clinical consulting case in urology we developed a software tool for determining nonlinear dose-response relationships. Unlike most existing statistical software packages, we directly compute and display analytical pointwise 95% confidence intervals for the prediction result. Furthermore, user-defined changepoints with 95% confidence interval can be calculated in order to estimate the dosage for a 50% response rate, for instance. This is necessary to compare the effect of different retinoids, tumor cell lines, etc. In this way we supplement the clinical software-equipment in our laboratory and encourage the evaluation of dose-response data. The numerical and computational problems arising with nonlinear regression, 4-parameter logistic as well as log-logit modelling and the respective confidence intervals are addressed in particular. Analysis of real data and an example data set demonstrate the approach. A demo version of the software tool can be downloaded from the first author's homepage.

1 Introduction

In the laboratory department of the Urologische Klinik und Poliklinik der Technischen Universität München, Klinikum rechts der Isar, the connection between doses of certain retinoids and response rates such as "cell kill" and "invasivity" of tumor cells are examined in vitro. The concentration is measured in μM, starting with small values and increasing accordingly. The response rates range from 0 (= 0% response) to 1 (= 100% response). For the target variable "invasivity" 0 equals to no invasivity of the tumor cells and 1 equals to 100% or full invasivity. For "cell kill" the response value 0 equals to no tumor cells left, i.e. 100% cell kill, whereas 1 equals to nothing happened or 100% cell survival, i.e. 0% cell kill. Fig. 1 displays an example file for a particular retinoid and tumor cell line. For low concentrations we have a limit of 100% response. Increasing concentrations

R.W. Brause and E. Hanisch (Eds.): ISMDA 2000, LNCS 1933, pp. 190–197, 2000.
© Springer-Verlag Berlin Heidelberg 2000

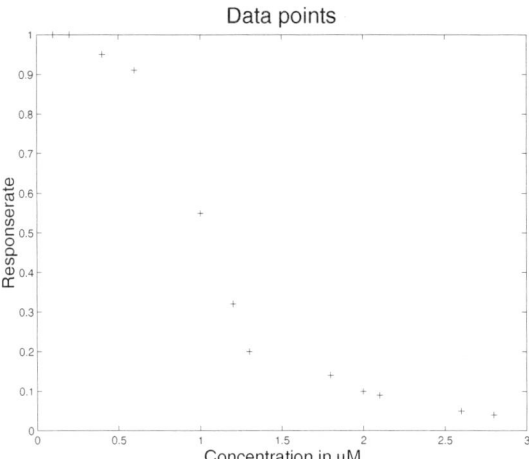

Fig. 1. Dose-response data (+) exemplifying laboratory measurements

yield decreasing response rates with a lower bound of 0% indicating a monotonic, nonlinearly decreasing relationship.

In general, ten or twelve dose-response combinations are determined in one trial. The response rates are obtained either by ELISA-reading for "cell kill" or counted manually within a reference field for "invasivity" of tumor cells. One aim is to estimate the underlying "true" dose-response relationship, which is a classical titration problem discussed in more detail e.g. in [1] and [2]. A common approach for exploring connections of the present kind with continuous doses and scaled binomial outcomes is the log-logit model. The 4-parameter logistic regression model is a generalized version where uncertainty about lower and upper bounds of response rates can be taken into account additionally. Moreover, confidence intervals are essential in order to compare retinoids and tumor cell lines from different trials. However, the software of the ELISA-reader described in [3] as well as most existing software tools for nonlinear regression display confidence intervals in their output only for regression parameter estimates, but not, although implicitly computed, for estimated response curves or predicted values, respectively. Some of the packages like standard SPSS (Statistical Package for Social Sciences) just do it on the grid of observed doses and not on the whole range of measured concentrations. Fig. 2 gives the estimated response curve of the ELISA-reader software for our example data in Fig.1.

Therefore, the task resulting from the laboratory consulting case was to provide a software tool for displaying the estimated response curve and the respective 95% confidence intervals simultaneously. Furthermore, a changepoint concentration should be detected indicating a significant decrease in the response rate. This we call our significant changepoint. The speed of decrease and the deceleration of the response curve at the changepoint are of interest, too. According to half-life periods of radioactive elements, concentrations with $y\%$ response rate

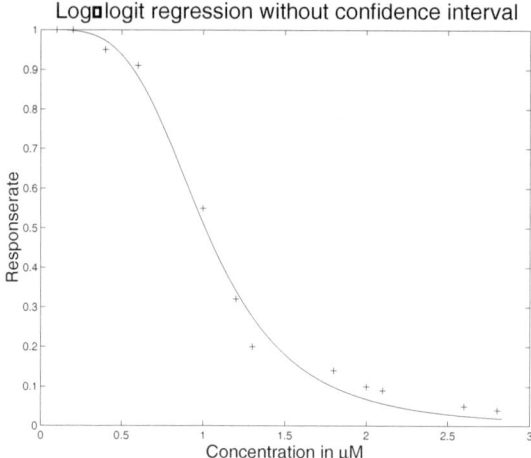

Fig. 2. Dose-response data (+) and estimated response curve (—) from log-logit model

also have to be estimated. We calculated these kind of changepoints for $y = 10$, 30, 50 and 70. The concentration with an estimated 50% response rate is called half-life concentration. Finally, we have to compute the 95% confidence intervals for the significant changepoint and the $y\%$ concentrations as measures of the accuracy of our estimates. Furthermore, the confidence intervals are essential in order to compare different tumor cell lines, retinoids, etc. for a series of trials.

The methods and routines applied are described in the next section. Results of the calculations for our example data file as well as a real data set are given in Sect. 3. Sect. 4 concludes.

2 Methods for Data Analysis

The log-logit model is a common way of analyzing monotonic, nonlinear dose-response relationships as given in Fig.1. It is a special case of the 4-parameter logistic model defined by

$$y = \frac{a - d}{1 + (\frac{x}{c})^b} + d \, , \tag{1}$$

where y is the estimated, predicted response rate at concentration x. As we have a 100% response (e.g. invasivity of tumor cells) for concentration $x = 0$ and no response for sufficiently high values of x in our case, a natural choice for a and d in (1) is $a = 1$ and $d = 0$. This yields the log-logit model underlying the statistical analysis of our example data. Note that we only have to estimates two parameters in this case: b describing how rapidly the curve makes its transition from the asymptotes to the center of the curve and c, the half-life concentration.

If the lower and upper bound of the resopnse rates cannot be fixed in advance as is common in real data problems, the use of the full 4-parameter logistic regression mode (1) is a natural choice.

In both cases estimation can be carried out by the method of least squares which is equivalent to likelihood estimation for the assumption of Gaussian errors, cf. [4], subsection 6.6.1. Because the regression function in (1) is nonlinear, a solution in closed form does not exist and iterative algorithms have to be applied, cf. [5] for details. We used the MATLAB procedure *nlinfit* described in [9], where the Gauss-Newton optimization method is implemented. A general description of nonlinear regression algorithms can be found in [6]. The most important methods are implemented in the optimization toolbox of MATLAB [7].

Special attention has to be drawn to badly-scaled data yielding singular matrices to be inverted within the nonlinear programming procedure. An indication of that problem are extremely high condition numbers as discussed in [8], subsection 4.5. Remedial measures can be taken by strictly monotonic increasing transformations of the concentration values. The log-function is a commonly used transformation in order to try come to a well-scaled problem. On the whole, the success of the nonlinear regression approach depends heavily on the scaling of the data. This is true for all available nonlinear regression tools.

To compute analytical 95% confidence intervals for the estimated response rates there are two ways, in principle. One is to impute the lower and upper confidence limit of the parameter estimates supplied by most of the usual software packages into formula (1). However, this is a heuristic approach and yields unsymmetric confidence intervals, in general. Moreover, a possible correlation between the likelihood estimates of b and c is not considered. Therefore we applied the δ-method described for example in [4], chapter 2, in order to get symmetric, pointwise confidence intervals. The necessary inverse of Fisher's information matrix is calculated from the score function stored in the Jacobian of the MATLAB function *nlinfit*, cf. [9]. A numerical stable implementation can be cribbed from the MATLAB procedures *nlparci* or *nlpredci* contained in the statistical toolbox cf. [9]. The relevant first partial derivatives of the log-logit function in (1) with respect to the regression parameters b and c can easily be obtained by symbolic differentiation in the symbolic math toolbox of MATLAB, cf. [10]. The toolbox is based on a MAPLE V kernel. An analytic formulation of the derivatives is given in the demo version of our software tool, procedures *geschw* and *beschl*. In the same way the first partial derivatives of (1) with respect to a and d can be calculated for the 4-parameter logistic model.

Exact confidence intervals in nonlinear regression as developed in [11] are not in common use. Bootstrap confidence intervals established in [12] would be a further choice if the analytical approach does not converge. However, in the setting of nonlinear regression they are extremely demanding with respect to computation time and power.

For computation of changepoints we have to devide between the $y\%$ concentrations and the significant changepoint. The $y\%$ concentration is easily obtained via the inverse formula of (1) given by

$$x = c\left(\frac{a-y}{y-d}\right)^{1/b} . \tag{2}$$

Again we have $a = 1$ and $d = 0$ for log-logit regression.

The significant changepoint is defined as the concentration value x where the upper limit of the regression curve confidence interval is instantly below a response rate of 1. This is the starting point for a significant reduction of the response rate. The respective confidence intervals for both types of changepoints are calculated by a grid search on the confidence limits of the response curve ensuring at least two valid figures after the decimal point. The speed of reduction of the response rate at the significant changepoint x_{sig} is defined as the first derivative of (1) with respect to x, evaluated at x_{sig}, and the deceleration is the respective second derivative. Again the symbolic formulation of the derivatives can easily be obtained from [10].

The previously discussed features together with the log-logit model (1) are implemented in our software tool "titration".

3   Results

Applying the software tool to the example data from Fig. 1 we get the regression curve estimate with 95% confidence interval within a graphic window as displayed in Fig. 3. Most of the data points lie inside the confidence region. As the 0 μM concentration is forced to have response rate 1 according to $a = 1$ in formula (1), the length of the confidence interval tends to zero in this area.

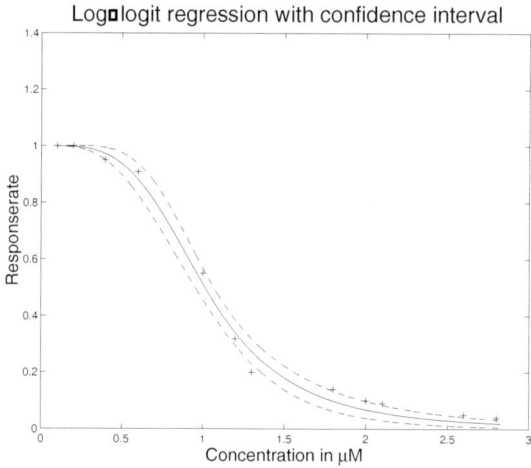

Fig. 3. Dose-response data (+) and estimated response curve (—) with pointwise 95% confidence interval (- -) from log-logit model

The respective regression parameter estimates for the model in (1), $y\%$ concentrations for $y = 10, 30, 70$, and the significant changepoint with its speed and response deceleration are obtained as text output summarized in Table 1. In particular, the confidence intervals are necessary to compare different retinoids, tumor cell lines, etc. for a series of trials.

Table 1. Estimates of regression parameters and changepoints with 95% confidence intervals from log-logit modelling of example data in Fig.1. Sig. refers to significant.

Parameter or changepoint	Estimate	95% confidence interval
Parameter b	3.8454	[3.0821 ... 4.6087]
Parameter c = half-life concentration in μM	1.0124	[0.9554 ... 1.0694]
70% concentration in μM	0.8122	[0.7412 ... 0.8762]
30% concentration in μM	1.2620	[1.1962 ... 1.3353]
10% concentration in μM	1.7928	[1.6242 ... 1.9846]
Significant changepoint in μM	0.1533	[0.1176 ... 0.3322]
Speed of decrease at sig. changepoint in %/μM	-0.0176	
Deceleration at sig. changepoint in %/$(\mu$M$)^2$	-0.3266	

Due to uncertainties in laboratory measurements, upper and lower bounds of response rates cannot be fixed in advance when evaluating real data sets. Therefore we apply the full 4-parameter logistic model in the following.

The real data set indicates the rate of cell kill for ten different concentrations of the retinoid 4-HPR for prostate tumor cell line DU145. Fig. 4 displays the estimated regression curve with 95% confidence interval on a semilog(x) scale. The measurement uncertainty is reflected by the width of the confidence interval at initial concentrations as well as the three upmost concentrations. Changepoints as indicated in the figure and regression parameter estimates of the 4-parameter logistic model are summarized in Table 2. The resulting point estimates in combination with their estimated 95% confidence intervals can be used for reasons of comparison with our example date, other prostate tumor cell lines like LnCaP, PC3, or different kinds of retinoids like 13cRA. For example, the half-life concentration of 4-HPR in Table 2 is significantly lower than the half-life concentration in our example data as the point estimate of c in Table 2 is below the lower bound of the 95% confidence interval of c in Table 1.

Further comparisons have to be left to a more extensive evaluation. At this stage, we want to demonstrate the usefulness and the necessity of comparisons of this kind for our application. Furthermore, we now have a basis for an automatic evaluation with our software tool "titration".

4   Conclusion

Initiated by a consulting case in urology, we developed a software tool for displaying estimated dose-response rates and their 95% confidence intervals simultaneously. Furthermore, a series of user-defined changepoints can be calculated together with respective confidence intervals. In this way, the effect of different

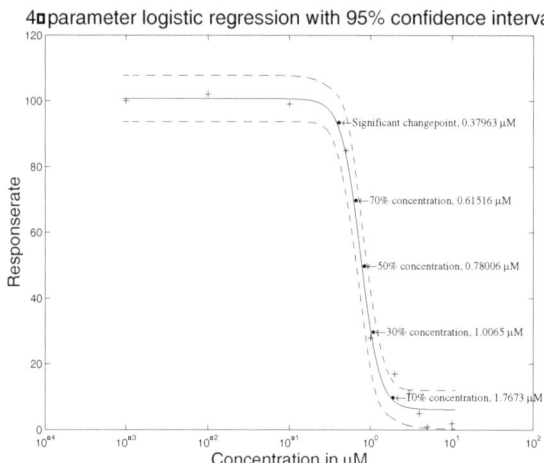

Fig. 4. Dose-response data (+) and estimated response curve (—) with pointwise 95% confidence interval (- -) from 4-parameter logistic model. Data: Response rate = cell survival = 1 - cell kill of DU145 tumor cells, concentration refers to 4-HPR on a semilog scale.

Table 2. Estimates of regression parameters and changepoints with 95% confidence intervals from 4-parameter logistic modelling of real data in Fig.4. Inf refers to infinity and sig. to significant.

Parameter or changepoint	Estimate	95% confidence interval
Parameter a	100.6533	[93.6089 . . . 107.6976]
Parameter b	3.6986	[2.0429 . . . 5.3543]
Parameter c = half-life concentration in μM	0.7500	[0.6265 . . . 0.8735]
Parameter d	6.1924	[0.3387 . . . 12.0461]
70% concentration in μM	0.6152	[0.5105 . . . 0.7211]
30% concentration in μM	1.0065	[0.8511 . . . 1.2078]
10% concentration in μM	1.7673	[1.2078 . . . Inf]
Significant changepoint in μM	0.3796	[0.0010 . . . 0.5224]
Speed of decrease at sig. changepoint in %/μM	-63.513	
Deceleration at sig. changepoint in %/$(\mu$M$)^2$	-359.1965	

tumor cell lines and retinoids can be compared for a number of trials. Special attention has to be drawn to numerical issues as badly-scaled problems may occure. The success of the underlying nonlinear regression procedure depends heavily on the well-scaling of the data.

A demo version of the software tool "titration" can be downloaded as ZIP-file from the first author's homepage at `http://www.imse.med.tu-muenchen.de/persons/wagenpfeil/index.html`. Please consider the readme_first.txt file. In order to run the program, MATLAB 5.0 Release 10 or lower, has to be installed.

References

1. Ortiz-Fernandez, M.C., Herrero-Gutierres, A.: Regression by least median squares, a methodological contribution to titration analysis. Chemometrics and Intelligent Laboratory Systems **27** (1995) 231–243
2. Chuang-Stein, C., Agresti, A.: Tutorial in Biostatistics: A Review of Tests for Detecting a Monotone Dose-Response Relationship with Ordinal Response Data. Statistics in Medicine **16** (1997) 2599–2618
3. Softmax Pro 3.0 User's Guide. Molecular Devices GmbH, Munich, 85737 Ismaning (1999)
4. Mardia, K.V., Kent, J.T., Bibby, J.M.: Multivariate Analysis. 8th printing, Academic Press, London, San Diego (1992)
5. Fahrmeir, L., Tutz, G.: Multivatiate Statistical Modelling Based on Generalizel Linear Models. 2nd edn. Springer-Verlag, Berlin Heidelberg New York (1996)
6. Dennis, J.E., Schnabel, R.B.: Numerical Methods for Unconstrained Optimization and Nonlinear Equations. Prentice Hall, Englewood Cliffs, New York (1983)
7. Coleman, Th., Branch, M.A., Grace, A.: Optimization Toolbox for Use with MATLAB, User's Guide, Version 2. 3rd printing, The Math Works Inc., Natick, MA 01760-1500, USA (1999)
8. Stoer, J., Bulirsch, R.: Introduction to Numerical Analysis. Texts in Applied Mathematics Vol. 12. Springer-Verlag, Berlin Heidelberg New York (1996)
9. Jones, B.: Statistics Toolbox User's Guide. 3rd printing, The Math Works Inc., Natick, MA 01760-1500, USA (1997)
10. Moler, C., Costa, P.J.: MATLAB Symbolic Math Toolbox, User's Guide, Version 2.0. 3rd printing, The Math Works Inc., Natick, MA 01760-1500, USA (1997)
11. Hartley, H.O.: Exact confidence regions for the parameters in non-linear regression laws. Biometrika **51** (1964) 347–353
12. Efron, B.: Bootstrap Methods: Another Look at the Jackknife. Annals of Statistics **7** (1979) 1–26

A Web–Based Electronic Patient Record System as a Means for Collection of Clinical Data

Lutz Fritsche[1], Kay Schröter[2], Gabriela Lindemann[2], Regina Kunz[1], Klemens Budde[1], and Hans–H. Neumayer[1]

[1] University Hospital Charité, Department of Nephrology
Charité Campus Mitte, Schumannstr. 20/21, D-10117 Berlin, Germany
email: Lutz.Fritsche@charite.de
[2] Humboldt University Berlin, Department of Computer Science,
Artificial Intelligence Laboratory, Unter den Linden 6, D-10099 Berlin, Germany
email: kschroet/lindeman@informatik.hu-berlin.de

Abstract. Availability of valid data is a prerequisite for medical data analysis. Traditional data collection (prospective studies, registries, use of administrative data) tends to be either expensive or inaccurate. By transferring the workflow of routine patient care to an electronic patient record(EPR), large amounts of detailed information are stored in a retrievable format, but the maintainance of EPRs in mainframe- or client/server–architecture is expensive. We therefore investigated the feasibility of an EPR based entirely on Web–Technology. The system is now operational since two years and has replaced the former paper–based patient records of the outpatient clinic completely (now 789 patients). With an average duration of access to all values of a specific laboratory day for a given patient taking 0.9s (SD:0.5s) and the automatic composition of a discharge letter taking 6.1s (SD:2.4s) the speed is adequate. We intend to enlarge the data pool by proliferating the system to other institutions.

1 Introduction

For innovative as for traditional methods of medical data analysis the availability of sufficient amounts of valid medical data is essential. The explicit collection of data for scientific purposes in registries, observational or experimental studies requires a dedicated effort and infrastructure and is therefore expensive[1]. With this approach the actual reporting of data at the point of care will often be added to the duties of the medical staff of the healthcare provider which may meet little enthusiasm leading to poor quality of the collected data. Hiring extra staff to do the reporting is a way to increase the data quality, but also increases the financial burden. To avoid these costs administrative data from health insurers have been used for many studies[2]. Administrative data are inexpensive to acquire and already computer readable. As many research questions can not be answered reliably due to the inferior quality of administrative data, a tradeoff — the credibility versus expense and feasibility — often results[1,3]. Furthermore in some countries like Germany the large number of independent health

R.W. Brause and E. Hanisch (Eds.): ISMDA 2000, LNCS 1933, pp. 198–205, 2001.

insurers and strict data protection laws make it difficult to obtain comprehensive healthcare data from administrative sources.

By whichever way medical data is collected, validation becomes nearly impossible once the information leaves the context of the patient's files[4]. Registries can run plausibility checks or generate queries, but are still depending on the assumption that the reported information is accurate. In observational and experimental studies the reported data can be verified by monitors visiting the premises of the healthcare provider. This again means financial endeavours that usually only pharmaceutical companies can afford.

A possible solution to this dilemma might be to give healthcare providers a tool that improves their normal work–flow while at the same time recording the medical data in a retrievable format. Repeated use of the stored information for actual patient care should help increase data validity as there is a good probability that wrong entries are discovered and corrected by the user[5]. Ideally all information pertaining to the patient should be collected in a kind of electronic file. The idea of an electronic patient record (EPR) is not new and has already been implemented in hospitals mainly in the United States[6]. These EPRs are mostly designed in the classic mainframe or client–server architecture. For these systems the maintenance effort rises parallel to the number of installed terminals or clients and a dedicated computer infrastructure is required[7,8,9]. The cost of installation and maintenance of such client–server EPRs can therefore hardly be met by the funds of scientific projects.

We feel, that for the collection of comprehensive and valid scientific medical data an EPR is required, that is

a) easy to install and maintain thus being less expensive
b) time–saving for the medical staff (users) in their daily work
c) able to store all medical information (including picture etc.) in a retrievable format
d) providing data validation by repeated use of the data in patient care.

The web–technology brought about by the internet allows the design of systems that are easier to install, use and maintain while more flexible and robust than traditional client–server applications. In a web–based system only a computer with a standard browser is needed on the user side. The communication with the central database is possible via different kinds of already existing lines (ethernet, telephone lines, ISDN), so that the actual location of the users is no obstacle.

We investigated the feasibility of designing and implementing an entirely web–based EPR that meets the requirements set forth above.

2   Materials and Methods

2.1   Design

We used the Internet Explorer (Microsoft Corp., Redmond, Wa.) at client side to present the user interface. Thus we can apply the extended design features of ActiveX Layout Control / Cascading Style Sheets and we can control other applications installed on user side, especially for the automatic generation of frequently used documents. The decision for a special browser type is no disadvantage in this case, as Windows PCs with Internet Explorer are readily available.

The Internet Information Server (IIS, Microsoft Corp., Redmond, Wa.) is the web–server for our application. For programming dynamic pages the ISAPI interface is used to exchange data between browser and server and to access resources on server side. This interface is custom–built for the IIS. Compared to the standard CGI interface it is faster and offers additional features like a session concept. As with other interfaces optimised for a specific web–server the application gains performance by loss of software independence.

By the adress of the requested page or by its location in a certain directory the web–server can distinguish whether a page is static or dynamic. Static pages are sent to the browser immediately upon request. Dynamic pages contain program code (server side script) that is processed at server side. These dynamic pages evaluate user input and query databases. Processing the code results in a new page that is generated and sent to the user.

The page that was sent can also contain scripts to be processed at client side in the web–browser. Client side scripts are mainly used for direct interaction with the user (support during data entry, context–sensitive advice and plausibility checks). Within the script functions can be defined and connected to certain elements in the page (e.g. push–buttons).

A user session starts when the user requests a page from the IIS for the first time. It ends after a predefined time without interaction (page requests) has expired. The session can also be ended by explicit termination order by the user. For each user an individual session is started. The session concept is realised via cookies. An encrypted cookie with the session ID is stored at user side. This cookie has a lifetime equivalent to the session time–out value. The session concept allows to define variables at server side, that can be accessed throughout the whole session. There is a separate variable space for each user. Thus it is possible to exchange data between the server side scripts of different dynamic pages.

Our system uses the Adaptive Enterprise SQL–Server (Sybase Inc., CA) as its central database. Data is accessed from the IIS via the standardised ODBC/OLEDB interface. Based upon this interface the ActiveX Data Objects technology (ADO) defines a set of objects that allow a comfortable database access from within the dynamic pages. Because only standard interfaces and languages are used our system can also run on all other standard SQL database systems. Most of the database tables satisfy the Boyce–Cod–Normal–Form (BCNF). The remaining tables fulfil at least the requirements for the second or third normal form. Triggers are used to guarantee that records referred to by foreign keys exist (referential integrity). For each table with reference to other tables a delete trigger is defined, that deletes all dependent records. The scripts in the dynamic pages take care of correct references on insert and update. Each table is sorted by its primary key (primary index). Further indices (secondary indices) are defined to support all searches initiated by the system. These indices are usually on dates, name and foreign keys.

The login page is the only dynamic page that can be accessed directly. All other dynamic pages first check whether the user has successfully logged in or not. Each user is identified by user name and password. The accessibility of patients and the actions within the database are restricted individually. After authentication the users rights are set at server side. User access can be limited to certain patients and actions (read, write, delete data) can be restricted. Each user gets the minimal necessary rights. A redundant check of these user rights is performed on the database level.

The user interface of our system is divided into two parts: In the smaller part at the left side of the browser window a navigation bar is shown (Fig. 1). The requested information is presented in the larger right part. The data items contained are grouped under semantic and medical aspects into several forms of different topics (e.g. administrative data, diagnoses, findings). The most important forms and functions can be accessed directly from the navigation bar. Before any information can be shown a patient must be selected. The patient selection form allows to scroll through the list of patients in alphabetic order, but also to search for names or birthdays. After a patient has been selected, the system jumps back to the last viewed topic. This makes it easier to compare data of different patients and to enter data of the same topic for more patients. All data shown in the different forms are of the currently selected patient. For a better orientation the name and birthday of the current patient is always shown at the top of the navigation bar.

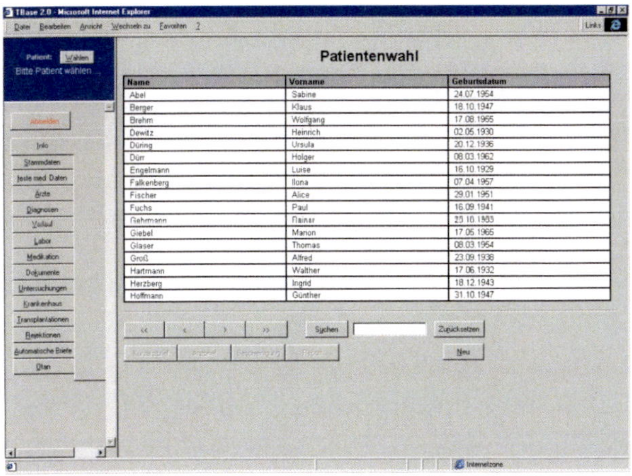

Fig. 1. User interface of the web–based electronic patient record. The navigation bar on the left is always displayed and indicates the selected patient and the current position within this patient's record. The patient selection form on the right allows to pick a patient's record by browsing or searching for name, birthday or patient number.

Buttons at the bottom of most forms allow to modify the data. The buttons are only active when the user has the rights required for this action. For certain topics it is not possible to show all the existing data within one page. In these cases an overview form is shown (e.g. list of dates of laboratory examinations) which contains links to more detailed information (e.g. results of laboratory examination.

For entering new data or changing existing data an input page is generated. The design of the input page is similar to that of the corresponding display page. While the input page is active the navigation bar is disabled. Thus the user can leave the input page only by saving his changes or by cancelling the input. The user is supported while entering new data by selection lists, suggestion of values, hints and error checks (presence of mandatory items, correct data types, value within a predefined range). After pushing the save button all data is written to an (invisible) HTML form and sent to another dynamic page. This page checks again whether the user is authorised for this action and the current patient. Then it generates SQL statements that translate the intended changes and sends them to the database server. Where appropriate the tables containing values for the selection lists are updated. Finally the user is redirected to a display page that shows the current data.

For some selection lists in the input pages too many items are to be transferred or the possible values depend on several other values. In these cases the list values are not transferred together with the input page. They are fetched later, when the values they depend on have been set or after the first letters of the list value have been entered. Thus it is possible to transfer just the much smaller number of items compatible with the part of the input that was already entered.

To ease the daily work of the users, it is possible to automatically generate documents and fill them with data from the electronic patient record. The OLE Automation Server technology allows to control a word processor (Word for Windows, Microsoft, Redmond, Wa.) on the user side. From within a HTML–page a client side script starts a new instance of Word with a pattern of the desired document. The script then automatically fills the gaps in the pattern with values from the database. The user can edit the resulting document or send it directly to his local printer (Fig. 2).

For encoding for users from outside the firewall–protected intranet the Secure Socket Layer protocol is already integrated within the browser and web–server. After an initial handshake with an asymmetric coding algorithm all data packages between the browser and the server are encoded with a session specific symmetrical key. The most secure algorithm both can cope with is chosen. Additionally on dial–in via phone line the telephone number of the user is verified.

2.2   Implementation

We implemented the pilot version of our system in a German kidney transplantation program. Kidney transplantation is a combined effort of many specialists caring for oft multi–morbid patients. Large amounts of medical information from

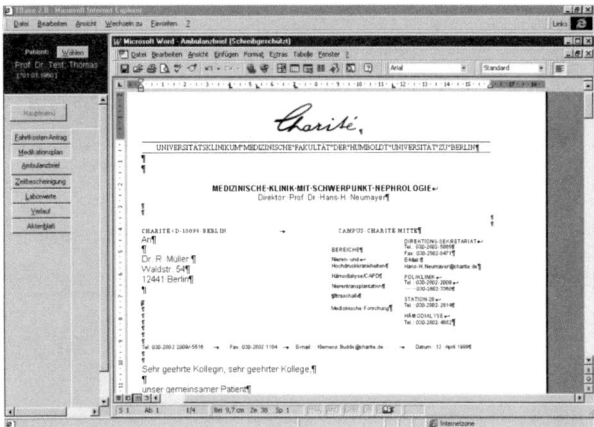

Fig. 2. Several word–documents can be generated directly with stored patient–related information. These documents can be modified, printed and saved on the user's computer. This is the pivotal feature in reducing the workload in routine patient care.

various sources result from this process. The German transplantation legislation compels transplant centres to record not only the information pertaining to the transplantation but also follow–up information for the whole life–span of the transplanted organ. Kidney transplantation therefore seemed well suited to test the limitations of an EPR system.

2.3   Testing

The main test to prove the feasibility of our approach was the implementation in the real–life situation of an academic transplantation program. Criteria to determine the outcome of this trial were

- amount of time required for instruction of new users (doctors, nurses, secretaries)
- degree of acceptance of the new system among the staff
- time of non–availability due to technical failure
- proportion of the workload transferable from the paper–based workflow to the new electronic system

One of the most important aspects in the comparison of the technical quality of our solution (web–technology) to more conventional architectures (mainframe or client–server) is the speed at which often used functions are performed. The EPR's access speed was tested with 50 repeated measurements of the duration of two key–functions:

1.) Display of all lab results for a given day and patient

2.) Automatic composition of a letter containing diagnoses, medication, notes and lab results (Fig. 2).

For the test a 233 MHz Pentium II Processor with 10 Mbit/s Ethernet connection (ping–time below 10 ms) over 2 hubs to the server (400 MHz Pentium II, 256 MB RAM) was used.

3   Results

The system is already fully operational since two years. The former paper–based patient records of the outpatient clinic have been completely replaced by the new EPR system. All patient encounters, their documentation and the composition of the resulting letter to the referring physician are performed with the EPR system.

At present about fifty users have access to the system. Instead of a formal instruction session new users are introduced by an experienced user with similar duties. After a brief overview about the system's functions the new user is encouraged to do self–directed exercises with the records of test patients. The instruction to enable new users to perform basic operations took less than two hours in all cases.

Within our hospital the staff of the various departments that treat patients during the preparation, transplantation phase and follow–up (on in–patient and out–patient basis) accesses the patient's EPR and records the diagnostic and therapeutic information in the EPR. More than thirty dialysis centres from six German states are supplying patients and taking part in their follow–up after transplantation. These dialysis centres can also access their patients EPR and contribute to the stored information.

The system now contains complete records of 798 transplant recipients with a total of 914 kidney transplantations and an average follow–up of 7.2 (SD : 5.7) years. The stored information comprises a total of over 1.2 million laboratory values, 40.000 records on medication, 30.000 records on clinical parameters like blood pressure and 10.000 diagnoses (together with their ICD–10 code). First analyses of this data set were performed and the results are being submitted for publication.

The average duration of access to all values of a specific laboratory day for a given patient takes 0.9(SD:0.5) seconds, the automatic composition of a discharge letter takes 6.1 (SD:2.4) seconds.

In order to increase the data basis we have invited other German transplant centres to adopt our system after the initial pilot phase. One further transplant centre is now in the process of implementing our system and four transplant centres have expressed their intent to do so in the near future. Joint data analyses with these centres will be performed by distribution of a common script that extracts anonymized data from each local database with consecutive pooling of the extracted data.

4   Conclusion

We demonstrated that design and implementation of a comprehensive EPR is
feasible with the application of recent web–technology. Large amounts of highly
detailed and valid data can be collected by this approach. As all information
is recorded in a retrievable format during and for routine patient care the need
for a separate collection of data for scientific purposes is obviated. The stored
information is repeatedly used in actual patient care increasing the likelihood
that incorrect information is discovered and corrected. The size of the data
pool can be multiplied for joint analyses by proliferating the system to other
institutions with similar patients.

References

1. L.I. Iezzoni. *Assessing quality using administrative data.* Ann.Intern.Med. 127,
   pages 666–674. 1997.   198, 198
2. R.A. Wayne. *Policy and program analysis using administrative databases.*
   Ann.Intern.Med. 127, pages 712-718. 1997.   198
3. J. Hornberger, E. Wrone. *When to base clinical policies on observational versus
   randomized trial data.* Ann.Intern.Med. 127, pages 697-703. 1997.   198
4. S.P. Pinfold, V. Goel, C. Sawka. *Quality of hospital discharge and physician data
   for type of breast cancer surgery.* Med Care.Jan. 38, pages 99-107. 2000.   199
5. W.R. Hogan, M.M. Wagner. *Accuracy of data in computer-based patient records.*
   J.Am.Med. Inform.Assoc. 4, pages 342-355. 1997.   199
6. C.J. McDonald. *The barriers to electronic medical record systems and how to overcome them.* J.Am.Med. Inform.Assoc. 4, pages 213-221. 1997.   199
7. S.H. Brown. *No free lunch: institutional preparations for computer-based patient
   records.* Proc.AMIA.Symp., pages 486-490. 1999.   199
8. M.C. Cupito. *Racing toward client-server solutions.* Health Manag.Technol. 19,
   pages 32-37. 1998.   199
9. S. Nakamura, K. Sakurai, M. Uchiyama, Y. Yoshii, N. Tachibana *UNIX based
   client/server hospital information system.* Medinfo. 8 Pt 1:400, page 400. 1995.   199

The InterAction Database: Synergy of Science and Practice in Pharmacy

Hilde Tobi, Paul B. van den Berg, and Lolkje T.W. de Jong-van den Berg

University of Groningen, Groninger University Institute of Drug Exploration, Department of Social Pharmacy and Pharmacoepidemiology, A. Deusinglaan 1, 9713 AV Groningen, The Netherlands
H.Tobi@farm.rug.nl
P.B.van.den.Berg@farm.rug.nl
L.T.W.de.Jong-van.den.Berg@farm.rug.nl

Abstract. In social pharmacy and pharmacoepidemiology the distribution, use and performance of medication after registration is studied. In both fields, the pharmacists are the main source of data on drug use. To increase the value of research, we think it important to exchange ideas and suggestions between scientific researchers and pharmacists who work in community pharmacies. Hence, the department of Social Pharmacy and Pharmacoepidemiology of the University of Groningen sought close collaboration with some community pharmacies in the region, resulting in the InterAction project. The pharmacists deliver data to the InterAction database and are explicitly invited to raise questions and issues from their practice, and to participate in research. Consequently, science and practice benefit from each other's input and expertise. This paper describes the architecture and contents of the InterAction project. Additionally, the first experiences with the database as a laboratory for social pharmacy and pharmacoepidemiology are discussed.

1   Introduction

The two fields social pharmacy and pharmacoepidemiology both study the use of drugs after registration in large populations. Social pharmacy focuses on the role of pharmacists in patient care, while pharmacoepidemiology focuses on drug use in the general population. The value of social pharmacy and pharmacoepidemiology for a safe and rational drug use is obvious and the limit of its potential is not yet reached. The pharmacy is the laboratory where ideas on social pharmacy and pharmacoepidemiology can be generated and put to the test [1]. Therefor, the fields of social pharmacy and pharmacoepidemiology depend on the input of pharmacists. Consequently, the department of Social Pharmacy and Pharmacoepidemiology sought a close collaboration with a number of community pharmacists in the northern part of the Netherlands. The pharmacists' motivations to participate were that they want to show their contribution to health care, and want to be actively and academically involved in the development of their profession. Specific concerns of the pharmacists were privacy of patients and doctors, and time management. The aim of this collaboration that started in 1998, is fourfold: Firstly, to construct a drugs-knowledge database for analyses in pharmacoepidemiology and social pharmacy. Secondly, to

R.W. Brause and E. Hanisch (Eds.): ISMDA 2000, LNCS 1933, pp. 206–211, 2000.
© Springer-Verlag Berlin Heidelberg 2000

stimulate pharmacy practice research. Thirdly, to offer scientific support to pharmacists and, fourthly, to enhance the learning environment for pharmacy students.

2   Design of the InterAction Database

2.1   Logistics

In the Netherlands, almost all patients obtain their prescription drugs from one community pharmacy. Every pharmacist keeps record of all prescribed medication in one of the available computerized pharmacy systems. The pharmacies involved in the InterAction project use either Euroned [2] or Pharmacom [3]. This software is meant to simplify reimbursement procedures and medication surveillance. When a patient is registered with a pharmacy, the involved pharmacy system checks every prescription with respect to dosage, co-morbidity, (pseudo) double medication, over-sensitiveness and co-medication. Each recipe results in one so-called patient-recipe line. All pharmacy systems can produce files with a uniform layout of patient-recipe lines. In the pharmacies, these files can be processed to aggregate prescription data for use in the pharmacotherapy audit with general practitioners.

The production of patient-recipe lines needs to be done at night to prevent impediment to patient care. The patient-recipe lines contain patient information that is, due to privacy legislation, not allowed to leave the pharmacy. Hence, an anonymity procedure has been developed that replaces the physician and patient codes by their own unique InterAction (IA) codes. The files are transferred to a PC to run the anonymity procedure. The file with the key for the IA codes remains in the pharmacy and is accessible to the pharmacist only. The resulting source files are compressed and sent to the University for entrance into the InterAction database.

2.2   Structure and contents

The database consists of four series of files: registration files, patient files, recipe files and the G-Standard [4]. The file registration system consists of a registration of the read source files (input from the pharmacies). Each file receives a unique number. The time period, total number of recipes and patients, as well as the number of recipes per Anatomic Therapeutic Chemical (ATC) group [5] are registered for each source file. The file registration number is also used in the patient files and recipes files.

There are three types of patient files. The first file consists of one line for each patient with patient number, date of birth, gender, first part of the ZIP code, general practitioner code and number of the first and last source file that contain the patient's number. The second patient file contains the patient's history with respect to variables in the first file, such as a new ZIP code due to moving house. The third series of files contain for each year and each pharmacy separately, the number of recipes a patient brought in.

For each year, the recipe lines are gathered containing patient number, drug number, date of delivery, quantity, daily dose, type of prescriber (GP, specialist, dentist or midwife), physician, pharmacy, insurance, statement of expenses, warnings, and number of the source file. The drug number is then linked to the G-Standard, the monthly updated database of all available drugs and related products in the Netherlands [4]. This linkage yields Anatomic Therapeutical Chemical (ATC) code, Number of Defined Daily Doses (NDDDs) and drug names.

Entries such as bandages and aids are also present in the recipe-file, but these do not have ATC codes.

3   Results

3.1 The InterAction database

All of the participating pharmacies except for two were able to retrieve their pharmacy data from 1994, so the database contains information from 1994 onwards (Table 1). When one wants to analyze the drug use in the general population, one needs to know to number of inhabitants in the service area of the pharmacies. However, the service areas of the pharmacies involved do not coincide with a geographic or administrative area, except for one pharmacy. This pharmacy delivered recipes to 33,643 registered patients in 1999. These patients constitute about 72% of the population as counted by the national Bureau of Statistics (Statistics Netherlands). The percentage of the population in this particular area that enters a recipe is used to estimate the total population (Table 2).

All recipe lines are entered into the database (see Table 1). More than 85% of the recipe lines are recognized immediately. The remaining recipe lines include non-drugs, pharmacy prepared drug formulation, pharmacy specific drug numbers and typing errors. After some detective work and programming, these are also recognizable in the database, leaving 4 % recipe-lines that can not be recognized at all.

Where data is incomplete, this may be because the information is not entered or because the information is irretrievable due to typing or coding error. For some important variables the completeness over the years is given in table 2.

To get access to the data, a researcher needs permission of the head of the department of Social Pharmacy and Pharmacoepidemiology and the architect of the database. After consent, the data-manager extracts that part of the database the researcher needs resulting in two files: a recipe file and a patient file. Depending on the research question, the resulting recipe file may contain all prescriptions for a certain newly marketed drug, or all prescriptions entered by senior citizens who use more than three drugs simultaneously. The matching patient file contains patient characteristics such as date of birth and gender.

Several practical problems have surfaced: It sometimes takes a dozen of phone calls and a few months patience to obtain the correct data from the pharmacies, due to difficulties with production of files, transfer of files, running the anonymity procedure, compression of files, and the transport to the university.

Table 1. Database and recipe line characteristics

	1994[1]	1995	1996	1997	1998	1999	Total[2]
Number of pharmacies	10	12	12	12	12	12	12
Total number of recipes	767,396	953,400	1,011,151	1,092,637	1,145,140	1,203,020	6,172,744
% recipes with ATC code	87.42	88.30	87.58	87.11	87.16	86.96	87.39
% recognized recipes, without ATC code	7.05	7.75	8.34	8.88	9.23	9.14	8.51
% not recognized recipes	5.52	3.94	4.07	4.02	3.60	3.90	4.10
% of recipes with known type of prescriber	93.95	94.14	93.18	94.59	96.99	96.54	95.03

[1] Start of the database
[2] From 1994 to 1999

Table 2. Completeness of data on patients who received at least one prescription

	1994	1995	1996	1997	1998	1999	Total
Number of patients	69,032	82,251	88,971	93,640	96,085	96,281	146,036
% with complete data	99.13	99.14	99.18	99.24	99.36	99.31	98.65
% date of birth missing or fault	0.42	0.39	0.36	0.34	0.32	0.34	0.51
% gender missing	0.00	0.01	0.01	0.01	0.007	0.009	0.02
% ZIP code (first 4 of 6) missing	0.49	0.55	0.49	0.44	0.33	0.38	0.91
Estimated population (nearest 5000)	95,000	115,000	125,000	130,000	135,000	135,000	

3.2   The database as a tool: exchange between science and practice

The InterAction project not only aims to yield a database but also to contribute to pharmacy practice research, scientific support to pharmacists and the learning environment for pharmacy students. The InterAction database is at the center of these goals. The pharmacists did raise questions, the department either did the research or helped the pharmacist to do the analyses and in all cases pharmacy students participated.

For example, one pharmacist wanted to verify his impression that methotrexate is sometimes prescribed without additional folic acid, which is against the guidelines. Methotrexate is a drug used for severe rheumatic arthritis. Adverse drug events associated with methotrexate include gastro-intestinal and hematological problems. These adverse effects can be reduced with folic acid, which is why according to the guidelines folic acid is prescribed simultaneously with methotrexate. Analysis of the InterAction data showed that patients who did not receive folic acid used methotrexate for a shorter period than patients who did receive folic acid, and often changed to an other medication because of the side effects of methotrexate. These results suggest that an increased awareness is needed to enhance adherence to the guidelines and give the pharmacists solid information for the pharmacotherapy audit with medical doctors.

Another project initiated by a community pharmacist aims to develop an instrument to detect patients having difficulties with their asthma medication. For example, when a patient uses his aerosol inhalator upside down he draws in propellant and not the actual medication. The inhalator will appear empty soon and the patient will return to the pharmacy too early. Also, a patient may use his maintenance medication not properly and consequently needs too often drugs that dilate the bronchial tubes immediately. These are frequently faced problems with asthma medication. The instrument aims to detect the patient so the pharmacist can make inquiries and act upon them either by giving the patient an instruction or alert the physician.

Examples of research initiated by the department are the use of Hormone Replacement Therapy by women in this region [6], the use of prescribed drugs by children in general [7], and more specifically the use of psychotropic medication in children over the past six years [8]. An example of research into adherence to guidelines is a study on the prescription of deptropine to children [9].

The involved pharmacists receive accredited points for postgraduate education. These points are earned by participating in the meetings that have scholastic as well as household affairs on the agenda. These meetings are held four times a year and topics on these meeting were, for example, measurements of agreement, and incidence *versus* prevalence.

4   Discussion

The InterAction database has proven to be a useful laboratory for research in the fields of social pharmacy and pharmacoepidemiology in the two years of its existence. Overall figures such as expenditure on specific ATC-code drug groups are comparable to other pharmacy-related databases in the Netherlands such as SFK [10], GIP [11] and Pharmo [12,13], despite the size of the InterAction database being relatively modest. An important advantage of the InterAction database over the other databases, is the fact that it is fastly up-to-date with a time lag of less than three months.

Some of the methodological issues that are common to pharmaceutical databases are yet unsolved. The main problem is a possibly imprecise estimation of the population size. In addition, the database contains passers-by and 'fake' patients, who are made by the pharmacist to manage supply. Often, the pharmacist is late or not notified when the family or one family member moves to another area, or when a patient dies. The above issues are now known and dealt with as far as possible.

An extension of the number of pharmacies involved in the Interaction project is anticipated changing the InterAction working group into a two-shell project: the outer shell contains pharmacists who deliver data, the inner shell contains pharmacists who contribute more than just data. The outer-shell is going to function as some sort of ante-chambre and the pharmacist in this ante-chambre can proceed into the inner shell after mutual agreement (the InterAction pharmacists, the other members of the InterAction working group and the individual pharmacist).

The InterAction database has raised interest from several institutes and industries and consequently a need has emerged to formalize the access to the database and to administer extracted data-files more extensively. Present developments include a migration from xbase to an SQL server with web access to assure safety and logging of activities. A library of tools to access and query the database will be included in the web-interface.

In conclusion, the exchange between scientists and community pharmacists centered on the InterAction database is fruitful for both science and practice. It has facilitated studies on adherence to guidelines, pharmacy practice research, as well as general studies on drug use.

References

1. de Jong-van den Berg, L.T.W.: Wetenschap en praktijk in synergy (Science and practice in synergy), Inaugural lecture. Groningen (1998)
2. Euroned. APCOS, Heerlen, The Netherlands, http://www.eurosys.nl
3. Pharmacom.   PharmaPartners   BV,   Oosterhout,   The   Netherlands, http:/www.pharmapartners.nl
4. G-Standard. Z-Index BV, The Hague, The Netherlands. Updated monthly. http://www.z-index.nl
5. Guidelines for ATC classification and DDD assignment. WHO Collaborating Centre for Drug Statistics Metholodoly, Oslo (1998)
6. van den Berg, P., Stuurman-Bieze, A., de Jong-van den Berg, L.: Informatie vooraf is essentieel. Het gebruik van hormoonsubstitutietherapie bij vrouwen. (Information in advance is essential. Utilisation of hormone replacement therapy in women) Pharmaceutisch Weekblad 135 (2000) 388-393
7. Schirm, E., van den Berg, P.B., Gebben, H., Sauer, P., de Jong-van den Berg, L.T.W.: Drug use of children in the community assessed through pharmacy dispensing data. To appear in: British Journal of Clinical Pharmacology.
8. Schirm, E., Tobi, H., van den Berg, P., de Jong-van den Berg, L.: Exponential growth of psychotropic medication in children: an American phenomenon? Submitted
9. Schirm, E., Gebben, H., Tobi, H., de Jong-van den berg, L.T.W.: Deptropine: wel uit de standaarden, maar nog niet uit de pen. (Deptropine: removed from the guidelines, but still being prescribed) Submitted
10. SFK Stichting Farmaceutische Kengetallen, The Hague, The Netherlands, http://www.sfk.nl
11. GIPeilingen, kengetallen farmaceutische hulp 1998 (GIP gauges, Index numbers pharmaceutical care 1998). Geneesmiddelen Informatie Project / College voor Zorgverzekeringen, Amstelveen (february 2000) http://www.cvz.nl
12. Herings, R.M.C.: Pharmo: a record linkage system for postmarketing surveillance of prescription drugs in The Netherlands, PhD thesis Utrecht (1993)
13. Herings, R.M.C., Panneman, M.J.M., de Graag, E.J.: Pharmo Report: Pharmacotherapie in beweging (Pharmacotherapy in motion). Pharmo Instituut, Utrecht (February 2000)

A New Computerized Method to Verify and Disseminate Medical Appropriateness Criteria

Maojo, V.[1]; Laita, L. [1]; Roanes-Lozano, E.[2]; Crespo, J. [1]; Rodriguez-Pedrosa, J. [1]

[1]Artificial Intelligence Laboratory and Department. School of Computer Science. Universidad Politecnica de Madrid. Madrid, Spain. Boadilla del Monte. 28660 Madrid.
vmaojo@fi.upm.es
[2]Dept of Algebra.Universidad Complutense de Madrid. 28040 Madrid.
eroanes@cucmos.sim.ucm.es

Abstract. In this article, we describe a new computerized method that we created, based on algebra, to check consistency in knowledge bases. We apply this method to sets of medical appropriateness criteria developed using the RAND method. An example of criteria tables for coronary bypass was used to test the method. Different computer tools were developed to facilitate this logical validation. A JAVA program was also developed to display criteria tables in a flowchart format, using any WWW standard browser. Thus, appropriateness criteria can be transformed into effective guidelines for medical practice.

1. Introduction

During the last decades there has been many efforts to stimulate the creation of evidence-based clinical practice guidelines and new methodologies for their creation, representation and routine use. In 1992, a panel study carried out by the Institute of Medicine in Washington, USA, defined Clinical Practice Guidelines as "systematically developed statements to assist practitioners and patient decisions about appropriate health care for specific clinical circumstances" [1]. The same study considered the differences between paper-based and computer-based guidelines.

Paper-based guidelines can be easily read and browsed, but they have various problems that limit their practical implementation. These problems include: (1) checking logical consistencies; (2) dissemination to professionals; (3) local adaptation to specific clinical settings; (4) difficult evaluation of their impact in medical care; (5) updating to adapt guidelines to new scientific discoveries, and (6) lack of feedback to guideline developers.

Computers can help to solve some of these constraints. Different approaches were considered to implement guidelines, which include the use of already existing models such as the ARDEN syntax or developing new formal specifications (e,g, Prestige, GEODE, GLIF). Some architectures were also developed or upgraded to link these specifications to medical records and different sources of medical information. For instance, researchers at Stanford have developed new architectures of PROTEGE to implement clinical protocols. Greenes and his collaborators at the Brigham and Women's hospital have also developed a clinical workstation, ARACHNE, that includes a module for practice guidelines, represented as graphical flowcharts [2].

Nevertheless, some of the problems remain unsolved. The most difficult one is to create a method for checking and ensuring the logical consistency of the medical

R.W. Brause and E. Hanisch (Eds.): ISMDA 2000, LNCS 1933, pp. 212–217, 2000.

knowledge embedded within the guidelines and protocols. We have developed a method, based on a logical algebraic model, to solve consistency in knowledge bases. This method is applied to medical appropriateness criteria, a evaluation method used in health services research that could be transformed and applied as practice guidelines to assist physicians in medical care.

2. Background and Rationale

Appropriateness criteria are commonly developed to evaluate retrospectively the use of medical procedures under specific clinical circumstances. According to the previously cited study of the Institute of Medicine, "appropriate care is conceptually defined as care for which the expected health benefit exceeds the expected negative consequences by a sufficient margin that the care is worth providing" [1]. Those sets can contain a few or even several thousand criteria. Thus, sets of criteria can be rather complex to apply. Evaluation is usually carried out by health services specialists, not being intended for assisting practitioners in decision making.

Several private insurers and health plans are using these criteria as a method to evaluate the quality of care, control costs, and reduce the variability of medical practice. Although their origin was initially centered in the USA, other entities at different countries in Europe are also working with appropriateness criteria.

The most commonly used methodology for developing appropriateness criteria was created by RAND Health Services/UCLA. This methodology has several phases: (1) systematic review and study of the scientific literature; (2) creation of a list of indications for analysis of the patient conditions under which a specific procedure can be used in clinical practice; (3) expert meetings, using panel techniques for reaching consensus; (4) subsequent meetings and refinement of the list of indications; (5) publication of results by means of sets of criteria [3].

To value the appropriateness of an indication, experts rates each indication using a scale ranging from 1 to 9. 1 stands for the lowest degree of appropriateness whereas 9 indicates the highest degree. Median and standard deviation of experts' ratings are calculated to label each indication as "appropriate", "inappropriate" or "uncertain". The criteria tables also indicate if the experts have reached a consensus, expressing "agreement" or disagreement". An example, developed for its use at the Spanish National Health System is shown below.

Moderad 2, ronda 2					ANEXO J, MODER A2.DOC, 26/02/97, pág 1
CAPÍTULO 1	Riesgo quirúrgico BAJO/MODERADO		Riesgo quirúrgico ALTO		
ASINTOMÁTICOS	Uso apropiado de Tto. méd. - Revasc.	Uso apropiado de ACTP · CAC	Uso apropiado de Tto. méd. - Revasc.	Uso apropiado de ACTP · CAC	Nº de indicación

A. CON PRUEBA DE ESFUERZO POSITIVA

1. Enfermedad de tronco común izquierdo

FEVI a) >50%	1 2 3 4 5 6 7 8 *• A : 9 ; 10	1 2 3 4 5 6 7 8 *••A : 9 1 9	1 2 3 4 5 6 7 8 *• A 4 6	1 2 3 4 5 6 7 8 *••A 1 1 1 7	(1-4)
b) >30% ≤50%	1 2 3 4 5 6 7 8 *• A : 9	1 2 3 4 5 6 7 8 *••A 1 1 6	1 2 3 4 5 6 7 8 *• A 1 1 7	1 2 3 4 5 6 7 8 *••A 1 1 9	(5-8)
c) >20% ≤30%	1 2 3 4 5 6 7 8 *• A	1 2 3 4 5 6 7 8 *••A	1 2 3 4 5 6 7 9 *• A	1 2 3 4 5 6 7 8 *••A	(9-12)

This is a section of a set of criteria developed to assess the appropriateness of coronary artery bypass surgery in heart disease patients. The indications are indicated with text and panelists' scores ratings are expressed numerically.

This methodology has several problems that constraint its efficiency. These problems have been widely known, and even the original RAND developers have acknowledged their importance. Those main problems are: (1) lack of methods to check the logical consistency of the criteria sets. Criteria are based on published evidences from different and sometimes contradictory studies and on experts' knowledge, elicited through panel meetings. Thus, it is rather common to find logical inconsistencies within these criteria, with contradictory indications. RAND specialists usually solve these inconsistencies by manually creating flowcharts containing the criteria and remeeting with experts. Both are inefficient, time-consuming, and expensive methods. (2) Appropriateness criteria are intended for retrospective analysis of medical practice. Thus, new methods are required for translating criteria into guidelines that can be routinely used by practitioners in medical care.

We have investigated two different approaches for solving these two major drawbacks. We will explore both methods in the sections below.

3. Methods

1. Detection of logical inconsistencies.

We have created a new logical method for verifying knowledge bases expressed by means of IF (premises)...THEN (consequences) rules. This method is based on Lukasiewicz' trivalent logic, using three values of truth: true, false and undetermined [4].

Appropriateness criteria can be easily translated into IF...THEN rules. In the angioplasty example inserted above, the whole table can be translated into rules. Our logical method can be applied to this rule-based knowledge base for checking consistency. A criteria table is inconsistent with respect to some given facts if and only if a logical contradiction or an integrity constraint is obtained when its rules are fired. Rules are transformed into algebraic expressions that can be mathematically verified. Using this method, it is possible t detect if the table contains anomalies and, once these have been corrected, extract new knowledge. The logical method has been described elsewhere [4].

2. Dissemination over Internet.

We created a model for representing practice guidelines as graphical flowcharts, with nodes representing state transitions in patient status and care. Each node is linked to multimedia information, such as text, video, sound, or graphics. We developed a preliminary version, with a new specification language, based on SGML, to represent clinical algorithms. Later, we chose a new approach, storing the guideline on Microsoft Access© (although any database management system can be used) [5]. We believe that it can facilitate acceptance from those users that are reluctant to use complex specification languages and computer tools.

Once a guideline is stored in a database file, it can be visualized using other different tools that we created, such as a JAVA program. This tool implements several functionalities for browsing, abstracting and zooming the algorithm. Users can browse different paths in the clinical algorithm, expanding nodes forward or contracting paths backwards with a mouse click, accessing text, tables, images, drawings, video and sound by using the links of each node. Other functions allow visualization of the graph, change of fonts, zoom of the whole graph, search and edition of text strings, accessing other guidelines simultaneously, or creating a report of the paths followed by any user. These tools can be reused for different applications.

4. Results

In a preliminary research we implemented several computer tools using C++ and the mathematical language CoCoA [6]. These programs translate rules into algebraic expressions that can be formally checked to find inconsistencies.

At this point, we considered that these kinds of programs could not be used by health practitioners or by health services specialists. Even computer programmers can have difficulties to understand the functioning of the system, since it is based on highly demanding knowledge of advanced logic. Thus, we thought that we should develop new tools, based on widely used applications such as M.S. Excel$^\circ$, M.S. Access$^\circ$, or any standard WWW browser (e.g., Netscape$^\circ$ or M.S. Explorer$^\circ$).

We have implemented a criteria table elaborated at the Spanish Institute of Health Carlos III for the study of appropriateness use of coronary bypass, similar to others carried out in different institutions (e.g., RAND). This table was created by a team consisting of panel and health services specialists as well as by 10 experts in coronary diseases. Several indicators were obtained and used: (1) symptomatic/asymptomatic patients; (2) positive/negative effort test; (3) 1, 2, or 3 vessels disease; (4) left common vessel disease, and (5) values of left ventricle ejection fraction.

Using integrity restrictions (experts' rules given by the panelists to control to ensure the logical consistency of the criteria), added to the original rules (transformed from criteria), our system was able to evaluate the logical consistency of 216 rules from the knowledge base in a few minutes. We used an average Pentium-based personal computer with 64 MB of RAM. Various rules were detected as inconsistent by the system, pointing out which knowledge needed to be reelaborated by the experts.

Several benchmark tests that we have carried out using other different knowledge bases show that the system is able to detect various types of logical inconsistencies. Thus, the system can be applied to different appropriateness criteria tables developed by the RAND/UCLA method or any other knowledge base represented by means of rules.

5. Discussion

Other research groups have previously reported methods to check the consistency of medical knowledge bases (e.g., ONCOCIN and similars) [7], or appropriateness criteria sets. The prior is based on traditional logical methods applied to medical informatics, and therefore just a few health practitioners can understand those methods. As far as we know, they have not been either applied to appropriateness criteria. The latter uses a method based on logic and decision tables to check the consistency of criteria tables [8]. Our tools implement a more comprehensive, automated, and faster method to check consistency in those criteria.

Regarding the user-interface, we adopted the convenience of using common off-the-shelves programs for creating the users interfaces. A M.S. Excel sheet is filled with the knowledge content of the criteria and M.S. Access forms are used to modify rules or check the consistency. These tools are connected to a CoCoA program [9], which is not shown to the average user. The other tool that we used is a JAVA program, accessible over Internet. With this tool, users can navigate in a graphical way through the knowledge of the criteria, transforming the original table in a standard flowchart with nodes linked to multimedia information. Thus, in a limited and small number of steps, health practitioners can browse the whole algorithm and choose the correct path to reach the conclusion regarding the appropriateness of a procedure [10].

Since appropriateness criteria were originally designed for retrospective analysis of clinical practice, our tools enhance those criteria for being used as an active aid in clinical decision making. The additional advantage of the JAVA-based program is that it can be accessed over Internet using any standard WWW browser. An example is shown below:

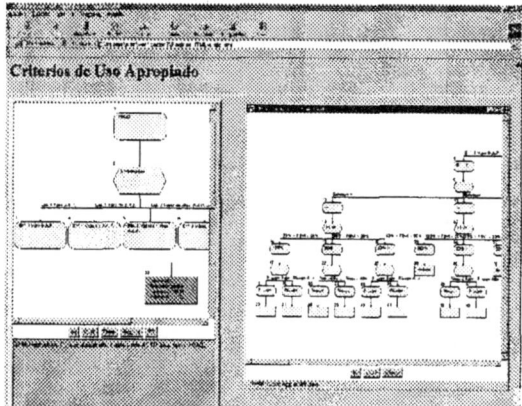

Figure 1. A Java tool to display appropriateness criteria in flowchart format

6. Conclusions and Future Directions

Computerized versions of practice guidelines and appropriateness criteria offer solutions to some of the main problems of paper-based versions. We tried to help practitioners with tools that solve two of the main problems associated to guidelines: a) checking consistencies, and b) transferring appropriateness criteria from retrospective analysis to prospective use in clinical practice.

We have chosen an approach to enhance the use of these evaluation procedures over Internet. With out tools it is also possible to adapt protocols, guidelines and criteria locally. An important reason for such question is variability in medical practice. For instance, practitioners at different medical centers might not accept a specific criteria. Users are able to modify contents and graphical displays to adapt the procedures to their specific clinical environments.

Our programs are not intended to access automatically patient data from medical records or hospital information systems. Such direction is being considered for future research.

Acknowledgements

We want to thank Sergio Corredor and David Caja for their contributions to the programming and development of some of the tools described in this paper. The Health Services Research Unit, Institute of Health Carlos III, Madrid, Spain developed the criteria tables used in this work, under the direction of Dr. Pablo Lazaro. This research has been funded by the Fondo de Investigación Sanitaria, Ministry of Health, Spain.

References

[1] Field M, Lohr K. (eds.). Guidelines for Clinical Practice (1992). National Academy Press, Washington, D.C.

[2] Liem EB, Obeid JS, Shareck EP, Shato L, Greenes RA. Representation of clinical practice guidelines through an interactive World-Wide-Web interface. SCAMC (1995) 19:223-227.

[3] Bernstein S J. (RAND):"Chairing an expert panel". Invited conference. Institute of Health Carlos III (1994) Madrid.

[4] Laita, L.; Roanes-Lozano; Ledesma, L.; Alonso, J. A Computer Algebra Approach to Verification and Deduction in Many-Valued Knowledge Systems. Soft Computing 3 (1999), 7-19.

[5] Maojo V; Herrero, C.; Valenzuela, F.; Crespo J, Lázaro P., and Pazos, A. A JAVA-based Multimedia Tool for Clinical Practice Guidelines. Proceedings of Medical Informatics Europe (1997) Porto Carras, Greece.

[6] Capani A, Niesi G."CoCoA User's Manual /v. 3.0b)". (1996) Dept. de Matemáticas, Universidad de Génova,.

[7] Buchanan, B., and Shortliffe, E.H. Rule-Based Expert Systems: the MYCIN Experiments of the Stanford Heuristic Programming Project (1984). Addison-Wesley, NY.

[8] Shiffman, R.N., and Greenes, R.A. Improving Clinical Guidelines with Logic and Decision-Table Techniques: Application to Hepatitis Inmunization Recommendations. Medical Decision Making 14-3 (1994) 245-254.

[9] Corredor S. "Aplicación para la creación y verificación de sistemas de conocimiento utilizando lógica trivalente". Unpublished Ltd. Dissertation (1997). Facultad de Informática, Universidad Politécnica de Madrid.

[10] Caja, D.; Rodriguez, J; and Maojo, V. Una herramienta para la visualización, edición y verificación de la consistencia de criterios de uso apropiado. Unpublished Ltd. Dissertation. (1998). Universidad Politecnica de Madrid.

Pharmacokinetic & -dynamic Drug Information and Dosage Adjustment System Pharmdis

Frieder Keller[1], David Czock[1], Michael Giehl[2], and Dietmar Zellner[1]

[1] Division of Nephrology, Medical Department, University of Ulm, Robert Koch Strasse 8, 89070 Ulm, Germany, frieder.keller@medizin.uni-ulm.de
[2] Benjamin Franklin University Hospital, Berlin, Germany

Abstract. Not only every patient is different, but also every drug. Drug dosage must be individualised, and adjusted to the patient's organ function (e.g. age, kidney) and severity of disease (e.g. intensive care, outpatient office). Within an European project, we are on the way to built up a drug information and dosage adjustment system. The essential components are available: the pharmacokinetic /-dynamic database NEPharm, calculation algorithms, a consensus on general pharmacokinetic concept, on dose adjustment rules, and on standard nomenclature (ATC code). A graphical user interface must be designed. The required components must be made interoperable, namely patient record, drug dictionary, pharmacokinetic /-dynamic database, calculation algorithms, graphical user interface. The dosage proposals made by the system must be clinically certified, and be compared to standard practice in an external environment to evaluate clinical applicability and reliability. Special versions of the system will be designed for the needs of our software partners. The integrated system will be implemented to establish an internet-based centre of excellence for individualised drug therapy.

1 Background

Fixed drug dosage can lead to serious adverse effects, especially in the sick and aged patients. This has first and convincingly been shown for digoxin and renal impairment [1]. Aminoglycosides haven even been advocated to be contraindicated in kidney patients because of dramatic oto- and nephro-toxicity [2]. This verdict until recently influenced standard practice not to treat cancer patients with anticancer drugs when kidney or liver function are impaired [3].

Three recent studies on computer-assisted drug dosage have shown that patient outcome can be improved by individualised drug dose calculations, namely chemotherapy [4], anticoagulation [5], and anti-microbial therapy [6]. The pharmacokinetic principles developed for these studies are applicable not only to methotrexate, dicoumarol, or gentamicin, but to all drugs in general. The specific pharmacokinetic parameters of the respective drug, and a general pharmacokinetic concept for the dosage calculations are required for this purpose.

R.W. Brause and E. Hanisch (Eds.): ISMDA 2000, LNCS 1933, pp. 218–224, 2000.

2   Approach

Four components are required. These requirements are available as single components, but must be made compatible within a common system.

1. pharmacokinetic database
2. pharmacokinetic calculation algorithms
3. hospital and/or office information system
4. the validation in real patients.

The final output will be a dosage proposal to every drug for every patient at every moment when any parameter is changing. That proposal must be given on a routine basis within the respective application.

All available sources must be made accessible, and the permanent maintenance of the database must be established. Electronic drug information is available on the server or the internet (e.g. RoteListe, Medline, PubMed). This information must be extracted by automatic text analysis tools. An appropriate parser must be designed for extracting numerical attributes of drug information systems (e.g. dose 10 mg every 12 hours).

According to our analysis of user needs, experts and practical doctors want three things: completeness, up-to-date information, and consistency with acknowledged standards (e.g. British Medical Formulary). The experts in the intensive care or nephrology units are aware of the problems, and frequently encounter situations where dosage adjustments must be done; they need a consultation system with access to the most recent information and individualised dosage proposals. The general practitioners are not aware of the problem, they rarely are dealing with critical dosage decisions; they need an automatic monitoring system providing warnings and unsolicited proposals.

2.1   Pharmacokinetic Concept

Drug dose adjustment can be derived from explicit functions provided that the pertinent pharmacokinetic, pharmacodynamic, patient related data, and clinical information is available. We have achieved a consensus on the theoretical basis of a pharmacokinetic/pharmacodynamic system. The most general pharmacokinetic correlation describes drug clearance as the mathematical product $(Clearance = Distribution \cdot Elimination)$ of corresponding distribution (Vd), and elimination parameters (Ke). The half-life $(T_{1/2})$ is the most intuitive elimination parameter $(T_{1/2} = 0.693/Ke)$. According to this concept, the pharmacokinetics of every drug can be recorded in a database with standardised format of corresponding distribution and elimination parameters

$$Cl = Vd \cdot Ke.$$

Pharmacokinetic parameters are influenced by disease, age, and body weight of patients. Drug clearance (Cl) explicitly depend on renal function [7]

$$Cl = Cl_{anur} + a \cdot CLCR, \qquad a = (Cl_{norm} - Cl_{anur}) / CLCR_{norm}.$$

For the case, where no data is published on pharmacokinetics in patients with functional anuric renal failure, the renal clearance in normal volunteers can be used (Cl_{ren})

$$a = (Cl_{ren} / CLCR)_{norm}.$$

Renal function can be estimated from the patient's age, weight and serum creatinine [8]. Also more complex urine-free methods are at hand [9]

$$CLCR = (140 - Age)\, BodyWeight / (0.8\, SerumCrea).$$

With repetitive drug administration $(i = 1, 2, 3 \dots)$, the peak concentration (C_{peak}) or trough levels (C_{trough}) are functions of dose (D), interval (τ), volume (Vd), half-life $(T_{1/2})$, or clearance (Cl)

$$C(t) = \sum_{i=1}^{\infty} D / Vd \;\; \exp[-0.693(t - i\tau) / T_{1/2}].$$

The parameters predicted for the average patient (X), can be individualised by the Bayesian objective function if one or more drug concentration measurements (C) are available [10]

$$\min \left(\frac{X_{ind} - X_{pop}}{SD_X} \right)^2 + \left(\frac{C_{ind} - C_{pop}}{SD_C} \right)^2 \longrightarrow X_{ind}.$$

2.2   Dose Adjustment Rules

Three different dose adjustment rules can be distinguished. The Dettli-rule (1), and the Kunin-rule (2) relate the individual dose to, and derive it from the normal standard dose (D_{norm}). Both rules need individual half-life $(T_{1/2})$ or clearance values (Cl), and nothing else. Standard dose (D_{norm}) and interval (τ_{norm}) form the all-available working basis for a dose individualisation.

$$D/\tau = (D/\tau)_{norm}\, Cl / Cl_{norm} \tag{1}$$

$$D/\tau = \frac{1}{2} D_{norm} / T_{1/2} \tag{2}$$

As an alternative to standard dosage, the target concentration approach (3) holds a better promise where such targets have been defined by clinical studies [11]

$$D/\tau = C_{target}\, Cl, \quad C_{target} = E \cdot CE_{50}/(E_{max} - E). \tag{3}$$

Accumulation kinetics allow to calculate target peak and trough levels. In addition, the Holford-approach (3) needs pharmacodynamic insight to define the

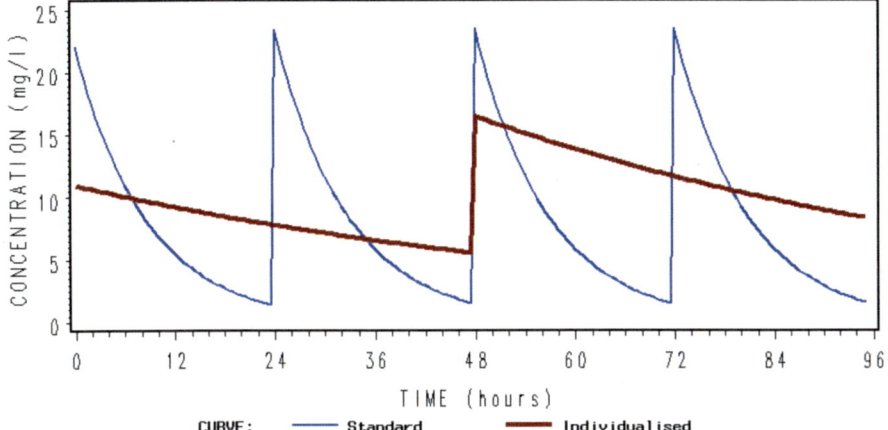

Fig. 1. Individualised dose for impaired drug elimination is a compromise between standard peak and trough concentrations.

target concentration under the condition of altered pharmacokinetics. The sigmoid E_{max} model can be fitted to sparse data to derive the pharmacokinetic and pharmacodynamic correlation

$$E = E_{max}/(1 + (CE_{50}/C)^H).$$

The most advanced dose adjustment rule can be derived from the area under the effect time curve (AUETC). The drug dosage is adjusted to keep the sumative effect constant, that is the area under the effect time curve. The AUETC is a function of the elimination half-life ($T_{1/2}$), dose interval (τ), peak concentration (C_{peak}), and trough concentration ($C_{trough} = C_{peak} \exp(-0.693\,t/T_{1/2})$). This function has a solution in closed form for most general linear one-compartment conditions [12]

$$AUETC = E_{max}\, 1.44\, T_{1/2}\,/H \, \ln\, \overset{\bullet}{(CE_{50}^H + C_{peak}^H)}/(CE_{50}^H + C_{trough}^H)^{\overset{\bullet}{}} .$$

The pharmacodynamic parameters are presumed constant, namely ($E_{max} = const$) and ($AUETC = const$). This dosing rule needs to know the concentration producing half-maximum effect (CE_{50}), and sigmoidicity coefficient (H). Both essential pharmacodynamic parameters are increasingly published, and can be extracted from the scientific literature.

2.3   Database

We have built-up a 9 MB database with pharmacokinetic and pharmacodynamic information from published literature.

NEPharm Database

       37 ... slots for parameter $(T_{1/2}, Cl, Vd, ...)$

   2496 ... generic drugs (acyclovir ... zidovudine)

   4318 ... primary citations (N Engl J Med, Drugs, ...)

 13824 ... statistically synthesised values

29945 ... primary extracted values

The values for parmacokinetic parameters are extracted from primary publications. Copies of the respective publications are collected in a physical archive. The data are recorded by a specially designed data-acquisition module.

3   Achievements

Statistical Synthesis: For maintenance of the database continuous updates of parameter must be recorded from published pharmacokinetic literature. The respective journals are regularly screened for appropriate articles, a photo-copy of the articles is taken, the articles are read by an expert to flag the relevant values of pharmacokinetikc parameters. From the marked copies the values are typed into our data-input module. From the input module the values are fed into the complete database and combined with pre-existing data. Within the database, a central value for each parameter (X) is calculated with parametric or non-parametric statistical methods as applicable to the respective set of data. Statistical standard solutions, and explicit calculations are programmed with high capacity statistical software (SAS).

Consistency: Plausibility tests are performed, where, for examples, the corresponding three parameters of distribution and elimination are available $(Cl = 0.693 \, Vd \, / \, T_{1/2})$. The statistically synthesised values are updated into the output module that gives access to the parameters in a structured format.

Parser: To built up a general database, the available information must be transferred into the standardised formats. The present information is available only in free text formats. A automatic text-analysis procedure must be developed to integrate the available information and systems into the common database.

Standardisation: We will use the ATC code as proposed by the WHO for drug classification, that is the anatomical, therapeutical, and chemical classification (ATC). Different specifications are associated with drugs [13]. Some specifications are numerical some semantic. For each classification and standardisation a specific format must be defined.

Evaluation: Recording of the clinical course of representative patients will be done. The data of interest are age, weight, creatinine, current medication, drug level measurements, and surrogate or essential outcome parameters (stay in hospital, complications, death). For this purpose a computerised patient recording system must be developed and designed based on the already available resources. Specific information must be incorporated manually, and later automatically. Drug level measurements are available for the most critical drugs (aminoglycosides, vancomycin, digoxin, digitoxin, phenytoin, carbamazepine, theophylline, cyclosporin, tacrolimus, mycophenolate). The recorded dosage practice is compared to the calculated dosage alterations as proposed from the system.

Navigator: For the internet-based version a navigtor must be designed. The navigator allows to find the way through the ubiqituous information. This must be specifically designed for drug-related, web-based systems. The user will need help with the available information either the Web-based [14] or the different systems (Drugdex, Micromedix, Medline). Navigators have been developed and should be implemented within our environment to provide this utility [15]. The unified database can be used to derive specified versions for each European country. For this purpose, a translation or interpreter function must be installed. Drug safety aspects must be solved before posing sensitive drug information into the internet [16].

Acknowledgement: PharmDIS is founded by the European Commission as CRAFT project BMH4-CT98-9548.

References

1. Beller GA, Smith TW, Abelmann HW, Haber E, Hood W. Digitalis intoxication: a prospective clinical study with serum level correlations. N Engl J Med **284** (1971) 989–996
2. Appel GB, Neu HC. Nephrotoxicity of antimicrobial agents. N Engl J Med **296** (1977) 722–728
3. Canal P, Chatelut E. Guichard S. Practical treatment guide for dose individualisation in cancer chemotherapy. Drugs **56** (1998) 1019–1038
4. Evans WE, Relling MV, Rodman JH, Crom WR, Boyett JM, Pui CH. Conventional compared with individualized chemotherapy for childhood acute lymphoblastic leukemia. N Engl J Med **338** (1998) 499–505
5. Poller L, Shlach CR, MacCallum PK, Johansen AM, Mnster AM, Magalhes A, Jespersen J, European Concerted Action on Anticoagulation. Multicentre randomised study of computerised anticoagulant dosage. Lancet **352** (1998) 1505–1509
6. Evans RS, Pestotnik SL, Classen DC, Clemmer TP, Weaver LK, Orme JF, Lloyd JF, Burke JP. A computer-assisted management program for antibiotics and other intiinfective agents. N Engl J Med **338** (1998) 232–238
7. Dettli L. Drug dosage and renal disease. Clin Pharmacol Therap **16** (1974) 274–279
8. Cockcroft DW, Gault MH. Prediction of creatinine clearance from serum creatinine. Nephron **16** (1976) 31–41

9. Levey AS, Bosch JP, Lewis JB, Green T, Rogers N, Roth D. A more accurate method to estimate glomerular filtration rate from serum creatinine: a new prediction equation. Ann Intern Med **130** (1999) 461–470

10. Sheiner LB, Beal SL. Bayesian individualization of pharmacokinetics: simple implementation and comparison with non-bayesian methods. J Pharm Sci **71** (1982) 1344–1348

11. Holford NHG (ed.). Taeschner W, Vozeh S, Bennett WM, Dettli L, Hebert MF, Begg EJ, Atkinson HC, Darlow BA, Holford NHG. Drug Data Handbook. Adis, Auckland (1998) 244 pages

12. Czock D, Giehl M. Aminoglycoside pharmacokinetics and -dynamics: a nonlinear approach. Int J Clin Pharmacol Therap **33** (1995) 537–539

13. Miller GC, Britt H. A new drug classification for computer systems: the ATC extension code. Int J Biomed Comput **40** (1995) 121–124

14. McMullin ST, Reichley RM, Watson LA, Steib SA, Frisse ME, Bailey TC. Impact of a Web-based clinical information system on cisapride drug interactions and patient safety. Arch Intern Med **159** (1999) 2077–2082

15. Ruan W, Burkle T, Dudeck J. An object-oriented design for automated navigation of semantic networks inside a medical data dictionary. Artif Intell Med **18** (2000) 83–103

16. Bloom BS, Iannacone RC. Internet availability of prescription pharmaceuticals to the public. Ann Intern Med **131** (1999) 830–833

Discrete Simulations of Cadaver Kidney Allocation Schemes

Dino Alberto Mattucci[1], Velio Macellari[1], Pietro Chistolini[1],
Gianluca Frustagli[1]

[1] Istituto Superiore di Sanita', Laboratory of Biomedical Engineering
Viale Regina Elena 299,
00161 Rome, Italy
{mattucci, velmac, chistol, gianfrus}@iss.it

Abstract The thesis of this study is that the use of discrete simulations is the most appropriate instrument to support the definition of any organs allocation procedure. We studied the influence of recipient pool size on the probability of obtaining a good match grade and the exchange rate between regional and/or interregional organizations for two different hypothesis of national allocation schemes. We also showed the potential of simulation methods at assessing the most appropriate adjustments for the optimization of any allocation scheme.

1 Introduction

The main objectives pursued in an organ allocation procedure are two: improve the probability of survival of the transplanted organs, and guarantee the patients in the waiting list a fair treatment. At the same time it is necessary to stimulate transplantation activity, which, in relation to the Italian situation, could mean a correct distribution of organs among the various transplantation centers within the regional and interregional organizations.

Therefore, The design of allocation criteria that will satisfy such requirements is an issue which has not straightforward solution. Whichever the allocation criteria chosen, it is not possible to foresee the rate of attainment of the prefixed objectives through analytical procedures.

The thesis of this study is that the use of discrete simulations [1] is the most appropriate instrument to support the definition of any organs allocation procedure. This approach has deserved considerable attention by an important supranational transplant organization like Eurotransplant [2]. Simulations offer the advantage to account for all the scientific knowledge available in the identification of the best algorithm and the formalization of objectives, and concurs to an estimation of the probability of the clinical outcomes. This is an extraordinary advantage over any approach based on the direct experimentation, which does not offer the possibility to optimize the adopted criteria or the attainable result.

R.W. Brause and E. Hanisch (Eds.): ISMDA 2000, LNCS 1933, pp. 225–233, 2000.

The effect of HLA matching on the outcome of cadaver kidney transplants has been already demonstrated [3]. It is possible to obtain both exact and qualitative information on how a variety of parameters influence the outcome of an HLA-oriented selection algorithm.

Mickey [4] studied the influence of recipient pool size on the probability of obtaining a good match grade. We have applied this kind of analysis to the Italian case; the data on 5492 donors were utilized to estimate the effect of pool size on match grade and on organ exchange rate between regional and/or interregional organizations for two different hypothesis of national allocation schemes. We should keep in mind that at present there is no national allocation scheme for the kidney.

Another aspect we explored regards to the two objectives of any organ allocation procedure: a good transplant follow-up and the fairness of treatment of the patients which is directly associated with the waiting time in list. Because of the shape of the frequency distribution of the clinical characteristics considered for the recipient selection, not all patients in the waiting list have "a priori" the same chance to receive a transplant in a reasonable time. For example, patients who possess rare HLA antigens have a lower probability of receiving a donor kidney if the selection is strictly determined by HLA matching. On the other hand, if the selection is based only on waiting times we obtain a significant decrease in the survival of transplants. Simulations can help minimize these effects and optimize the allocation algorithm with well suited adjustments.

2 Materials and Methods

Two methods were used to simulate the organ allocation process, both developed with "Mathematica" by Wolfram research [5]:

2.1 Method 1: Steady-State Simulation

In brief [2], one donor is taken from the pool; the others are considered to be potential recipients. For each donor the number of HLA-A, -B. -DR mismatches is calculated in relation to every patient in the waiting list. The procedure is repeated for all the patients in the list. The probability of mismatch is computed for different waiting list sizes RWL using elements of combinatorial calculus. If WL is the dimension of the simulation pool and M_k the number of possible recipients for a donor with $\geq k$ mismatch (with $0 \leq k \leq 6$) in this pool, the probability p_k to find at least one patient with $\geq k$ mismatch on a waiting list of size RWL (with RWL $\leq$ WL) is

$$p_k = \frac{\binom{M_k}{RWL}}{\binom{WL}{RWL}}. \tag{1}$$

The probability P_k to find at least one patient with k mismatch is then $P_k=p_k-p_{k+1}$ for k < 6 and $P_k=p_k$ for k=6. The mean of P_k for all donors is the k mismatch probability for the first kidney of an average donor. There are two methods currently used in Italy to calculate the mismatch grade. In the method herewith called "O" the blank values are considered to have the same value as the not blank one, and in the method herewith called "E" the blank values are assumed to have a value which is always different from the antigens considered for mismatch grade evaluation.

To estimate the organs exchange rate among the Italian regional and interregional (composed by two or more regional bodies) organizations, we assigned the waiting lists these representative dimensions: 100, 500 and 1000 for the regional list, 2000 for the interregional list and 5492 for the national list.

The two national algorithms tested were both strictly HLA oriented. The first to receive a transplant are patients with 0 mismatch, then patients with 1.0.0 or 0.1.0 or 1.1.0 mismatch (for instance 1.0.0 means 1 mismatch in locus A and 0 mismatch in locus B and DR), defined as second band criteria hereafter.

Algorithm A: Organs are first allocated with 0 MM (mismatch) at the regional level; if no patients are found, the algorithm searches for patients with the same condition at the interregional level, and then on the national waiting list. The same steps are followed for the second band. If no patients are found through these criteria, the organ is allocated within the regional list.

Algorithm B: Organs are first allocated with 0 MM or following the second band criteria at the regional level. If no patients are found, the algorithm goes on to search only for patients with 0 MM at the interregional level and then on the national waiting list. If this should fail, the algorithm detects the organs responding to the second band criteria. If again no patients are found with these latter criteria, the organ is allocated within the regional list.

This means that algorithm B attempts the highest number of organs within the regional waiting list. We give an estimation of the effect of this features when applied to the Italian situation.

2.2 Method 2: Dynamic Simulation

In this case our goal was to have complete control over the variables of the simulation and we, therefore, created a virtual waiting list whose statistical characteristics were coherent with real ones.

By this method we studied the waiting list and its temporal evolution as a function of the transplants carried out with a fixed criterion of allocation. We first describe how the waiting list has been generated. The single virtual patient is represented by two variable, the same as those introduced in the allocation algorithm:
1.   waiting time (in months)
2.   six values relative to the first and the second antigen A, B and DR.

All values were generated developing a procedure known as "Robin Hood" 's algorithm [6] which generates random values following any given discrete distribution of frequencies or probabilities.

The list generated was of 6000 patients which is approximately the dimension of an hypothetical national waiting list for kidney transplant. It is worth noting no correlation term has been introduced between the six antigens values, but the ensuing error is negligible. On the initial waiting list we entered the patients with a waiting time of 0 to 60 months (with a negative exponential distribution). No significant influence of the initial waiting time distribution on the results was found after several simulations.

Both transplants and new patients in list were simulated with a relative probability equal to the unit, which means that, in average, for every transplant there was a new entry in list. Therefore we ran simulations constraining the dimension of the waiting list to be constant in time. Robin Hood generated the virtual donors with the same statistical properties of the patients. Obviously this is not necessarily true for real transplant, but with this approximation we have avoided other factors of difficult interpretation. Moreover, after every transplant or entry in list, the waiting time grew of a constant amount equal to 1 month every 100 transplants/new entry. Several tests were made before obtaining a certain stability in the results.

The tested criterion of allocation defines a transplant priority score:

$$\alpha(NM) + \beta(TA) = Pt, \ 0 \le Pt \le 100 \quad \alpha + \beta = 1 \tag{2}$$

Where α and β are the weights assigned to the patient/donor mismatch score and to the waiting time score, respectively; the final score will always be a number between 0 and 100. NM indicates the mismatch score that is:

$$NM = (6 - (number \ of \ mismatch)) \times \frac{100}{6} \tag{3}$$

As for the score assigned to the waiting time we have:

$$TA = (waiting \ time \ in \ months) \times \frac{100}{(largest \ waiting \ time \ in \ the \ list)} \tag{4}$$

To obtain statistically reliable results we simulated cycles of 20000 transplant/new entry events.

It is important to emphasize that the first method uses real data because it is prediction oriented, and that the second method is designed on well defined mathematical models because its seeks an optimization of the algorithm [7].

3 Results and Discussion

Steady-state simulations give the theoretically attainable match grade which is in general higher than the actual ones for two reasons: i) we used donors as recipients and this means that the data had already gone through some sort of selection, ii) we did not estimate the effects of the differences between donor and recipients population on these data. In view of the direct proportionality between mismatch grade and first year graft survival [8], Tables 1 and 2 show the strong influence of waiting list size on transplant success. In the case of the method "O" almost 85% of transplants can be done with 0 or 1 mismatch on a waiting list of 5492 patients, in contrast to only 32% on a list of 100 recipients. There is also a big difference between the methods "O" and "E" as far the match grade attainable on a waiting list of a fixed size; this is particularly evident for transplants with 0 MM, which means that in average the data we used had only one blank in either locus A or B or DR. Anyway, the results obtained demonstrate the necessity of a rigorous formalization of the evaluation of mismatch grade when an organ is transplanted in Italy.

Table 1. Distribution of the probability of a transplant with a fixed mismatch grade evaluated by method "O" for different pool sizes in Italy: result of a steady-state simulation. CTS- Data from a 1993 report about Western Europe transplants by the Collaborative Transplant Study.

Pool size	0MM	1MM	2MM	3MM	4MM	5/6 MM	1.0.0-0.1.0-1.1.0	Others 1MM and 2MM
5492	25.75	59.50	14.73	0.02	<0.01	0	72.85	1.38
3000	21.14	60.40	18.40	0.05	<0.01	0	76.65	2.15
2000	18.06	59.79	22.04	0.11	<0.01	0	78.93	2.90
1500	15.98	58.65	25.18	0.18	<0.01	0	80.27	3.61
1000	13.25	56.04	30.33	0.39	<0.01	0	81.35	5.01
500	9.25	49.18	40.23	1.34	<0.01	0	80.30	9.11
200	5.37	37.36	51.89	5.38	<0.01	0	71.26	17.99
100	3.42	28.70	57.13	10.75	<0.01	0	60.79	25.04
50	2.19	22.12	59.66	16.02	<0.01	0	51.42	30.36

Table 2. Distribution of the probability of a transplant with a fixed mismatch grade evaluated by method "E" for different pool sizes in Italy: result of a steady-state simulation. CTS- Data from a 1993 report about Western Europe transplants by the Collaborative Transplant Study.

Pool size	0MM	1MM	2MM	3MM	4MM	5/6 MM	1.0.0-0.1.0-1.1.0	Others 1MM and 2MM
5492	7.10	54.34	36.85	1.71	<0.01	0	73.96	17.22
3000	4.99	51.13	41.72	2.15	<0.01	0	74.96	17.89
2000	3.83	47.62	45.91	2.64	<0.01	0	75.03	18.50
1500	3.13	44.49	49.22	3.15	<0.01	0	74.67	19.04
1000	2.32	39.34	54.13	4.20	<0.01	0	73.38	20.09
500	1.34	29.54	61.54	7.52	<0.01	0	68.07	23.02
200	0.61	17.58	64.73	16.86	0.20	<0.01	54.00	28.30
100	0.34	10.94	61.35	26.93	0.43	<0.01	40.85	31.45
50	0.19	6.63	56.46	36.05	0.66	<0.01	29.84	33.25

Using the data of Tables 1 and 2 we have been able to evaluate the kidney exchange rate at the national level between the different Italian interregional organizations; figure 1 shows the percentage of kidneys shared by a regional organization at the national level according to algorithm A and B for methods "O" and "E". The results obtained ranged from a 25% of a list of 100 patients to 7.5% of a list of 1000 patients.

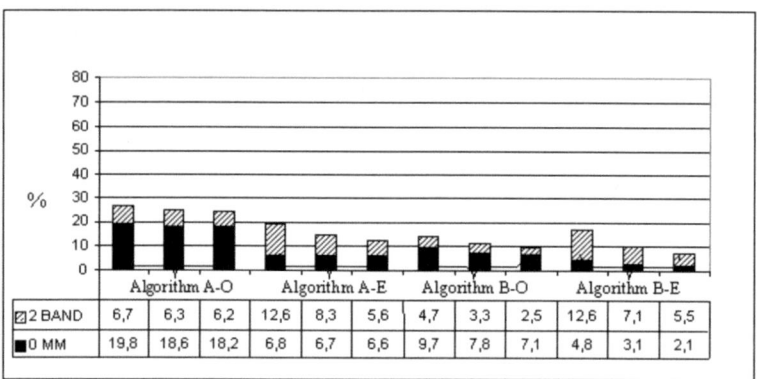

Fig. 1. Percentage of kidneys shared at the national level by three regional waiting lists (sized from left to right: 100, 500 and 1000 patients) according to algorithms A and B following methods "O" and "E" for mismatch grade evaluation.

Figure 2 reports the total percentage of organs transplanted with 0 mismatch. The differences estimated are important: with method "O" this percentage is twice as high for algorithm A when compared to algorithm B. This entails a substantial variation in transplant survival rate.

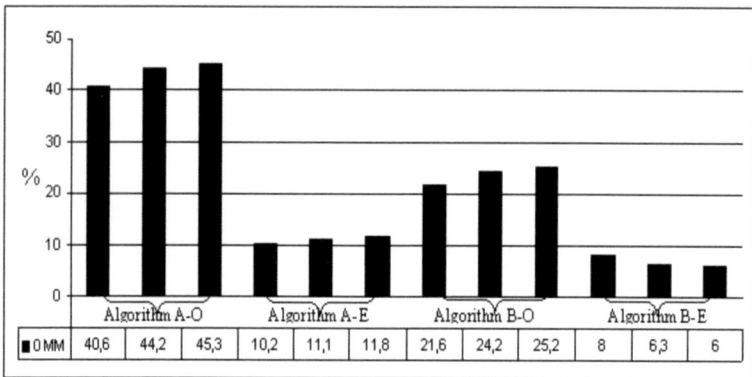

Figure 2. Total percentage of kidneys transplanted with 0 mismatch by three regional waiting lists (sized from left to right: 100, 500 and 1000 patients) according to algorithms A and B following methods "O" and "E" for mismatch grade evaluation.

The two algorithms differ depending on the method been used for counting the number of mismatch. The difference between algorithm A and algorithm B is clearer when applying method "O", with method "E" this difference is less overt, and the initial dimension of the regional list influence the percentage of shared organs.

We used the dynamic simulation to weigh the influence of waiting time and mismatch grade, on the statistical characteristics of the waiting list and the transplants carried out. The goal of this procedure is to optimize the algorithm itself. The results are analyzed as a function of the relative weight α given to score assigned to the number of matches. The first result we expected is shown in Figure 3: the higher the value of α , the higher the average value of the match in the simulated transplants. This also means that the overall graft survival increases. Every value in the graph is the result of a dynamic simulation of approximately 10000 transplants, having adopted an allocation criterion in which the indicated value of α is the number reported in abscissa.

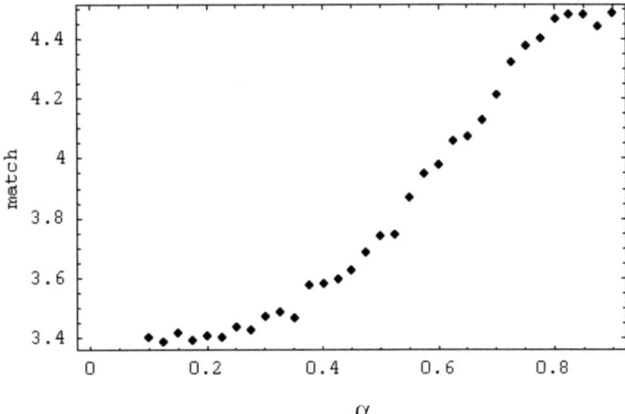

Fig. 3. Average value of match in about 10000 simulated transplants as a function of the parameter α : results of dynamical simulation.

All the simulations we ran to obtain the data reported in Figure 3 used the same initial or time zero waiting list. In Figure 4 we show the value of the average waiting time for the patients in list at the end of simulation. The more the allocation scheme weights the number of mismatches the longer the average waiting time. The reason for this is the non-uniform distribution of HLA phenotypes in the population of recipients and donors. The patients with frequent HLA-A, -B and –DR antigens have a better chance to obtain a transplant within a limited time if the value of α is higher: i.e., in the list, the percentage of a patients with rare phenotypes grows and the overall effect is an increase in the average waiting time.

Figure 5 shows the two previous results in the same graph: the average match grade attained by the simulated transplants as a function of the final average waiting time. Considering the directed correlation between the values of match and the probability of survival of the transplant it is evident that an allocation algorithm implies a compromise between the probability of survival of the transplant and a fair distribution of the waiting times among the patients in list; where one variable increases the other one decreases and "viceversa".

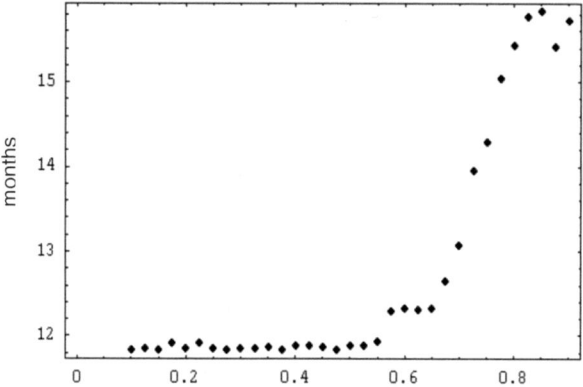

Fig. 4. Average value of waiting time as a function of parameter α for the patients on the list at the end of the simulation

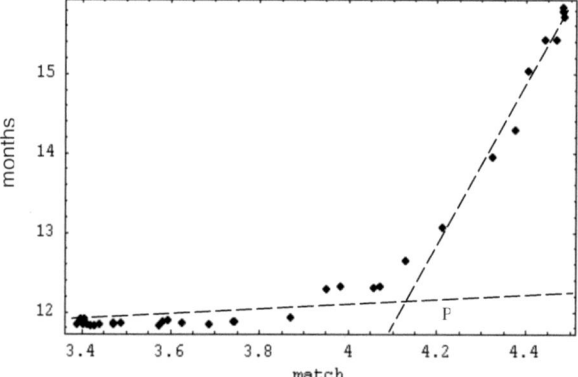

Fig. 5. Average value of waiting time for the patients in the list after the simulation as a function of average match grade in the transplants. Point P is the intersection of two linear regressions which best fit the first and the final trend of the experimental data.

From the data reported in Figure 5 we could make an estimation of the value of parameter α for which the increase in average waiting time is kept low and the survival of the grafts is still good. As a point of fact we observed that the trend of the experimental curve reveals sort of a threshold value for which the growth of the average waiting time is remarkable. Fitting the initial and the final part of the curve in Figure 5 with two linear regressions we obtained a threshold value of α equal to 0.65 which does not differ greatly from a value reported by G.Opelz [9].

4   Conclusions

The study of the effects of an allocation algorithm on the statistical properties of the waiting list and the transplants carried out is a complex issue, as it probably follows a chaotic dynamics with stocastic properties. This is the reason why simulations are the only tool we have to make predictions in this field. The influence of waiting list size on a "good" match grade ratio has been shown. These results, along with the knowledge of the magnitude of organ exchange among the different interregional organizations supported the first proposal for a national kidney allocation scheme in Italy.

We also showed the potential of simulation methods at assessing the most appropriate adjustments for the optimization of any allocation scheme. In the future we intend to focus on the characteristic times of the system as we believe they present very interesting clinical [10] and statistical aspects to be investigated.

References

1.   C. Cassandras, and S. Lafortune: Introduction to discrete event systems. Academic Publishers, (1999).
2.   T. Wujack e G. Opelz: Computer analysis of cadaver kidney allocation procedures, *Transplantation*, (1993).
3.   Opelz G.: The role of HLA matching on surival of second kidney transplants in cyclo-treated recipients, *Transplantation*, (1989).
4.   M. Mickey: Recipient pool sizes for prioritized hla matching, *Transplantation*, (1989).
5.   Hal R. Varian: Computational economics and finance: modelling and analysis with Mathematica, *editor TELOS/Springer-Verlag*, (1996).
6.   Hal R. Varian: Computational Economics and Finance: Modeling and Analysis with Mathematica, editor TELOS/Springer-Verlag, (1996).
7.   Goldberg, D. E.: Genetic algorithms in search, optimization and machine learning, *Reading, Mass: Addison-Wesley*, 1989.
8.   Terasaki PI Toyotome A. Mickey M.R. et al: Patient, graft and functional survival rates: an overview, *Clinical Kidney Transplant*, 1985.
9.   T. Wujack e G. Opelz: A proposal for improved cadaver kidney allocation, *Transplantation*, dicembre 1993.
10.   Yakowitz S: Computational probability and simulation, *Addison-Wesley, Reading, Mass.*, 1977.

Bootstrap and Cross-Validation to Assess Complexity of Data-Driven Regression Models

Willi Sauerbrei[1] and Martin Schumacher[1]

[1] Institut für Medizinische Biometrie und Medizinische Informatik, Universitätsklinikum Freiburg, Stefan-Meier-Strasse 26, D-79104 Freiburg
wfs@imbi.uni-freiburg.de

Abstract. The number of potential variables included into a regression model is often too large and a more parsimonious model may be preferable. Selection strategies are widely used, but there are few analytical results about their properties. To investigate problems as replication stability, model complexity and selection bias we use bootstrap and cross-validation methods. For stepwise strategies, we discuss the importance of the predefined selection level. The methods are illustrated by investigating prognostic factors for survival time of patients with malignant glioma in the framework of a Cox regression model.

1 Introduction

In the application of regression models, data analysts are often faced with many predictor variables which may have an influence on an outcome variable. In the following $\mathbf{X}=(X_1,...,X_k)$ denotes the vector of predictor variables under consideration and $g(\mathbf{X})=\beta_1 X_1+...+\beta_k X_k$ a linear function. A linear regression model with a vector of regression coefficients $\beta=(\beta_1,..., \beta_k)$ is given by

$$E(Y|\mathbf{X})=\beta_0+g(\mathbf{X}) \qquad \text{with var } (Y|\mathbf{X})=\sigma^2.$$

For possibly censored survival times, Cox's proportional hazards model is usually chosen [7]. The influence of predictors is modelled through the hazard rate

$$\lambda (t|\mathbf{X})=\lambda_0 (t)\exp\{g(\mathbf{X})\},$$

with $\lambda_0(t)$ denoting an unspecified base-line hazard rate.

If the number of variables is large, a parsimonious model involving fewer variables may be preferable. One aim of the analysis is the selection of the subset of `important' predictors, i.e. the variables which have an influence on the outcome. For this task, sequential strategies, such as forward (FS), stepwise (StS) or backward elimination (BE) procedures, or all subset selection with different optimization criteria, such as Mallows' C_p, the information criterion of Akaike (AIC) or the Bayesian Information Criterion (BIC) are often used [8]. As there are only few analytical results about their properties their usefulness is discussed controversially.

R.W. Brause and E. Hanisch (Eds.): ISMDA 2000, LNCS 1933, pp. 234–241, 2000.
© Springer-Verlag Berlin Heidelberg 2000

If several predictors are available the 'correct' model, which includes all important and no noise variables, is unlikely to be selected. In the linear regression model, elimination of variables with influence on the outcome results in biased estimates for the selected parameter set (omission bias), except for the special case of orthogonality between the selected variables and the nonselected important variables [8]. Underfitting increases the error sum of squares and the estimate of the error variance σ^2, complex models with many variables may overfit the data. Apart from difficulties in interpreting the contribution of each predictor, overfitting increases the estimates of the variance for each regression estimate and increases the variance of the prediction. The increase depends on the amount of multicollinearity. These problems usually transfer to more general regression models, in which additional problems may also occur. A penalty term per variable can be used in order to control the complexity of a final model derived by all subset selection procedures, and a suitable selection level may be chosen for sequential strategies. However, in many publications the selection level of the sequential strategy is not even stated explicity.

Depending on the aim of a study, the severity of potential biases induced by model selection may be considered differently. For a predictive model, the main concern may be its overoptimism. A 'complex' model may be tolerated and the contribution of each individual variable is hardly considered. In medical applications the effect of a single variable, and whether it should be included in a final model, is also often of additional interest.

With increasing computational power, resampling methods such as crossvalidation and bootstrapping [5] are becoming more popular for investigating problems caused by data-driven model building. Although the theoretical basis is often not well developed, these approaches do offer possibilities for such investigations where results based on asymptotic theory are scarce. This will be shown by investigating potential prognostic factors for patients with a brain tumor in the framework of a Cox regression model. Using backward elimination with different selection levels, cross validation and bootstrap resampling, emphasis is placed on the choice between simple and complex final models.

In chapter 2 we will discuss several problems caused by variable selection. We will propose variable selection within bootstrap samples to investigate stability of selected models and crossvalidation to estimate shrinkage factors for coping with selection bias. In chapter 3 we will investigating the prognostic values of factors for patients with malignant glioma in the framework of a Cox regression model with special emphasis on the complexity of selected models. We will illustrate the possibilities of the resampling approaches. Based on their results we will argue in the discussion for greater simplicity of final regression models.

2 Resampling Approaches to Investigate Problems Caused by Variable Selection

When the same selection procedure as for the original data is used in an 'ideal' validation study, e.g. on a population defined by the same inclusion and exclusion criteria, then (nearly) the same variables should be selected. This is sometimes called 'replication stability'. Differences between selected variables in two populations may increase when procedures selecting more complex models are used. Using bootstrap data sets, replication stability can be investigated for regression models. For survival data, the records of patients with complete observations (predictors, outcome and a censoring indicator) can be used as the sampling units. Sauerbrei and Schumacher [11] took 100 bootstrap samples and selected with the same stepwise procedure as in the original analysis a final model in each of the replications. Generally, important variables should be included in most of the replications and the inclusion frequencies may be used as a criterion for the importance of a variable. Sauerbrei and Schumacher [11] extended earlier approaches [4] concentrating on demonstration of the instability of selected final models. They considered the inclusion frequencies of all possible pairs of variables to cope with the problem of correlated variables where often only one 'representative' is selected in each bootstrap replication. They proposed two different selection strategies depending on whether only strong factors are of interest, or whether weak factors should also be included in a final model.

If estimation of regression parameters is based on the same data which were used to select the final model, selection bias can be a central problem [8]. Motivated by the PRESS (predicted residual sum   of squares) approach, where $\beta_{(-i)}$ denotes the regression coefficient of a variable when the ith observation is eliminated, a (leave-one-out) crossvalidated log likelihood (l*) approach was proposed to investigate this issue for generalized linear models and survival time models by van Houwelingen and le Cessie [16], and extended by Verweij and van Houwelingen [17]. They proposed the crossvalidated loglikelihood (l*(1)) as a measure of the predictive value of the model and maximising this likelihood gives a (global) shrinkage factor. This factor may be used to reduce the bias of parameter estimates caused by model building. Their shrinkage factor shrinks each component of the vector of regression coefficients by the same constant amount. As selection bias is mainly a severe problem for weak factors [9], [12], this global shrinkage factor may 'overcorrect' and bias towards zero the effect of a strong variable. Hence Sauerbrei [10] proposed parameterwise shrinkage factors (PWSF) for each component of the $\beta_{(-i)}$ vector as an extension by maximising the crossvalidated loglikelihood as a function of the individual components.

3 Glioma Study

A randomized trial to compare two chemotherapy regimes included 447 patients with malignant glioma. At the time of analysis, 293 patients had died and median survival time from randomization was about 11 months. Besides therapy, 12 variables (age, three ordinal and eight binary variables) which might influence survival time were considered. The three variables measured on an ordinal scale (Karnofsky index, type of surgical resection and grade of malignancy) were each represented by two dummy variables, resulting in a total of 15 predictors denoted by X_1, ..., X_{15}. More details about the study and various strategies for analysis can be found in Ulm et al [15]. In contrast to the analysis by Sauerbrei and Schumacher [11] we use only the data of 413 patients (274 events) with complete data. For the calculation of shrinkage factors the predictors are standardized to mean 0 and standard deviation 1; this standardization does not have any influence on the results of the variable selection procedures used here. The standardized regression parameter estimates in the model with all variables indicate that some strong predictors are present (Table 1). The absolute values of the standardised regression coefficients of X_5 and X_8 are around 5 and X_3 has a value of about 3. Several other variables seem to have a weaker effect on survival time, of which X_6 is significant if a selection level of 5% is chosen. For backward elimination we chose this 'usual' level and the stronger 1% criterion in addition; the level 15.7% was chosen because of its similarity to the AIC criterion in the all subset approach [13]; [10]. At the 1% level a model with four variables was chosen, one variable was added at the 5% level and another four variables at the 15.7% level. Variables selected can be identified by the results for the parameterwise shrinkage factors in the right part of table 1. The increase of the selection level usually results in models with additional factors, however, it may also happen that a variable is deleted and replaced by two or more other variables. As known from statistical theory the log likelihood values ($l(1)$) increase if variables are added to a model, however, the cross-validated log-likelihood ($l*(1)$) of the models selected by BE are already larger than the corresponding value from the full model. The shrinkage factor gives also an indication that the complex model may overfit the data. The parameterwise shrinkage factors of the models with 4 or 5 variables indicate that bias in the estimate of the regression parameters is no serious issue. However, bias is more serious for the additional 4 variables selected at the 15.7% level. PWSF from the full model are difficult to interpret. Negative values or values much larger than 1 may be caused by estimating too many shrinkage factors in the corresponding model. They should not be used as multiplicators in the usual way, but we consider them as strong indicators that estimation of the individual regression parameters is associated with serious problems because the model considered is too complex.

Using BE (0.05) as the selection strategy in 100 bootstrap samples the (in-)stability of the selected model can be shown. Only X_5 and X_8 are selected in all replications, X_3 in more than 90%, but altogether the variability of the models is obvious. The variables X_2, X_7 and X_{13} were selected in 20 respectively 5 replications, the corresponding regression parameter estimates had partly a negative and partly a positive sign. We consider this as an indication that these variables have at most a weak influence on the outcome and should be eliminated from a 'sensible' model. There is no model which was selected in a larger percentage of the replications. The bootstrap selection strategy of Sauerbrei and Schumacher [11] for strong factors selected only X_3, X_5 and X_8. The strategy for weak factors selected additionally X_6, X_9, $X_{11,}$ X_{12} and X_{14}. For more details see Sauerbrei [10].

Table 1. Glioma study: Log-likelihood without (l) and with (l*) cross-validation and a global shrinkage factor for the full model and three models selected by using backward elimination (BE) with selection levels 0.157, 0.05 and 0.01 – for individual variables standardized parameter estimates, parameterwise shrinkage factors and bootstrap inclusion frequencies are given.

Variables	All Variables			Selected Model		
				BE (0.157)	BE (0.05)	BE (0.01)
Number of Variables	15			9	5	4
l(1)	-1332.1			-1334.3	-1340.3	-1342.6
l*(1)	-1350.7			-1345.0	-1345.6	-1346.9
Shrinkage[0]	0.825			0.894	0.943	0.952
Variables	$\hat{\beta}$/SE	BIF[1]	PWSF[2]	PWSF[2]		
X_1	-1.36	30	0.20			
X_2	-0.91	20[3]	-0.31			
X_3	3.18	92	1.12	0.97	0.96	0.96
X_4	1.35	33	0.70	0.76		
X_5	5.75	100	0.97	0.98	0.98	0.98
X_6	-2.27	63	1.47	0.84	0.84	0.85
X_7	-0.23	5[3]	-16.23			
X_8	-4.90	100	1.04	0.97	0.94	0.94
X_9	-1.55	34	0.74	0.54		
X_{10}	0.69	11	-0.63			
X_{11}	1.89	59	0.77	0.70		
X_{12}	-1.80	52	0.90	0.78	0.81	
X_{13}	0.49	20[3]	-1.99			
X_{14}	1.53	49	1.10	0.52		
X_{15}	-1.08	22	-0.14			

[0] Global Shrinkage Factor
[1] BIF= Bootstrap Inclusion Frequency using BE(0.05)
[2] PWSF= Parameterwise Shrinkage Factor
[3] Negative and positive signs of the corresponding regression parameter estimate

4 Discussion

In the analysis of observational studies, statistical models are often determined by data-driven selection methods. These methods usually have only a heuristic basis and their statisitical properties are not satisfactoryly understood. Only asymptotic results for complex selection procedures are available in special situations, e.g. in the linear regression model for the asymptotic significance level of all subset procedures for the decision concerning one additional variable [13]. Their results indicate the similarity between all subset selection using AIC or C_p and backward elimination with a selection level 0.157. This is confirmed by some simulation results from Sauerbrei [9]. For sequential procedures the predefined selection level can be chosen by the investigator, but this important aspect is often ignored in practice. The aim of a specific study should have a strong influence on the choice of this level [10].

Data splitting has been proposed to investigate some of the problems of data-driven variable selection methods, but has several important disadvantages. With increased computer power resampling methods offer new insights into problems caused by complex model building procedures. They are useful tools and should complement the analysis of the original data, though for the investigation of complex relationships their theoretical background is not well understood yet. It has to be stressed that they are only heuristic proposals; several alternatives are possible and may be useful [12]. To demonstrate possibilities for the investigation of the stability of selected models and to assess the bias of parameter estimates caused by data-driven variable selection we used an analysis of survival data in the framework of a Cox regression model as an example.

In the full model the proposal to estimate parameterwise shrinkage factors suffers the problem of too many parameters to estimate. This results in difficulties in interpretation and they cannot sensibly be used in the usual context of shrinking the effect of a factor which is estimated. However, they indicate that some variables should definitively not be included in a model. This can be seen as a strong argument against the full model. In the models selected by backward elimination the estimated PWSFs seem to indicate the amount of selection bias caused by variable selection. Multiplying the regression parameters with the corresponding PWSFs may result in useful predictors. Our proposals to shrink an estimate after variable selection can be seen as an alternative to the Garotte approach of Breiman [1] and the Lasso approach of Tibshirani [14] in which shrinkage and variable selection are performed simultaneously.

Besides severe difficulties in the interpretation of complex models the behaviour of the cross-validated likelihood gives another strong argument for the preference of simpler models. The resampling approaches demonstrate the instability in the selection of weak factors and indicate a more serious selection bias in the estimated regression coefficients for weak factors. As the resulting indices from more or less complex models are often highly correlated we see the result of our investigation as an additional argument for greater simplicity of final regression models. This can be controlled by the predefined selection level or by the penalty term in all subset procedures.

Using the bootstrap, a statistician will recognize the instability in the model selected, especially when a complex model including several weak factors is chosen. In our example a different model was selected in nearly every replication. There are several explanations for this result. A weak factor has only a low power to enter the final model and will be included in only some of the replications. From correlated weak factors usually only one will be selected to represent the corresponding effect of the variables from the 'correlated cluster' of several variables [11]. If the effects are of a similar size the specific 'representative' selected in a bootstrap replication depends on chance. Furthermore variables without influence on the outcome are selected with a probability depending on selection level. If several are considered in the study, the probability that at least one of them is included in the final model is high. The stability of the selected model decreases with an increase in the number of candidate variables. First approaches to incorporate 'model uncertainty' in the data analysis more formally have been proposed and are the subject of ongoing investigations [3]; [2], [6].

Incorporating these issues in model building can reduce the over-confident inferences as they will show that approaches ignoring investigations on bias of regression estimates after selection, stability and uncertainty of selected models will lead to 'decisions that are more risky than one thinks they are' [6].

References

1. Breiman, L.: Better Subset Regression Using the Nonnegative Garotte. Technometrics **37** (1995) 373-384

2. Buckland, S.T., Burnham, K.P., Augustin, N.H.: Model Selection: An Integral Part Of Inference. Biometrics **53** (1997) 603-618

3. Chatfield, C.: Model Uncertainty, Data Mining and Statistical Inference (With Discussion). J. R. Statist. Soc. A **158** (1995) 419-466

4. Chen, C.H., George, S.L.: The Bootstrap and Identification of Prognostic Factors via Cox's Proportional Hazards Regression Model. Stat. Med. **4** (1985) 39-46

5. Efron, B., Tibshirani, R.J.: An Introduction to the Bootstrap. Chapman and Hall, London (1993)

6. Hoeting, J.A., Madigan, D., Raftery, A.E., Volinsky, C. T.: Bayesian Model Averaging: A Tutorial. Stat. Science **14** (1999) 382-417

7. Marubini, E., Valsecchi, M.G.: Analying Survivial Data from Clinical Trials and Observationals Studies. W. Chickster (1994)

8. Miller, A.J.: Subset Selection in Regression. Chapman and Hall, London (1990)

9. Sauerbrei, W.: Comparison of Variable Selection Procedures in Regression Models - a Simulation Study and Practical Examples. In: Europäische Perspek-

tiven der Medizinischen Informatik, Biometrie und Epidemiologie (eds. J. Michaelis, G. Hommel and S. Wellek) pp. 108-113. Munich (1993), MMV Medizin Verlag

10. Sauerbrei, W.: The Use of Resampling Methods to Simplify Regression Models in Medical Statistics. Appl. Stat. **48** (1999) 313-329

11. Sauerbrei, W., Schumacher, M.: A Bootstrap Resampling Procedure for Model Building: Application to the Cox Regression Model. Stat. Med. **11** (1992) 2093-2109

12. Schumacher, M., Holländer, N., Sauerbrei W.: Resampling and Cross-Validation Techniques: a Tool to Reduce Bias Caused by Model Building? Stat. Med. **16** (1997) 2813-2827

13. Teräsvirta, T., Mellin, I.: Model Selection Criteria and Model Selection Tests in Regression Models. Scand. J. Stat., **13** (1986) 159-171

14. Tibshirani, R.: Regression Shrinkage and Selection via Lasso. J. R. Statist. Soc. B **58** (1996) 267-288

15. Ulm, K., Schmoor, C., Sauerbrei, W., Kemmler, G., Aydemir, Ü., Müller, B, Schumacher, M.: Strategien zur Auswertung einer Therapiestudie mit der Überlebenszeit als Zielkriterium. Biometr. Inform. Med. Biol. **20** (1989) 171-205

16. Van Houwelingen, J.C., le Cessie, S.: Predictive Value of Statistical Models. Stat. Med. **9** (1990) 1303-1325

17. Verweij, P.J.M., Van Houwelingen, H.C.: Crossvalidation in Survival Analysis. Stat. Med. **9** (1993) 487-503

Genetic Programming Optimisation of Nuclear Magnetic Resonance Pulse Shapes

Helen Frances Gray[1], Ross James Maxwell[2]

[1]Computer Science Department, City University, Northampton Square, London, UK
H.F.Gray@city.ac.uk
[2]Gray Laboratory Cancer Research Trust, Northwood, Middlesex HA6 2JR, UK
maxwell@graylab.ac.uk

Abstract. Genetic Programming is used to generate pulse sequence elements for a Nuclear Magnetic Resonance system and evaluate them directly on that system without human intervention. The method is used to optimise pulse shapes for a series of solvent suppression problems. The method proves to be successful, with results showing an improvement in fitness of up to two orders of magnitude. The method is capable of producing both simple and novel solutions.

1   Introduction

Nuclear Magnetic Resonance (NMR) techniques have a wide range of applications from the identification of chemical compounds (with NMR spectroscopy) to the diagnosis of cancer (with (N)MR imaging). Improvements in techniques to acquire NMR data can lead to simplifications in the analysis of that data. Apart from the choice of sample and details of hardware, the main feature determining the information obtained from the NMR measurement is the choice of pulse sequence. In general, an NMR pulse sequence comprises a series of radiofrequency (RF) pulses, applied magnetic field gradients, delays and data acquisition events. However, a simple case of NMR spectroscopy requires only a single RF pulse followed by a period of data acquisition. Considerable effort and expertise has been used in designing and implementing NMR pulse sequences for specific purposes. The present study investigates the possibility of using GP to evolve one or more NMR pulse sequences elements and, ultimately, entire pulse sequences. If this is possible, it will allow collection of data to be tailored to allow for more straightforward analysis.

   Genetic Programming (GP)[1] is an evolutionary computation technique which uses a tree structure rather than a vector (e.g. as genetic algorithms do) to describe an individual or candidate solution to a problem. Techniques such as GP operate on a population of candidate solutions. They often use a generational model whereby the population is replaced by new individuals; some of which will be the same as in the previous generations and some of which will have changed through the use of the genetic operators crossover and mutation. The aim is to improve the fitness of the population as a whole, which will lead to improvement of the best individual.

R.W. Brause and E. Hanisch (Eds.): ISMDA 2000, LNCS 1933, pp. 242–249, 2000.

GP methods have previously been used with data from NMR systems including classification and feature selection of tumour data collected by NMR spectroscopy [2] and image enhancement [3]. In addition, evolutionary methods have been shown to be useful in range selection in spectroscopic infrared imaging [4], shaping of laser pulses [5] and to generate pulses for NMR spectroscopy [6]. The latter study used a subjective fitness function, interactively judging fitness.

NMR spectroscopy involves one or more radiofrequency pulses to detect the presence and quantity of different substances in a sample or region of interest. The output is displayed as a spectrum with different substances giving rise to peaks at different frequencies. It is often the case that some peaks (such as water) may dominate the spectrum and it may be desirable to suppress these or enhance others. This is especially a problem for *in vivo* NMR spectroscopy where the water concentration (about 40 M) is substantially greater than that of all biochemical compounds of interest. Elevated lactic acid concentrations are a common feature of several diseases (such as in stroke and solid tumours) but even in such cases a concentration of 1-10 mM is typical, i.e. about 10000-fold lower than that of water. The selective suppression or excitation of NMR signals can be achieved using shaped pulses with frequency selective properties. The pulse shape is described by a sequence of values of phase, amplitude and duration.

The design of such pulse shapes can be done on a theoretical basis [7]. However, for many purposes, only approximate solutions are obtained. In addition, hardware errors or deviations are not taken into account. It may be the case that new pulse shapes are variations on existing successful ones and that it may be difficult to find novel sequences. Evolutionary techniques, such as GP, offer a way of developing pulse shapes which explore a wider range of possible solutions.

There are advantages to running candidate solutions directly on an NMR system rather than in simulation. Hardware features can be incorporated into the fitness measure without needing to be explicitly programmed. This means that novel solutions that overcome hardware limitations may be discovered.

The work detailed in this paper uses GP to generate pulse sequence elements and automatically evaluate them on an NMR system without human intervention.

2   Methods

2.1 GP Parameters

The GP system used is lil-gp [8]. The functions available to the program are addition, subtraction, multiplication, protected division (returning 1.0 to a division by zero) and `writepf`. This constrains its two arguments to the ranges –360.0 to +360.0 and 0 to 1023.0 and writes them to a text file as phase and amplitude values. The duration value is set to be 1.0 for each pulse sequence element in all experiments. `writepf` also returns the value of its first argument. The terminal set consists of random real numbers in the range –1.0 to +1.0. The fitness function is as follows;

$$\text{Standardised fitness} = 1\text{-}((\text{nmr\_fit} +(3* \text{no\_lines}))/10000) \,. \qquad \textbf{(1)}$$

nmr_fit is the value returned by the NMR system and is a ratio between two of the peaks, one to be suppressed, the other detected. The value of 10000 is an arbitrary one (and thus standardised fitness is not used as a test of success). no_lines is the number of lines in the pulse file generated by the individual. This term is included to encourage the development of longer pulse files. The factor of three was included so that the term is relatively significant in early generations where raw fitness values are small and becomes relatively less significant as raw fitness values increase.

2.2   NMR Setup

The NMR system involves a 4.7 Tesla magnet and a Varian NMR spectroscopy/imaging system running VNMR (version 6.1) software (Varian, Palo Alto, CA, USA). The sample used in the experiments is 255 mM trimethylsilyl-2,2,3,3-tetradeutero-propionate sodium (TSP) dissolved in a 1:2 mixture of water and dimethylsulphoxide (DMSO). This was contained in a 30µl spherical bulb, placed in the centre of a 13mm diameter two-turn coil tuned to the ^{1}H NMR resonance frequency (200 MHz). This sample gives three signals in the ^{1}H NMR spectrum: the DMSO and TSP signals are 370 Hz and 900 Hz upfield, respectively, of the water signal.

Matlab (The Mathworks, Natick, MA, USA) is used for receiving and copying the files and for displaying results.

2.3 Experimental Setup

At each generation of the GP run each individual is evaluated, producing a pulse shape in text format (referred to as a pulse file). The pulse file is made available to the NMR system which then activates the pulse-acquire sequence with a pulse width of 200-2000 µs (fixed for any given GP run). The offset frequency of the pulse is set to be the same as the water resonance frequency. The resulting spectrum is received by the NMR system. Calculations of peak heights and ratios take place there and the resulting value (nmr_fit) is returned to the GP program to allow for fitness calculation. The evaluation of each new pulse occurs every five to eight seconds.

The aim of the first experiment was to maximise the ratio between DMSO and water. The second was to maximise the ratio of TSP to water. In both of these cases the task was therefore to suppress the signal (water) at the pulse carrier frequency compared to off-resonance signals (DMSO or TSP). The third experiment was to maximise the ratio of TSP to (DMSO + water).

All experiments were run with a population of 50 over 50 generations. The replication and mutation rates were each set to 0.1 and the crossover to 0.8. Initial depth of trees was between two and six with a maximum depth of 20. Each experiment was run three times with different random number seeds.

Results of the second experiment were compared to several known pulse shapes and to sets of 2550 random pulse shapes (i.e. the same number of pulse shapes were tested in the random runs as in the GP runs).

3   Results

The results from the first set of experiments showed an increase in mean fitness of the population as well as an increase in the fitness of the best. The best individuals had fitness values more than 100-fold better than the mean fitness value seen in the initial (random) generation. Figure 1a shows the increase in mean fitness in one run.

The spectra produced from experiments can be compared with that produced by a square pulse. The square pulse shape is produced by values [0.0, 1023.0, 1.0] describing phase, amplitude and relative duration, respectively. The resulting spectrum is shown in Figure 1b.

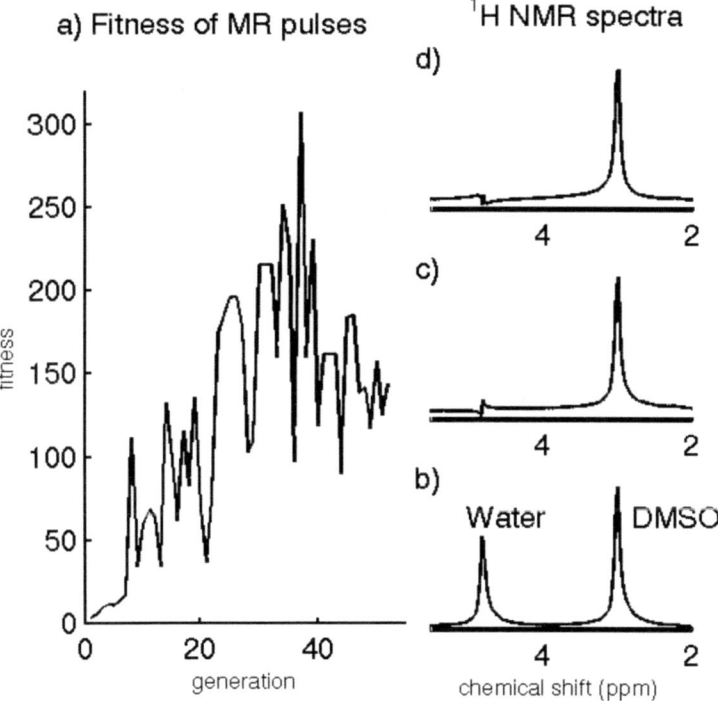

Fig. 1. Results of the experiment to maximise the ratio between DMSO and water. a) mean fitness changes during GP run ; ^{1}H NMR spectra with b) square pulse c) 1-1 like pulse from GP run and d) best pulse from GP run.

Running experiments on the NMR system directly has the effect that identical runs will not always produce identical results, although the differences are small. For this reason all the results in this paper are shown with the baseline fitness (i.e. the fitness score for a one-element square pulse shape) set to 1. This calculation was performed at the end of GP runs and allows a more meaningful comparison between runs and between experiments. An individual in generation five produced the following pulse file [179.94, 100.0, 1.0; 0.0, 95.39,1.0]. The spectrum from this is shown in Figure 1c. This is very close to simple 1–1 pulses (i.e. pulses with two elements of equal amplitude and 180^0 phase difference) which are well known for their solvent suppression properties. The 1-1 pulse is the simplest of the family of binomial selective excitation pulses and pulses approximating another binomial pulse (1-3-3-1) have also been produced in GP runs.

Later generations contained individuals producing higher fitness. The best in one run, from generation 26, had a fitness of two orders of magnitude higher than the base line value. The spectrum produced from this individual is shown in Figure 1d.

The second set of experiments was also successful, again showing improvements in fitness in the region of two orders of magnitude. Table 1 compares the results from the GP runs to pulses obtained by other methods. The pulses used were a non-selective square pulse, three binomial pulses and a BURP pulse. The BURP pulse was calculated using 'Pandora's Box' software included in the Varian NMR programme based on the method described in [7]. The pulse was defined as having a bandwidth of 2250Hz (corresponding to 2000 μs pulse width) and the off-resonance excitation optimised (to –1900Hz) to give the maximum fitness value. Figure 2 shows the spectra from these pulses.

Table 1. Comparison of GP with other pulse shapes for suppressing the water peak in relation to TSP (a-f correspond to the NMR spectra in Figure 3)

Pulse shape	Fitness
a) Square (24 μs)	1
b) 1-1 binomial (2000 μs)	3
c) 1-3-3-1 binomial (2000 μs)	41
d) 1-5-10-10-5-1 binomial (2000 μs)	335
e) BURP (2000 μs)	19
f) GP (2000 μs)	91
Best random pulses (2000 μs)	5

It can be seen that the best pulse obtained by GP performed better than the 1-1 and 1-3-3-1 binomial pulses and the BURP pulse. The 1-5-10-10-5-1 gave the best performance although from Figure 2 it can be seen that water suppression is virtually as effective with the GP pulse (f) as with the 1-5-10-10-5-1 (d). The latter pulse is also very effective in suppressing the DMSO signal but this factor was not used for the fitness calculation in these experiments. The BURP pulse performed relatively poorly. The comparison is not entirely fair as one of its features (avoiding phase distortions) is not evaluated here because signal phase is not taken into account (magnitude spectra are used). The best pulses found by random search of the same number of pulses tested in the GP runs showed only a 5-fold improvement in fitness compared to non-selective pulses.

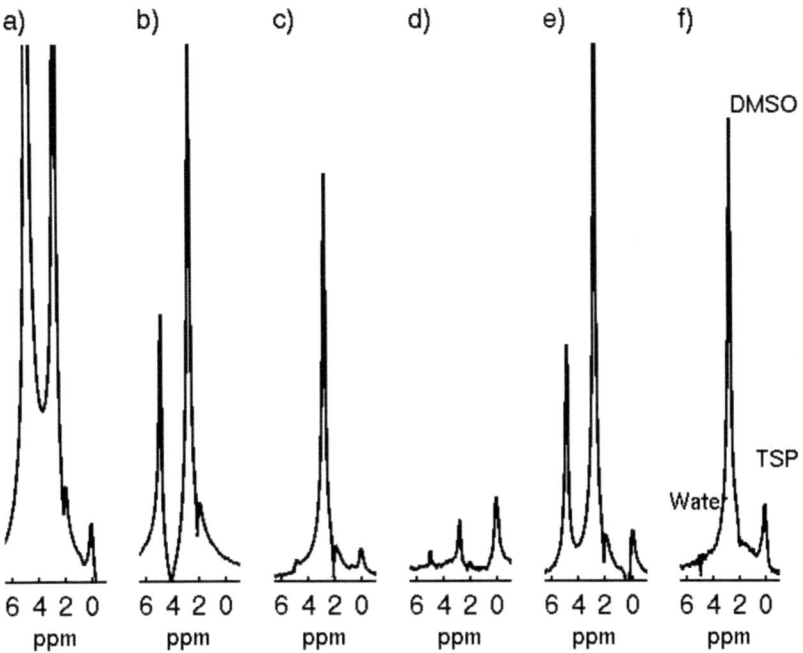

Fig. 2. Improvements in ratio between TSP and water. a) square pulse, b) 1-1 binomial, c) 1-3-3-1 binomial, d)1-5-10-10-5-1 binomial, e) BURP, f) GP

The third experiment is the hardest and improvements over 50 generations are smaller. Improvements of fitness in the order of five times as high as baseline have been found. These pulses tend to be relatively good at suppressing the water peak and relatively poor at suppressing the DMSO peak.

4   Discussion

The discovery of 1–1 pulses in the first experiment was interesting as, although not novel, they were discovered with little prior knowledge built into the system (The only assumptions made are in defining the GP fitness function and function set which are expected to be sufficient to find a solution). Later generations produced more complex pulse shapes with much higher fitness. The emergence of novel solutions argues the case for this type of method.

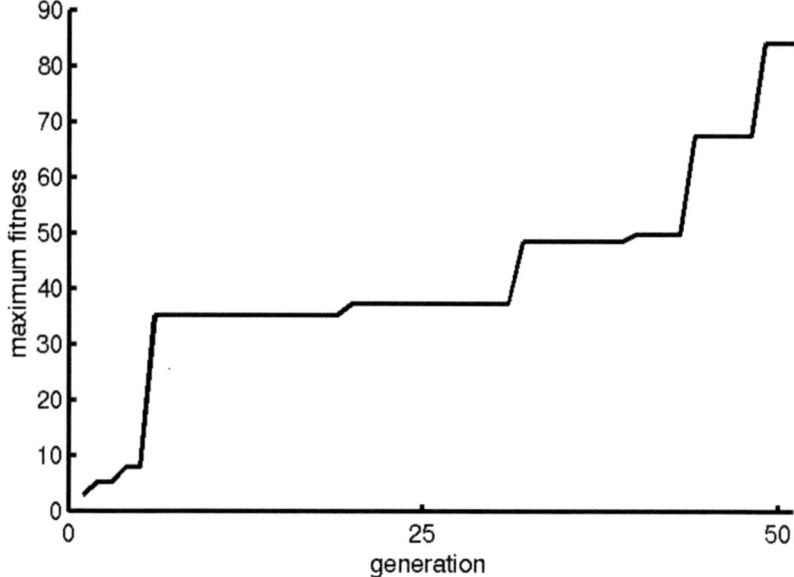

Fig. 3. Improvement in maximum fitness in each generation for pulses optimising TSP signal compared to water signal.

An advantage of techniques such as GP that work on a population of candidate solutions is that multiple solutions can be found. Although analysis of successful pulse shapes and the GP trees that produce them has not been undertaken in this work, it may be, as with [3], that there are underlying features to these that can be exploited by further experimentation or other optimisation methods.

The advantage to running experiments on hardware is that the results are optimised for the hardware. Features and limitations of the hardware are taken into account, either explicitly, as when setting up limits to values in pulse files, or implicitly as e.g. effects of non-standard lineshapes and eddy-currents should be compensated for. The main disadvantage to running directly on hardware is time. A typical experiment with 2500 individuals takes between six and eight hours to run. Taking human intervention out of the experiment has meant that it has been possible to have larger populations and a greater number of generations than previous studies e.g. [3, 6]. However, it is still a heavy time burden. There are possible ways of speeding the process up, one of which is to operate the acquisition stage in batch mode, where all pulse shapes produced by a generation could be run in one step.

The success of the method of evolving pulse shapes allows for the possibility of co-evolving more than one pulse sequence element with the final aim to evolve a complete pulse sequence. This could then be used to aid data analysis.

5   Conclusions

GP has been used to automatically generate NMR pulses and evaluate them directly on an NMR spectroscopy/imaging system.   This GP approach has automatically evolved solvent suppression pulses. Both simple and novel pulses have been obtained with virtually no prior knowledge (using only the restrictions described in the methods).

Although it is not proposed that GP necessarily is the best way of finding solvent suppression pulses, the approach does offer a number of advantages. The existence of a population of candidate solutions allows for the discovery of novel solutions and may prove to be useful in discovering common underlying features in the more successful pulses.

A second potential advantage of this approach is that RF pulses are evaluated on the NMR system itself such that hardware limitations or features are intrinsically taken into account. An additional advantage of the automatic evaluation of pulses without human intervention (compared to previous implementations of evolutionary computation [3,6]) is that a much larger number of pulse shapes can be tested.

References

1.   Koza, .J.: Genetic Programming: On the Programming of Computers by Means of Natural Selection. MIT Press, Cambridge, Massachusetts (1992)

2.   Gray, H., Maxwell, R., Martinez-Perez, I., Arus, C., Cerdan, S.: Genetic Programming for Classification and Feature Selection: Analysis of ^{1}H Nuclear Magnetic Resonance Spectra from Human Brain Tumour Biopsies. NMR in Biomedicine 11 (1998) 217-224

3.   Poli, R., Cagnoni, S.: Genetic Programming with User-Driven Selection: Experiments on the Evolution of Algorithms for Image Enhancement. In Koza et al (ed.), Genetic Programming 1997: Proceedings of the Second Annual Conference (1997) 269-277, Morgan Kaufmann

4.   van den Broek, W., Wienke, D., Melssen, W., Buydens, L.: Optimal Wavelength Range selection by a Genetic Algorithm for Discrimination Purposes in Spectroscopic Infrared Imaging. Applied Spectroscopy 51:8 (1997) 1210-1217

5.   Assion, A., Baumert, T., Bergt, M., Brixner, T., Kiefer, B., Seyfried, V., Strehle, M., Gerber, G.: Control of Chemical Reactions by Feedback-Optimized Phase-Shaped Femtosecond Laser Pulses. Science 282 (1998) 919-922

6.   Freeman, R., Wu, X.: Design of Magnetic Resonance Experiments by Genetic Evolution. Journal of Magnetic Resonance 75 (1987) 184-189

7.   Geen, H., Freeman, R.: Band-Selective Radiofrequency Pulses. Journal of Magnetic Resonance 93 (1991) 93-141

8.   Zongker, D., Punch, B.: Lil-gp User's Manual. Michigan State University (1996)

Application of a Genetic Programming Based Rule Discovery System to Recurring Miscarriage Data

Christian Setzkorn[1], Ray C. Paton[1], Leanne Bricker[2], and Roy G. Farquharson[2]

[1] Department of Computer Science, University of Liverpool, Chadwick Building, Peach Street, Liverpool L69 7ZF, United Kingdom
Email: chris@csc.liv.ac.uk (Setzkorn), rcp@csc.liv.ac.uk (Paton)
[2] Miscarriage Clinic, Liverpool Women's Hospital, Crown Street, Liverpool L8 7NJ, United Kingdom
Email: lbricker@dial.pipex.com(Bricker)

Abstract. This paper introduces a rule inference system based on the paradigm of genetic programming. Rules are deduced from a medical data set related to recurring miscarriage. A rule consists of an IF-part (antecedent) and a THEN-part (consequent). The system has to be supplied with the consequent and works out antecedents. An antecedent classifies the predictive class which is represented by the supplied consequent. The antecedents produced take the form of a tree, where Boolean operations such as AND, OR and NOT represent nodes, and Boolean expressions represent the leaves. Boolean expressions can be built from nominal and numeric attribute values, which makes the system very versatile.

1   Introduction

This paper introduces an approach developed during collaboration between the Computer Science Department of the University of Liverpool and the Recurrent Miscarriage Clinic (RMCL) of the Liverpool Women's Hospital. The approach uses the paradigm of Genetic Programming (GP) building upon the work of Freitas [3] [13]. The work can be described as an attempt to perform a generalised classification task for one prediction class which is represented by the consequent. The generalised classification task, also referred to as dependency modelling, has the goal of seeking to discover a few interesting rules called knowledge nuggets [13].

The objective of this collaboration was to produce computer-aided support tools that would help medical practitioners at the RMCL in their aim to gain new insights into the causes and unknown associations of an unfortunately common condition referred to as recurring miscarriage. Over the last ten years the staff at the RMCL have collected data from patients suffering from this

R.W. Brause and E. Hanisch (Eds.): ISMDA 2000, LNCS 1933, pp. 250–259, 2000.

condition and stored it as a spreadsheet; or rather a data matrix. In the data matrix a row contains data regarding a particular patient and the columns represent specific attributes. The attributes depict demographic details, information regarding previous pregnancies, other pertinent medical details, and observations made subsequent to referral to the RMCL.

The developed GP system has the capability of rule inference from data in the described data matrix form. The rules take the form of IF-THEN. The THEN-part (consequent) has to be supplied to the system and corresponds to a predictive class within the supplied data. The IF-part (antecedent) is evolved so that it classifies the predictive class as precisely as possible. An antecedent takes the form of a tree whose nodes may consist of Boolean operators: AND, OR and NOT. Boolean expressions represent the leaves of the tree. Examples of possible Boolean expressions are: $Age \geq 30$, $Blood\ Value\ X = abnormal$ and $Occupation\ Level = High$.

This form of rule inference is a promising approach to evolve rules which have high prediction accuracy and represent new and interesting knowledge. In addition, evolved rules can be easily understood by users [5]. This, and the fact that the system can cope with nominal and numeric data, makes this approach especially attractive.

2 Genetic Programming - A Brief Introduction

John R. Koza introduced GP in 1987 with the objective of "enabling computers to solve problems without being explicitly programmed" [6] [7]. Numerous candidate solutions for a given problem are summarised and evolved within a population in a biologically inspired manner similar to genetic algorithm (GA) [8] [9] [10]. This allows a parallel search through the given problem domain in order to find one or more satisfactory solutions to a given problem.

Candidate solutions are also referred to as representation schemes or individuals, and are usually represented in the form of a tree with changeable size. A tree consists of so-called functions, which represent the nodes, and terminals representing leaves. Functions and terminals, available for building an individual, are respectively summarised within a function or a terminal set. The chosen sets must be suitable to the problem.

The more sophisticated tree representation scheme for GP reflects a crucial difference with GA's, where the representation scheme is normally unchangeable in size and form. This makes GP a more attractive and powerful candidate for the task of data mining due to the effectiveness of GP in searching very large spaces. On the other hand, the structure of a GP system itself is very similar to those of a GA. Figure 1 shows one such possible structure.

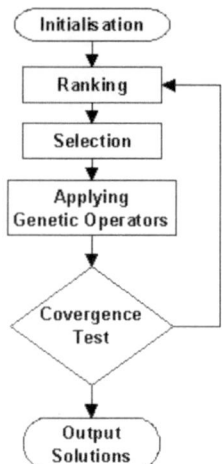

Fig. 1. Structure of a genetic algorithm.

During step 1 an initial population of candidate solutions is produced randomly. In step 2 each individual in this current population is evaluated with respect to its capability of representing a good solution for the given problem. An individual capability of solving the given problem is referred to as *fitness* and is calculated using an externally imposed fitness function, appropriate to the given problem. Step 3 consists of selecting individuals for the next generation according to their fitness. The selection process enables fitter individuals to be selected with a higher probability in comparison to individuals with lower fitness. There exist several selection processes such as roulette wheel selection, tournament selection, and ranking. [11] provides a summary and comparison of selection processes. Step 4 consists in employing the so-called genetic operators, such as crossover and mutation. The latter was not used in Koza's original form of GP. Figure 2 illustrates mutation in the case of GP.

Each individual, or rather its parts, has a specific probability of undergoing a mutation, determined by the parameter *mutation probability*. A random generator is used to decide whether or not a particular part of an individual undergoes mutation. If the value produced by the random generator is less than or equal to the *mutation probability* then the part of the tree is created anew using the supplied function and terminal set. Figure 3 illustrates crossover.

Two individuals are required in order to perform crossover in its simplest form. One possible implementation of crossover is to build a sub-population by randomly removing individuals from the current population. The choice of an individual for that sub-population works on the same principle as described for mutation, by using a random generator. Whether or not an individual is chosen is determined by the parameter *crossover probability*.

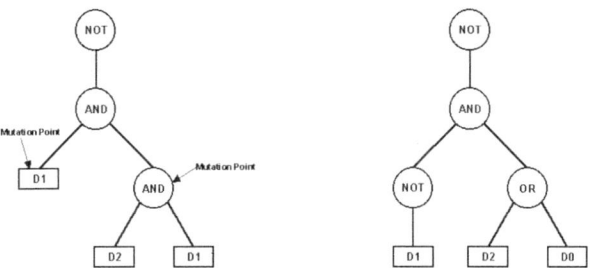

Fig. 2. Example of genetic operation mutation for genetic programming. On the left is an individual before mutation (parts to be mutated are marked), on the right of the figure is the result of the mutation.

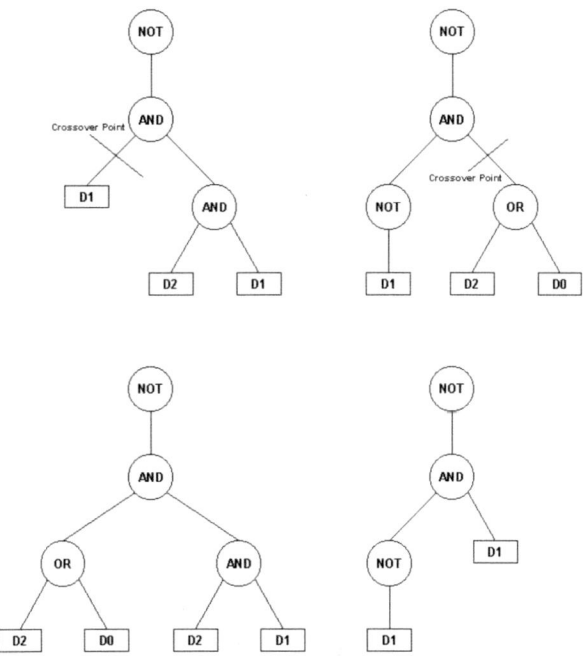

Fig. 3. Example of genetic operation crossover for genetic programming (D0 - D2 represent terminals).

Note, that it must be ensured that the sub-population has an even number of individuals. Consequently, individual pairs are taken from this sub-population, undergo crossover and are returned to the original population. For each individual a so-called crossover point is randomly determined, as shown at the top of figure 3. The parts below each crossover point are exchanged between the two individuals. The bottom of the same figure shows the result of crossover.

The next step is to perform the convergence test, which determines whether or not the system terminates and presents the individuals in the current population as solutions to the given problem, or evolves the population further by repeating steps 2 to 5 (see figure 1). A termination criterion may be a specific number of iterations or a specific fitness level to be achieved by the fittest individuals.

3   Details of the Implemented GP System

This section supplies some details of the implemented GP system. More information is available in [4].

Representation Scheme: An individual takes the form of a tree, where the function set may consist of three Boolean operations: *OR; AND; NOT.* The terminals take the form of Boolean expressions built depending on the supplied data set. A Boolean expression is composed of an attribute name, relational operator, and an attribute value. Three conditions are introduced which must be fulfilled during the creation of a tree: (1) Each attribute from the supplied data set can only be used once to build a Boolean expression. (2) The attribute(s) used to build the consequent must not be used to build a Boolean expression. (3) The depth of the tree is limited by the number of available attributes within the supplied data set minus the attribute(s) used for building the consequent. The user also can limit the depth of a tree.

These conditions and the nature of the supplied data set determine the composition of a Boolean expression. The composition is divided into three steps. The first step is determination of the attribute (name). The second step is random selection of one attribute value from all available values for the chosen attribute. The final step is the determination of the relational operator, which is constrained by the chosen attribute value. Obviously, if the available attribute values consist of nominal values, only the relational operator '=' would be appropriated. In a case where the attribute consists of numbers, other relational operators such as: $<; \leq; >; \geq; =$ are appropriated. However, there are two special cases. For numbers representing the smallest or greatest possible values of a particular attribute, the use of relational operators: $<; \leq$ and $>; \geq$ respectively would not be sensible.

Genetic Operators: Two genetic operators, crossover and mutation, were implemented in this study. These operators work on the same principle as described above. However, the maximum depth of a tree represents a restriction for crossover because insertion and/or exchange of sub-trees may cause an individual taking part in crossover to exceed its maximum depth. Also the inserted/exchanged sub-tree must not contain any attributes already contained within the recipient tree. Mutation can take place on functions and terminals. If a terminal mutates, it may create a new terminal (Boolean expression) or another function (Boolean operation) if the tree did not reach its maximum depth. Naturally, the building of a new Boolean expression (or several, if the terminal changes to a function) has the same restrictions as described above.

Fitness Measurement: The employed fitness function is based on the so-called *J-measure* [12]. The higher the *J-measure* for a particular individual, the higher its fitness. There are some weak points in the original *J-measure* as described in [13]. Due to this fact, this work used only the modified version of the *J-measure*. The modified version is presented as follows and referred to as *J1measure*.

$$a = \frac{|P|}{N}$$

$$b = \frac{|C\&P|}{|C|} \tag{1}$$

$$J1measure = \frac{|C|}{N} \; b \cdot log \; \frac{b}{a}$$

Here C represents the number of cases in which the antecedent of a particular rule is fulfilled, whereas P describes the number of cases which fulfil the consequent. The expression $C\&P$ stands for the number of cases in which both the antecedent and the consequent are fulfilled at the same time. The resulting fitness function is:

$$fitness = \frac{w_1 \cdot (J1) + w_2 \cdot \dfrac{n_{pu}}{n_T}}{w_1 + w_2} \tag{2}$$

Where n_T is the number of attributes within the antecedent, n_{pu} is the number of potential useful attributes within the antecedent, and $J1$ corresponds to the modified *J-measure*. An attribute is potentially useful, if the Boolean expression built from it, and the consequent, are fulfilled for at least one data entry at the same time. The values for w_1 and w_2 are user-defined weights and are assigned values of *0.6* for w_1 and *0.4* for w_2, as suggested in [13].

Selection: Three different selection mechanisms were implemented: roulette wheel selection, rank selection, and tournament selection. All three selection mechanisms produced similar results.

The Structure: The structure of the implemented GP system is the same as depicted in figure 1.

4   Experimental Investigations

The data set utilised during these experiments consisted of 353 complete cases (individual patients) and 13 attributes. These were obtained from the original data set consisting of many more cases (904) and attributes (50). Only specific attributes were selected. These were assumed to be valuable for the discovery of new knowledge regarding the causes and associations of recurring miscarriage. No feature selection has been employed so far. Since the original data set also contains incomplete cases, the number of actually available complete cases depends on the choice of attributes.

The data set was split into a training set and test set. The former contained two-thirds of the available cases and the latter the remaining third. It was ensured that each class was properly represented in both data sets. This is also referred to as stratification [16].

Figure 4 contains one example rule evolved for the consequent *Outcome Code* = *B*. It should be noted that the meaning of the presented rules and their Boolean expressions, cannot be explained in this paper. However, the data dictionary supplied in [4] can serve as a reference.

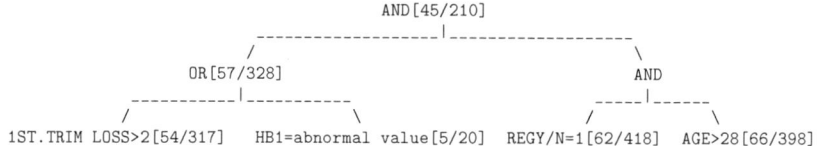

Fig. 4. Antecedent evolved for consequent **Outcome Code = B**.

In order to generate such a tree structure, a freely available program [15] was used since the rules produced by the implemented GP system were in form of s-expressions. S-expression are not easily comprehensible, but had to be used here due to lack of space.

Each node and leaf of the presented tree contains two numbers. The first number indicates how often the logical expression built by the particular part of the tree and the logical expression built by the consequent are fulfilled in respect to the supplied data set at the same time. The second number indicates how often this is the case without considering the logical expression built by the consequent. These numbers are thought to be an additional comprehensible judgement of the quality of the particular tree and its parts.

Table 1 contains some of the best rules evolved by the GP system. A particular rule, in form of a s-expressions, was applied to the training and test data set and the value for a and *J1measure* (see formula 1 are supplied. In addition, the fitness achieved by a particular individual is also shown. The value of a is also referred to as *confidence factor* [13] and serves as a simple judgement of the performance of a particular rule applied to the unseen test data. The number *consequent hits* contains the number of cases in which the particular consequent is fulfilled in respect to the supplied data set.

Table 1. Certain results in the form of s-expressions.

Supplied Consequent	S-Expression	Fitness	J1measure	b	Consequnet Hits
APS = 0	(OR [139/200] (AND [48/64] (T4 1 = normal value [220/331]) (REG Y/N = 0 [53/71])) (AND [112/166] (OP1 = P [118/174]) (TSH 1 = normal value [219/329])))	0.4111	0.0186	0.695	234
	(OR [61/78] (AND [23/26] (T4 1 = normal value [100/144]) (REG Y/N = 0 [24/27])) (AND [49/66] (OP1 = P [51/71]) (TSH 1 = normal v alue [102/144])))	0.4241	0.0401	0.7821	112
APS = 1	(AND [94/259] (OR [110/322] (OP1 = S [63/179]) (2TL = 0 [96/284])) (REG Y/N = 1 [101/282]))	0.4118	0.0197	0.3629	119
	(AND [30/80] (OR [30/93] (OP1 = S [27/88]) (TSH 1 = abnormal value [5/15])) (REG Y/N = 1 [44/132]))	0.4269	0.0449	0.375	47
REG Y/N = 0	(AND [52/73] (OR [60/345] (TSH 1 = normal value [66/329]) (OP1 = S [34/179])) (DTNP1 = 0 [52/74]))	0.5118	0.1863	0.7123	71
	(AND [23/30] (OR [27/154] (TSH 1 = normal value [26/144]) (OP1 = S [13/88])) (DTNP1= 0 [23/30]))	0.5308	0.2180	0.7666	27
REG Y/N = 1	(AND [255/272] (NOT [260/279] (DTNP1 = 0 [22/74])) (OR [276/345] (TSH 1 = normal value [263/329]) (OP1 = S [145/179])))	0.4694	0.1156	0.9375	282
	(AND [120/124] (NOT [125/129] (DTNP1 = 0 [7/30])) (OR [127/154] (TSH 1 = normal value [118/144]) (OP1 = S [75/88])))	0.4694	0.1157	0.9677	132

5   Conclusions and Further Work

The results demonstrated in this paper, yielded from the data set and the positive feedback obtained from the medical practitioners, led to the generation of conclusions regarding the system's practical potential. The presented results show that the rules perform well on unseen test data. Further research may reveal additional improvements in the quality of rules evolved by the system, and the system's performance.

Parallelisation of the GP system, as suggested in [13], is planned for future work. As well as enhancing the system's performance this may also lead to the discovery of qualitatively superior rules by using, for example, an *island model* as suggested in [2].

Furthermore, alternative fitness evaluation may prove more successful. In some cases the GP system is prone to developing rules of low interest value and thus truism knowledge. Ways to overcome this problem are suggested in [14].

Another possibility for improving the systems capability could be offered by *feature selection*. It results in an appropriate choice of features (attributes) for the current prediction class and thus a smaller search space for valuable rules.

More elaborated genetic operators might also prove to be more successful, as described in [4]. Other data sets have already been used to validate the developed system and proved its practical potential.

6   Acknowledgements

We would like to thank Dr. Alex A. Freitas for his support during the development of this approach.

References

1. Alex A. Freitas, Heitor S. Lopes, and Dieferson Luis Alves de Aranjo (1999). *A Parallel Genetic Algorithm for Rule Discovery in Large Databases.* Available at http://www.ppgia.pucpr.br/~alex/papers.html.
2. John R. Koza and David Andre (1995). *Parallel Genetic Programming on a Network of Transputers.* Available at ftp://elib.stanford.edu/pub/reports/cs/tr/95/1542/
3. Alex A. Freitas, Heitor S. Lopes, and Celia C. Bojarczuk (1999). *Discovering comprehensible classification rules using Genetic Programming: A case Study in a medical domain.* Available at http://www.ppgia.pucpr.br/~alex/papers.html.
4. Christian Setzkorn (2000). *Investigation into the Application of Artificial Intelligence Methods to the Analysis of Medical Data .* Available at http://www.csc.liv.ac.uk/~chris /Publications.html.

5. U. M. Fayyad, G. Piatetsky-Shapiro and P. Smyth (1996). From data mining to knowledge discovery: an overview. In: U. M. Fayyad, G. Piatetsky-Shapiro, P. Smyth and R. Uthurusamy (eds.), Advanced in Knowledge Discovery & Data Mining, 1-34, AAAI/MIT

6. John R. Koza (1993). *Genetic Programming I.* MIT Press London

7. John R. Koza (1994). *Genetic Programming II.* MIT Press London

8. Lawrence Davis (1991). *Handbook of Genetic Algorithm.* Van Nostrand Reinhold; ISBN: 0442001738

9. Thomas Baeck (1999). *Evolutionary Algorithm in Theory and Practice.* Inst of Physics Pub; ISBN: 0750306653

10. K.F. Man, K.S. Tang, and S. Kwong (1999). *Genetic Algorithm.* Springer-Verlag Berlin

11. Tobias   Blickle   and   Lothar   Thiele   (1995).   *A   Comparison   of Selection   Schemes   used   in   Genetic   Algorithm.*   Available   at http://www.handshake.de/user/blickle/publications/index.html

12. Smyth P., Goodman R. M. (1991). *Rule induction using information theory.* In Piatetsky-Shapiro G. and Frawley J. *Knowledge Discovery in Databases* MIT Press

13. Alex A. Freitas, Heitor S. Lopes, and Dieferson Luis Alves de Aranjo (1999). *A Parallel Genetic Algorithm for Rule Discovery in Large Databases.* Available at http://www.ppgia.pucpr.br/~alex/papers.html.

14. Edgar Noda, Alex A. Freitas, and Heitor S. Lopes (1999). *Discovering Interesting Predictive Rules with a Genetic Algorithm.* Available at http://www.ppgia.pucpr.br//~alex/papers.html.

15. Available at: http://www.dai.ed.ac.uk/daidb/students/chrisg/

16. Ian H. Witten and Eibe Frank (2000). *Data Mining: Practical Machine Learning Tools and Techniques with Java Implementations.* Morgan Kaufmann Publishers; ISBN: 1558605525

Detecting of Fatigue States of a Car Driver

Roman Bittner [1], Karel Hána [2], Lubomír Poušek [2], Pavel Smrčka [1],
Petr Schreib [2], and Petr Vysoký [3]

[1] Czech Technical University in Prague, Faculty of Electrical Engineering, Dept. of
Cybernetics, Technická 2, 166 27 Prague 6, Czech Republic
Bittner@cbmi.cvut.cz, Smrcka@lab.felk.cvut.cz
[2] Czech Technical University in Prague, Centre for BioMedical Engineering,
Bílá 91, 166 35 Prague 6, Czech Republic
{Hana, Pousek, Schreib}@cbmi.cvut.cz
[3] Czech Technical University in Prague, Faculty of Transportation Sciences, Dept. of
Automation in Transportation, Konviktská 20, 110 00 Prague 1, Czech Republic
Vysoky@fd.cvut.cz

Abstract. This paper deals with research on fatigue states of car drivers on
freeways and similar roads. All experiments are performed on-the-road. The
approach is based on the assumption that fatigue indicators can be derived from
driver+car system behaviour by measuring and processing appropriate factors.
For our experiments we designed an array of devices to measure selected
physiological and technical parameters. On the basis of experiments already
performed and described in the literature, we selected signals that carry
appropriate information about fatigue states of a driver. Two data sets are
compared: the first set was obtained from alert drivers, and the second one from
provably sleep-deprived drivers. We are trying to calibrate "fatigue states" of
the driver through trained rater estimates, and to extract reliable symptoms from
the measured signals; we are seeking relations between the symptoms and raters
fatigue estimates. The results of experiments already performed indicate that the
values of symptoms evolve in cycles, which is essential to take into account
during design of classifiers in the future.

1   Introduction

Most human manual activities dealing with regulation and control have nowadays
been substituted by automatic control. However, there is one major area where
manual control by a human operator is still utilized: driving various kinds of vehicles,
especially automobiles. In fact, this is one of the most-performed of all human
activities. According to a rough estimate [1], people world-wide devote over 10
million man-years each year to driving automobiles, and this figure is constantly
increasing.

The human operator as a controller is very flexible and can learn and adapt to
changing ambient conditions, etc. This ability to change his/her properties is a great
disadvantage in the case of repeating monotonous activities. During any long-term
monotonous activity a human being becomes tired, loses motivation, and his
effectiveness as a controller deteriorates considerably. In critical situations his control

R.W. Brause and E. Hanisch (Eds.): ISMDA 2000, LNCS 1933, pp. 260–274, 2000.

function diminishes – he/she may fall into a microsleep. Not only long periods of driving can cause this negative phenomenon, but it may also result from initial conditions, or from previous activities. Previous physical activity or sleep deprivation, in particular, has a negative effect. A set of other factors such as age, sex, daytime or night-time driving, driver's circadian rhythms, etc., play an important role [2].

During long periods of driving or as a result of above-mentioned initial conditions, motivation for steering declines, reaction time extends, short-term memory deteriorates, attention drops, variability of control actions as a response to the same impulse increases, important signals are ignored, decision errors and short-term failures of memory occurs. In extreme case a microsleep comes on. This can have fatal consequences. It is very difficult to prove that an accident was caused by driver fatigue, but the US National Transportation Safety Board estimates that it is the cause of more than 10% of all traffic. 28% of these accidents are fatal. Taking into account the total number of accidents, the losses caused by them reach tens of billions of dollars.

The economic and safety reasons mentioned above have led to an attempt to solve this problem by all possible means. Technical means are possibly the most promising. More advanced technological means include automatic freeways and intelligent cars. The intelligent car is assumed to be equipped in such a way that it is capable of analysing the drive signals or physiological signals of the driver, and can warn him in advance that his ability to drive has distinctly worsed due to fatigue, or that he could fall asleep. This is the main motivation underlying our research. We do not suppose that we will able to use the measured data as a basis for predicting the driver will fall asleep, but we aim to provide a warning against enhanced risk, probability or possibility of this event.

2   What is the Fatigue?

In our introduction, we mentioned some manifestations of fatigue. What, in fact, is fatigue? First of all it should be stated that fatigue is very a vague concept used as an umbrella term for phenomena caused by many different factors. Driver's activities can be divided into perception (distinguishing his course, obstacles, signs, optical and acoustical signals, etc.), cognitive activities (decision on appropriate behaviour) and his motorics (his/her control actions, steering movements, braking etc.). All these activities, including functions connected with memory, are influenced by fatigue to a varying extent.

This concept has been referred to by various terms that are more less mutually interchangeable in the research literature. (Loss of alertness or vigilance, fatigue, drowsiness). There is no significant difference between "loss of alertness" and "drowsiness".

Let us try to define the concept of fatigue. Distinctions are often made between physical and mental fatigue, subjective and objective fatigue. Our interest is focused especially on mental (or central) fatigue. Mental fatigue often follows from physical fatigue, and both are very probably caused by the same physiological mechanism. There is no commonly accepted physiological explanation of the origin of mental fatigue. However, there are hypotheses supported by experimental evidence.

Much more is known about physical (muscular) fatigue. This kind of fatigue is caused by exhausting the sources of energy in the muscles. We know much less about the origin of mental fatigue, which is closely connected with physical fatigue. (Physical fatigue leads to mental fatigue in the case of long-term load.) This connection is carefully explained by a hypothesis of central fatigue [3] which, indeed, is supported by a number of positively proved facts.

Briefly, this central fatigue hypothesis claims that a higher level of free tryptophan in conjunction with a lower level of branched chain amino acids increases the level of serotonin in the blood, which is the main cause of central (mental) fatigue.

Central fatigue decreases the number of active motoric units and decreases the frequency of nervous impulses stimulating the motoric units. Further, it diminishes the activity of those parts of the cortex which participate not only in motorics but also in decisive processes. It also leads to a number of other changes which are not really substantial from our point of view.

These facts indicate that most probably, there exists no single measure providing comprehensive information on the degree of fatigue. Online measurement of a driver's tryptophan or serotonin concentration is scarcely possible. Since there are at least five types of membrane receptors for serotonin, its increased concentration may be manifested quite differently in distinct parts of the nervous system. However these facts indicate where we may find indicators carrying most information on fatigue. Changes in the neuro-motoric system will be most distinctive on the most innerved muscles i.e., eyelid muscles and muscles for eye movement. Changes in cortex activity will be followed by changes in EEG activity, and both will cause secondary changes in the function of autonomous control loops such as heart rate variability.

It is clear that degree of fatigue is measurable only indirectly, on the basis of measurement of a lot of signals carrying any information about fatigue. All symptoms extracted from these signals will be called the [4] fatigue indicators.

3   Indicators of Fatigue

This section provides a brief overview of measures carrying information about driver fatigue. These measures are related either to the physiological state of the driver or to dynamic properties of the driver + car system or his/her behaviour. For more references see [4], [5].

Promising measures found in the literature. Many physiological measures have been examined in earlier studies as predictors or indicators of driver's fatigue. An enhanced percentage of *eyelid closure* in one of the most reliable predictors of the onset of sleep. However, a camera and demanding eye-tracking software must be used to measure this percentage. As the driver's drowsiness increases the *eye movements* slow down, sometimes accompanied by characteristic rolling movements. Eye blinking is also slower and more frequent with increasing level of fatigue. The type and speed of these eye movements can be determined on the basis of analysis of vertical and horizontal electrooculogram (EOG).

Human consciousness and psychological states (among which fatigue belongs) are closely related to *brain activity*. Variations in the subject's alertness cause changes in both the temporal and the frequency domain of the EEG signal. It is a well-known fact that states close to sleep are characterized by increasing alpha and theta activities and diminishing amplitude of beta activity. Spectral EEG analysis is the most appropriate method for detecting the onset and different stages of sleep – but automatic evaluation of drowsiness via EEG analysis failed. The EEG of an alert person has proved be very individual, and influenced by many psychological phenomena.

The correlation between changes of heart rhythm and fatigue is still an issue of controversy. Some authors take it for granted, while others reject it. Some sources mention a dependence between *skin potential level* (SPL) and alertness, but no reliable relation was found, because SPL varied significantly with the subject's mood, his body activity and temperature. It has been found that *facial muscle activity* changes according to alertness and drowsiness, but not enough research has been performed in this field.

Measures characterizing the quality of driving performance reflect the driver's driving skills also affected by fatigue. These measures are obtained via sensors installed in the car. The properties of these measures were thoroughly investigated by Wierwille et al. *Lane-related measures* are computed from the relative position of the car to the lane border. They include, for example: lane deviation, standard deviation of the lane position, the global maximum lane deviation and the mean square of lane deviation. The last of these is considered to be a reliable measure for detection of fatigue. Another group of measures is derived from the steering wheel position – *steering-related measures*. The main interest is focused on small steering wheel movements compensating the direction of the moving car. A drowsy driver shows worse sensitivity to small movements and, as a result, the number of micro-wheel adjustments decreases. Steering velocity was found to be highly correlated with eye movements. *Heading/lateral acceleration related measures* have similar properties as the two previous groups. Global maximum yaw deviation, yaw deviation variance and mean yaw deviation were found as a good predictors of fatigue. The accelerometer's signals are disturbed by the high level of high-frequency noise caused by vibrations of the fast moving car.

Long distance driving affects the *behaviour-related measures* of the driver. Shortly after beginning his drive, the driver frequently looks into his rear view mirror and side window mirrors, and actively watches the road. After 30-60 minutes this activity decreases: the driver prefers to move his eyes rather than turn his head when checking mirrors, and stretches his body when he feels tired. With increasing fatigue he yawns, bends his head to the left or right, takes deep breaths from time to time, and so on. These epiphenomena must be recorded by a camera inside the cabin – and can hardly be evaluated automatically.

4 Methods

4.1 Design of the Experiments

A large number of experiments are required for a systematic investigation of the relationship between fatigue and the recorded measures. Ideally, each age group is examined, men and women separately. And hundreds hours of data from on-the-road experiments are necessary to prove the accuracy of the evaluating algorithms.

In order to start working on and testing hypotheses, we had to choose a certain age group, although we were aware of the shortcomings of such an approach. We chose the group of young men between 20-27. This part of the population shows the highest accident risk. All experiments will take place on-the-road and will be restricted to freeways, where the risk of the driver falling asleep is higher than in city traffic or on smaller roads. No simulators are intended, and the same car will be used in all experiments. The Prague-Pilsen and Prague-Brno freeways seem to be suitable for the purpose, both having 2 lanes and similar traffic density. Further, in the first stage of our research we limit ourselves to one type of fatigue only – fatigue caused by sleep deprivation, which can easily be ensured and quantified. Other types (caused by physical/mental workload) are not being examined.

Our aim is to record and compare 2 data sets: a) from fully alert drivers, and b) from maximally tired drivers. The alert driver undertakes the experiment first, and after 24 - 48 hours of sleep deprivation he drives the same route again. Through correlation, factor and statistical analysis of both data sets we expect to extract measures carrying significant information about fatigue.

In order to determine how a particular measure correlates with fatigue, we need to know about the degree of driver fatigue at the same moment. This is the key problem of experimental methodology, and the whole of section 4.3 is devoted to it.

The course of each experiment is written down in a protocol containing data about the driver, passengers, route, time, weather conditions (rain, crosswind, visibility), etc. Before and after the drive, the driver records the degree of his subjectively estimated fatigue in the protocol. For safety reasons, a fully alert co-driver must be on board.

4.2 Technical Equipment for Experiments

The technical equipment for the experiments consists of a Škoda Octavia measuring car, provided for this project by the Škoda Auto (Volkswagen AG) Company, and internal equipment enabling scanning and storing of all the measures recorded during the drive. The whole measuring array was designed and developed with respect to the possibility of making a synchronous digital record in real-time, with a record length of several hours, mechanical and electrical resistance, proper placing inside the car from point of view of safety and control, and, last but not least, resistance to a range of disturbance sources. The final version of the measuring array in use is shown in fig 1. The technical equipment for the experiments was developed and produced in our workplace (CBME CTU in Prague) within a six-months period.

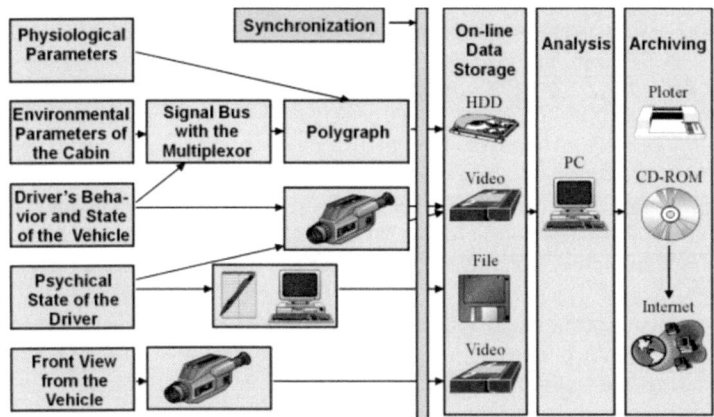

Fig. 1. Block structure of measuring equipment

Currently, the following signals are routinely recorded using a polygraph: EEG, ECG, EOG (i.e., physiological signals), temperature, noise level, light level (environmental signals inside the cabin), steering wheel positions, longitudinal and lateral accelerations (driving performance measures). Two video cameras (Sony DCR-TRC10, DCR-TRV310) scan the driver face and behaviour as well as the situation in front of the car.

Physiological signals are recorded through the an M&I BrainScope (Czech republic) polygraph. Inputs are sampled at 256 Hz with a 14-bit AD converter. The environmental and driving performance measures are recorded through the signal bus with multiplexor, and are stored on the hardisc using the polygraph synchronously with the physiological signals. Finally, the two video-camera recordings are digitized and stored on CD-ROMs for further analysis.

4.3 Multi-rater Fatigue Estimate

As mentioned above, the concept of "fatigue" belongs to category of measures that are very difficult to quantify. Every attempt to express fatigue numerically necessarily suffers from subjective evaluation that is impossible to verify in an exact way. No "gold standard" (ethalon) of fatigue exists to serve as the key position for calibrating an automatic detector of fatigue. Nevertheless, for our purposes we need to develop a reliable method which might provide this calibration (reference) signal for us.

Principally, this method can be based on: 1) an introspective fatigue estimate provided by the driver himself, 2) analysing measures with a precisely known relationship to fatigue, 3) an estimate made by a group of independent observers. Each approach has its imperfections. The introspective estimate can scarcely provide a quality estimate in short time intervals (e.g. every minute). While the driver is engaged in the introspective observation, he is also performing a mental workload, and thus the experiment is distorted. It is a well known fact that a subject gives an imprecise evaluation of his own state when tired. Ad 2) Short note only: we don't know this relationship, but are seeking it. Wierwille [5] examined the way of evaluating degrees of fatigue using a group of independent raters – a so-called mutli-rater estimate. In our work we developed this approach in grater details.

The fatigue estimate is performed by a group of 10 psychologically trained raters on the basis of analyzing a video-recording of the drivers's face. The camera fixed on the car panel scans both the driver's face and part of his body, so the rater can see the tired driver fidgeting, stretching, having heavy eyes, etc. After the experiment the video-recording is digitized and cut by special software into 1-minute segments. It is then screened for the group of raters in random sequence. They evaluate the video-recording using a questionnaire and record their scores into table.

In each segment the raters look for fatigue-related features and determine how intensely the feature is present. The questionnaire contains 7 features, including the time of eye opening (this feature reflects prolonged blinks / bursts of blinks), regular breathing (yawns / deep breaths), the head position of the driver (head bent to the left or right / falling head), the rater's subjective evaluation. The last mentioned is scored on a 5-level scale, while the other features are scored on a 3-level scale only. The fatigue degree related to a certain video-segment evaluated by the rater i is expressed as:

$$e_i = f(\{a_1, w_1\}, \{a_2, w_2\}, \dots, \{a_7, w_7\}),$$

where a_j is the rater's scoring (feature intensity) and w_j is its weight. The resulting fatigue degree of video-segment k depends on the reliability r_i of each rater:

$$MEX_k = g(\{e_1, r_1\}, \{e_2, r_2\}, \dots, \{e_{10}, r_{10}\}).$$

In this work, f represents the min-max aggregate function and g is the weighted average value of each contribution. The time course of parameter $MEX \in <0, 5>$ is depicted in fig. 4 (bottom).

4.4 Data Processing and Methodology

This section briefly describes the methodology of data processing of selected signals measured by the equipment proposed in the section 4.2 is shortly described. It is supposed (section 3) that the used signals provide information about the "fatigue" states of the driver.

Selection and Categorization of Used Signals

1. All signals were divided into 2 disjunctive subsets: **A.** Set of *reference signals*, which includes especially the EEG, EOG and video-recordings of the driver's face. The results of detailed analyses of these signals show which "fatigue" state the driver is in (see, e.g., section 4.3 for details). These reference signals are relatively hard to access and complicated to analyze – it is difficult to imagine a fully operational driver with more than 30 electrodes on his body and cables connected to a "magic device". The main idea is to replace these signals by other, much more accessible signals – subset **B.** – such as longitudinal and lateral car acceleration, small steering wheel movement, etc. The two subsets are in mutual interaction (generally non-linear) and it is necessary to verify the existence of any relationship at all, and to find out more details about the characteristics of the relationship under different conditions.

2. The signals were (virtually) divided in accordance with the "fatigue" state in which the experiment was performed: the first set contains signals obtained by the

alert driver + car system, and the second set contains signals obtained by the tired driver + car system.

3. Currently, the only selected subset of all signals measured by our equipment (see 4.2) is analyzed as follows:

  - EEG, international 10-20 system;
  - EOG, 1 vertical channel, bipolar lead located on right side;
  - Video-recording of the driver's face;
  - Small steering wheel movements;
  - Video-recordings from the external video-camera and the cabin inside temperature are partially consulted.

The volume of obtained data is enormous, the size of the data file is approximately 40 MB per one hour (excluding video-recording). Detailed examination of these *source data* leads to the conclusion that

- all signals are strongly noised with unprecedented quantity of artefacts, which can significantly damage the useful information, therefore radical *pre-processing* is necessary. For these purposes, the DFILT program (section 4.5) was used.

- no significant differences in basic statistics (such as mean value, variance, etc.) were found between alert and tired drivers, i.e., rather more sophisticated parameters must be extracted from the source signals.

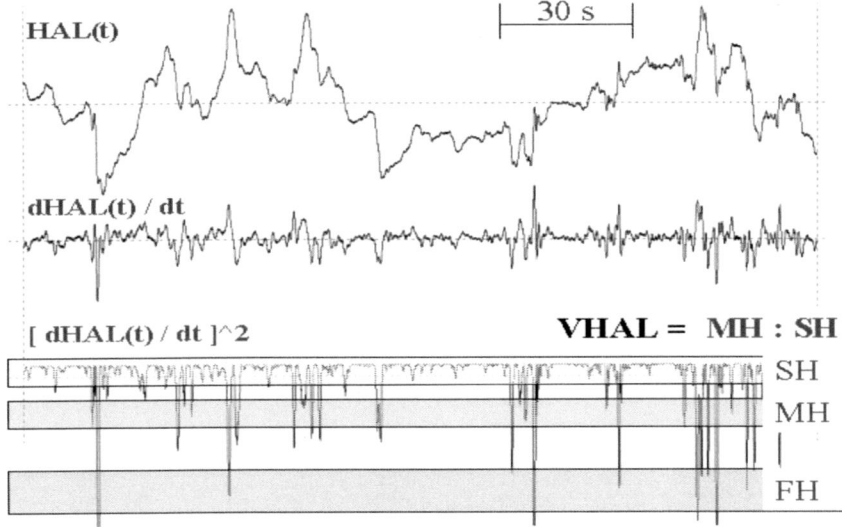

Fig. 2. Extraction of VHAL index

Extraction of Parameters

A brief description of the extraction process used for computing the discriminative parameters follows. The length of time-window for parameter extraction is of 20 sec. in all cases. **EEG-related parameters: *EAB index.*** EAB = EA/EB, where EA is the energy of the α-band (8-12 Hz in this case) and EB is the energy of the β-band (14-30 Hz in this case). Since the time-window for extraction is 20 s, the shortest episodes are averaged. **Steering wheel-related parameters: *VHAL index.*** The extraction process is shown in fig. 2. Its fiducial signal is the quadrate of the first derivative of the steering wheel position, i.e the velocity of the steering wheel movements. The MH:SH ratio is computed, where MH is the number of fast movements and SH is the number of slow movements. The band limits are selected in such a way that the index will remain in the <0,1> interval in the given experiment. **Vertical EOG-related parameters:** *NOF index*, number of blinks per minute. We obtained this parameter by manual counting of blinks from the computer screen. *VOCU index*, averaged velocity of activity in the electrooculogram. The extraction process is similar to the *VHAL* index: if the velocity is greater than the given limit, the *VOCU* is incremented. The limit is given by the 5% quantile. *NOX index*, number of special graphoelements - non-standard eye movements and eyelid movements. This parameter is manually counted from the EOG series on the computer screen. **Parameters derived from video-recording of the driver´s face.** See section 4.3 for details. The *MEX* parameter projecting the average level of rater's fatigue estimate is used. This parameter ranges in the <1,5> interval, value 5 indicates a dangerously tired driver.

4.5 Used Software Tools

As mentioned above, data processing is performed off-line and the volume of processed data is enormous. For the purposes of visualization and pre-processing it was necessary to prepare some special software tools. A list with brief descriptions follows:

DFILT: a program for linear filtration of very large multichannel data files. Until now 9 kinds of FIR and IIR filters have been implemented. Algorithms are optimized for fast-running.

DCSA: this program computes FFT, cross correlation functions and averaged mutual information of delayed time series. The computation runs on sequence of floating windows, e.g. in FFT mode we obtain Compressed Spectral Arrays (CSA).

DVIZ, DCSA: simple programs for visualization of long multi-channel data files which enable the user to observe both time and frequency series

DataViewer7: a user-friendly program for visualization of long multi-channel data files which enables the user to observe both time-series and digitized video-sequences synchronously.

5 Discussion

There is evidence of some (quasi)periodicity in all the mentioned parameters obtained from the data sequences in all measurements completed hitherto. There are at least *3 different dynamics* in the data sequences: **(1)** *short-time* (a) 1-30 s episodes, which probably sometimes contain, e.g., microsleeps, etc., and (b) 30–180s cycles. Currently we are not interested in short-time dynamics. We have focused our attention on **(2)** *medium-time* dynamics, which contains 10-20 min. cycles, and finally **(3)** *long-time* dynamics, which includes the trend in fatigue evolution and on which the medium and short-time dynamics are superposed. The median filter (length 5-15 samples) and the moving average (length 10-15 samples) were applied to data sequences of all extracted parameters in order to accent the medium-time dynamics.

EEG-related parameters: It's supposed [8] that the multi-channel EEG signal provides a great deal of information about fatigue. Unfortunately, it's a very complicated signal and can lead to major problems: for example, it has very significant interpersonal variability and it is also highly nonstationary and responds to some hardly detectable stimuli. In our work we start from the widespread assumption that sleep deprivation causes a rapid increase in the total rate of α and θ activities in selected leads. This assumption is partly well-founded; we can demonstrate it in fig. 3 which shows two sequences of Compressed Spectral Arrays (CSA) for the same person: the left part is obtained from the alert driver and the right part is obtained from the sleep-deprived driver (one second time-window per one spectral array, T4 lead). Increase of α-activity is evident.

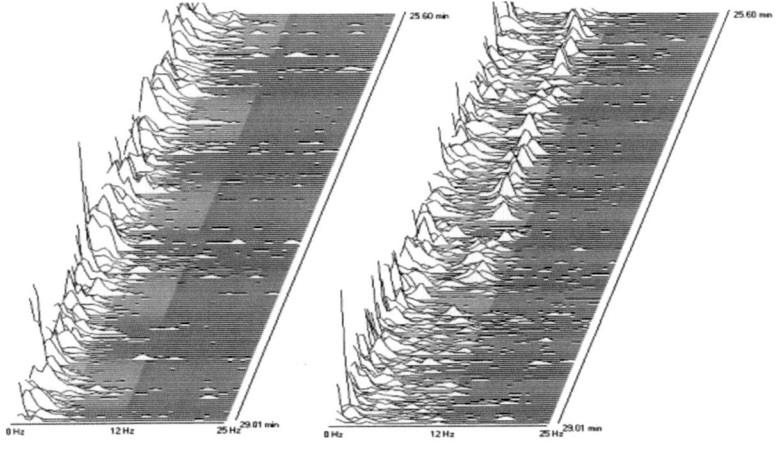

Fig. 3. Compressed Spectral Arrays (CSA)

The mentioned *EAB index* increases during sleep deprivation, but not significantly (e.g., arbitrary mental activity avoids an artefact on the *EAB index*). **Steering wheel-related parameters:** the basic idea is that a tired driver selects an easy driving strategy, i.e., he compensates only large regulation deviations which can be detected from steering wheel movements. An example of the *VHAL* time series is shown in fig. 4. (top). The bottom curve of the same figure illustrates the *MEX* – the averaged raters estimate of fatigue level. It can be seen that, in approximately the fifteenth minute the courses of the two parameters become very similar, both in shape and in phasing (it seems that the first 15 - 20 minutes is the time necessary for the driver to adapt to the given freeway and the appropriate driving style). The *VHAL index* value decreases with increasing fatigue (as can be seen in the mentioned medium-time periods and long-time trend). **The vertical EOG-related parameters,** namely the *VOCU* and *NOF* indices: an example of time series of the *VHAL* and *VOCU* parameters is shown in fig. 5. – there is again clearly good agreement. The *VOCU* index decreases in fatigue states. All presented figures provide evidence of the mentioned medium-time 10 - 20 minute cycles superimposed on the basic long-time trend, which can be separated by averaging (more than 40 minutes). Differences in the mean value of the *VOCU*, *VHAL* and *MEX* indices between alert and tired drivers are more than 10 - 20 %, i.e., these indices are our first candidates for sufficiently discriminative parameters. However, the *NOF* index increases non-specifically, and probably interacts with, e.g., light conditions.

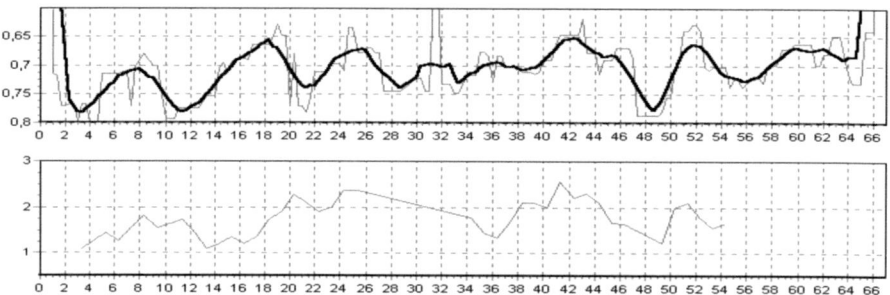

Fig. 4. Time series of *VHAL* (top) and *MEX* (bottom) indexes. The horizontal axis is in minutes.

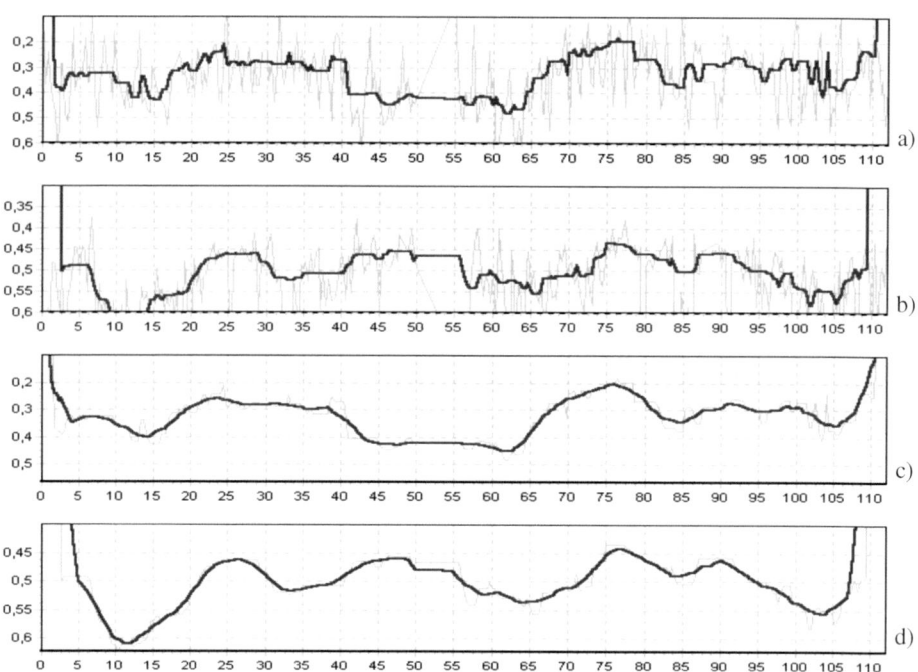

Fig. 5. Time series of *VHAL* (a),(c) and *VOCU* (b),(d) parameters. (a),(b) - original series (thin line) and median filtered series (thick line). (c),(d) - median filtered series (thin line) and series smoothed by the moving average (thick line).

In this phase it is necessary to quantify the relations between parameters more exactly. We can use the classical correlation coefficient and measure linear dependence or utilize averaged mutual information, which can detect both linear and nonlinear interactions. Let us divide the time series of the *VHAL* and *MEX* on fig. 4 into two equal sections (approximately 30 minutes). The correlation coefficient of the first section is 0.12, and that of the second section is 0.54. In both cases we can reject the hypothesis about their zero values (α=5 %). The synchronization of the two time series in the second section is evident. When testing the independence of random measures using averaged mutual information we will use a special transformation which transforms mutual information into series with roughly χ^2 distribution, [10]. The hypothesis of independence based on averaged mutual information can be rejected (α=5 %) in both mentioned sections. The number of quantization levels was 3; the number of samples was small, but still theoretically sufficient.

All results mentioned here are preliminary, and much more work will be done in the near future in order to verify many hypotheses. We can already predict that:

- a classifier based on some mentioned (or other much more reliable) parameters will be adaptive, with an adaptation time of not less than 40-60 minutes: the first approximately 15 - 20 minutes are necessary for the driver to adaptation to driving under the given conditions, and the driver must undertake at least two 10-20 sec. medium-time cycles, which can be seen in all measured parameters.

- such a classifier cannot be principally combinatorial because, as has been shown, a situation can occur when the current (short-term) value of a parameter on the classifier's output is in such a position within the medium-time cycle that, e.g., a tired driver can be classified as alert (or vice versa). This fact is particularly important. We suspect that the slight inconsistency in the results of previous studies (section 3) may be caused by this fact (known as aliasing).

Now we will present a very brief description of an approach that can help to solve the mentioned problems: a **fuzzy automaton** (fig. 6) as a terminal unit.

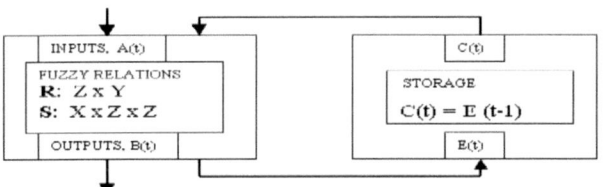

Fig. 6. Block scheme of the fuzzy automaton. A=<X,Y,Z,R,S> , working frequency 60 s.
X ... set of input states, Y...set of output states, Z ...set of internal states

The main idea of this approach is based on the belief that most biological and bio-technical systems go through some "fuzzy" states during their lives. This means that the system must be in at least one state at the moment, but it can also be more or less in some other states (with another order of membership in "fuzzy" terminology). The current output of the fuzzy automaton depends on the past state and the current input through state-transition and output relations. Both fuzzy relations are represented by matrices and a simple max-min composition is used. In our case, specially modified values of the mentioned parameters (*VHAL*, *VOCU* etc., paragraph 4.4) are used as input values of the fuzzy automaton. In our present simplified version, "special modification" means application of static threshold criteria and fuzzification. However, a much more sophisticated adaptive classifier can be used in this place. The state-transition and output relations can be adjusted so as to obtain output states which correspond closely to the real evolution of the "fatigue states" of a driver (for example, if the automaton has passed the state which means a "high risk" of fatigue it cannot in the near future return to the "no risk" state, and must also in some higher state be not far from the "high risk" state). The number of internal states is not higher a 5; a major problem is that no exact method is available for determining the suitable state-transition relation. There are also some other problems with the functionality of the fuzzy automaton, e.g., the max-min composition that is used causes "bruising" of the fuzzy states, the setting of correct initial values to the fuzzy automaton is not easy, etc. On the other hand, software simulation of the fuzzy automaton is quite easy and fast (no more than 30 lines of C source code) and, likewise, the fuzzy automaton simulates the well known behaviour of many natural systems.

6 Conclusion

Because of small number of experiments performed up to now we can not make generalized and definitive conclusions. To some extent, we repeated the experiments carried out by other authors, but with an important difference: our experiments took place on the road. Very interesting (and promising) results were achieved by analyzing micro-wheel adjustments. On the other hand, the analysis of changes in eye-blinking frequency caused by fatigue gave sceptic results.

We have proved the existence of (quazi)periodicities in different bands. We have also verified that the medium-frequency component of wheel adjustments is always present, and does not depend on the driver nor the route. Nearly identical periodicities occured in the multi-rater estimate, frequency of eye-blinking and micro-wheel adjustments signals as well as. At this time, another measurements are carried out to provide material for serious statistical analysis.

References

1. Rothery, R.W.: Car following models. In: Gartner, N.H., Messer, C.J., Rathi, A.K. (eds.): Monograph on traffic flow theory. US Department of Transport, Transportation Research Board, Washington (1997)
2. Freund, D.M., Knipling, R.R., Landsburg, A.C., Simmons, R.R., Thomas, G.R.: A holistic approach to operator alertness research. Transportation Research Board, Annual meeting 1998, Washington (1998)
3. Gandevia, S.C. et al (eds.): Fatigue: Neural and muscular mechanisms. Plenum Press, New York (1995)
4. Knipling, R.R., Wierwille, W.W.: Vehicle-based drowsy driver detection. Current status and future prospects. Proc. IVHS America Fourth Annual Meeting, Atlanta (1994)
5. Wierwille, W.W., Ellsworth, L.A., Wreggit, S.S., Fairbanks, R.J., Kirn, C.L.: Research on Vehicle-Based Driver Status/Performance Monitoring; Development, Validation, and Refinement of Algorithms For Detection of Driver Drowsiness. U.S. Department of Transportation, National Highway Traffic Safety Administratlon. DOT HS 808 247, Final Report (1994)

6. NCSDR/NHTSA Expert panel: Drowsy driving and automobile crashes. National Highway Traffic Safety Administration, Washington (1998)
    http://152.119.106.101/people/perform/human/Drowsy.htm
7. Vysoký, P.: Calibration of the Driver's Fatigue Estimator with Help of Fuzzy Aggregation Functions, Proc. Biosignal 2000, Brno, Czech Republic
8. Makeig, S., Jung, T.P.: Changes in allertness are a principal component of variance in the EEG spectrum, Neuro report **7** (1995) 213-216
9. Juang, T.P., Makeig, S., Stensmo, M., Sejnowski, T.J.: Estimating alertness from the EEG power spectrum. IEEE Trans. BME, Vol. 44 (1997) No. **1**, 60-69
10. Reinke, W., Diekmann, V.: Uncertainty analysis of human EEG spectra. Biological cybernetics, Vol. 57 (1989) No. **6**, 379-387
11. Adlassnig, K.P., Steimann, F.: Clinical monitoring with fuzzy automata. Fuzzy Sets and Systems **61** (1994) 37-42

Operator Method of Fuzzification

Arkady Bolotin

Epidemiology and Health Services Evaluation Department
Ben-Gurion University of the Negev, P.O.B. 653, Beersheba 84105, Israel

Abstract. This paper presents a contribution to elaboration of theoretical methods of fuzzification. This is a very important problem, which was so far tackled from the side of probability and/or metric (topological) methods. A new method based on Hermit's operators of quantum mechanics is proposed in this paper. The paper is illustrated with two examples of life sciences systems: an interval of normal concentrations of physiologically active blood substances and a set of old persons.

Usually it is considered that the only condition a membership function must really satisfy is that it must vary between zero and one. The function itself can be an arbitrary curve whose shape can be defined as a function that suits the aims of modeling from the point of view of simplicity, convenience, speed, and efficiency. By this "arbitrary" approach, however, the membership function proves to be a purely mathematical construction, an abstract fiction that represents nothing in the world of reality.

In this paper, trying to fix this "drawback", we attempted to elaborate (at least partially) a new "theoretical" method of constructing membership functions. This method is based on a similarity between fuzzy and quantum-mechanical logic and suggests using the mathematical apparatus of quantum mechanics (Hermit's operators and wave functions) for the purpose of fuzzification. Indeed, the Hermit's operators and their sets of eigenvalues are an ideal analogy of linguistic variables and their fuzzy sets. Therefore, advancing this analogy, we put the Hermit's operators in correspondence with the linguistic variables, which characterize a fuzzy system.

Our main assumptions are as follows. A membership function μ associated with an analyzed fuzzy system may be determined by the module (amplitude) of the corresponding wave function Ψ obtained from the generalized Schrödinger's stationary wave equation:

$$\left[\hat{\mathbf{P}}^2 + \mathbf{U}(\hat{\mathbf{Q}}) \right] \Psi = L\Psi \quad , \tag{A.1}$$

where $\mathbf{U}$ is the quasi-potential function, L is the eigenvalue of the generalized Hamiltonian. The generalized momentum and coordinate are mutually non-commuting operators

$$\left\{ \hat{\mathbf{P}}, \hat{\mathbf{Q}} \right\} \equiv i \left(\hat{\mathbf{P}}\hat{\mathbf{Q}} - \hat{\mathbf{Q}}\hat{\mathbf{P}} \right) = \text{const} \neq 0 \quad . \tag{A.2}$$

We draw attention to the fact that assumption (A.2) is actually a mathematical reflection of fuzziness.

Let us show how this operator method of fuzzification works in different cases.

1. Quantum-Mechanical Systems

In case of quantum mechanics we can simply use Cartesian coordinates x and regular momenta p as generalized variables $\mathbf{Q}$ and $\mathbf{P}$:

R.W. Brause and E. Hanisch (Eds.): ISMDA 2000, LNCS 1933, pp. 274–281, 2000.
© Springer-Verlag Berlin Heidelberg 2000

$$\begin{cases} \hat{Q} = x \quad , \\ \hat{P} = \dfrac{1}{\sqrt{2m}} \, \hat{p} \quad . \end{cases} \tag{1.1}$$

Then the commutation relation (A.2) will be of the form

$$\{\hat{p}, x\} = \text{const} = \hbar \quad . \tag{1.2}$$

Within the scope of the operator method of fuzzification, this means that fuzziness of quantum mechanical systems arises just because of the Planck's constant $\hbar$. From (1.2) follows

$$\hat{p} = -i\hbar \frac{\partial}{\partial x} \quad , \tag{1.3}$$

and, therefore, the membership function $\mu(x)$ associated with the given quantum system

$$\mu(x) \propto |\Psi(x)| \tag{1.3}$$

will be determined by the equation

$$\left[-\frac{\hbar^2}{2m} \frac{\partial^2}{\partial x^2} + U(x) \right] \Psi(x) = L\Psi(x) \quad . \tag{1.4}$$

2. Statistical Mechanics Systems

In case of statistical mechanics, we will use the following expressions as generalized coordinates $\mathbf{Q}$ and momenta $\mathbf{P}$:

$$\begin{cases} \hat{Q} = x + \hat{\varepsilon} \quad , \\ \hat{P} = \dfrac{1}{\sqrt{2m}} (p + \hat{\theta}) \quad , \end{cases} \tag{2.1}$$

where the operators $\hat{\varepsilon}$ and $\hat{\theta}$ represent the influence of the system's environment on the position x and physical momentum p. Substituting (2.1) into the commutation relation (A.2) we get

$$\{p + \hat{\theta}, x + \hat{\varepsilon}\} = \{p, \hat{\varepsilon}\} + \{\hat{\theta}, x\} + \{\hat{\theta}, \hat{\varepsilon}\} = \text{const} \neq 0 \quad . \tag{2.2}$$

Therefore, according to the operator method of fuzzification, fuzziness of the statistical mechanics system is accounted for by the uncontrolled influence of the system's environment.

Assuming that

$$\{p, \hat{\varepsilon}\} = \{\hat{\theta}, x\} = 1 \quad , \quad \{\hat{\theta}, \hat{\varepsilon}\} = 0 \quad , \tag{2.3}$$

(here we use the dimensionless system of unit $[p] = [x] = 1$), we find

$$\hat{\varepsilon} = i \frac{\partial}{\partial p} \quad , \quad \hat{\theta} = -i \frac{\partial}{\partial x} \quad , \tag{2.4}$$

and then obtain the formula

$$\left(H - i\left[H\,,\,\right] - \frac{1}{2m}\cdot\frac{\partial^2}{\partial x^2} + \sum_{n=2}\frac{1}{n!}\cdot\frac{\partial^n U}{\partial x^n}\cdot i^n\frac{\partial^n}{\partial p^n}\right)\Psi(x, p) = L\Psi(x, p)\,, \qquad (2.5)$$

where H stands for the classical Hamiltonian, and $[H\,,\,]$ is the Poisson's bracket. Considering $\Psi(x, p)$ as a real function of x and p and asserting that the following inequality is true

$$\left|\frac{\partial U(x)}{\partial x}\cdot\frac{\partial\Psi}{\partial p}\right| >> \left|\frac{\partial^3 U(x)}{\partial x^3}\cdot\frac{\partial^3\Psi}{\partial p^3}\right| \qquad , \qquad (2.6)$$

we get an expression:

$$\left[H(x,p)\,,\,\Psi(x,p)\right] = 0 \qquad . \qquad (2.7)$$

A wave function $\Psi(x, p)$, which simultaneously satisfies the equation (2.7) and the boundary requirement

$$0 \le \left|\Psi(x, p)\right| \le 1 \qquad , \qquad (2.8)$$

is of the form:

$$\Psi(x, p) = \exp\left(-\frac{1}{2T}\cdot H(x, p)\right) \qquad , \qquad (2.9)$$

where T is the absolute temperature of the system. Consequently, the operator method of fuzzification gives us that with the certain potential $U(x)$, which meets the condition

$$\left|\frac{\partial U}{\partial x}\right| >> \frac{1}{mT}\left|\frac{\partial^3 U}{\partial x^3}\right| \qquad , \qquad (2.10)$$

the membership function $\mu(x, p)$ of the thermal equilibrium can be represented by the formula analogous to Gibbs distribution:

$$\mu(x, p) = \mu(p)\times\mu(x) = \exp\left[-\frac{p^2}{4mT}\right]\times A_x\cdot\exp\left[-\frac{U(x)}{2T}\right] \qquad , \qquad (2.11)$$

where the constant A_x can be found from the equality

$$\mu_{max} = A_x\cdot\exp\left[-\frac{U_{min}}{2T}\right] = 1 \qquad . \qquad (2.12)$$

3. Life Sciences Systems

In case of biological systems, we will use system parameters q and their time derivatives as generalized coordinates $\mathbf{Q}$ and momenta $\mathbf{P}$:

$$\hat{Q} = q \quad , \quad \hat{P} = b\cdot\hat{\dot{q}} \quad , \qquad (3.1)$$

where b are certain dimensional coefficients. Substitution of (3.1) into the commutation relation (A.2) produces the following:

$$\left\{\hat{\dot{q}}, q\right\} \ne 0 \qquad . \qquad (3.2)$$

Expression (3.2) implies that the time derivative $\hat{\dot{q}}$ cannot be a function of q

$$\hat{\dot{q}} \ne F(q) \qquad . \qquad (3.3)$$

Hence, (unlike the case of a "crisp" system) it is not enough to know the parameters q of a biological (or physiological) system in order to predict how the system's state will be changed in the course of time. Thus, according to the operator method of fuzzification, fuzziness of life sciences systems is conditioned by lack of complete information regarding the state of these systems.

Assuming that

$$\{\hat{q}, q\} = a \tag{3.4}$$

(where a are some non-negative constants), we get

$$\hat{q} = -ia \frac{\partial}{\partial q} \quad . \tag{3.5}$$

Eq.(3.5) gives us the form of the generalized Schrödinger's wave equation for the case of a biological system:

$$\left[-a^2 b^2 \frac{\partial^2}{\partial q^2} + U(q) \right] \Psi(q) = L \Psi(q) \quad . \tag{3.6}$$

Thus, to determine the "objective" (theoretical) membership function $\mu(q)$ associated with a given biological system we only need to compose the system's quasi-potential $U(q)$. We will illustrate the use of equation (3.6) with two simple examples, following bellow.

Example 1. Normal Concentrations of Physiologically Active Blood Substances

We will start with a rule *"if the concentration of every physiologically active blood substance is normal then the condition of endocrine system is good."* It is known that at least two mechanisms govern the concentration of any physiologically active blood substance (PABS); these mechanisms are *PABS secretion* and *utilization*. Both mechanisms behave in a different way for different PABSes, though they have general traits that are true for every PABS:

1. The secretion mechanism is responsible for production of a PABS and its injection into the blood stream. A work of the secretion mechanism is inversely proportional to the current PABS concentration q: the smaller q, the greater quantity of the PABS is produced and injected into the blood, and vice versa.
2. The utilization mechanism is responsible for removal of a PABS from the blood via the PABS utilization or disintegration. Its work is proportional to concentration q: the higher q, the greater quantity of the PABS is utilized or disintegrated. However, when concentration q gets up to some level q_C, the work of the utilization mechanism reaches a *plateau*.

In order to build a fuzzy model of the system regulating the concentrations q, we assume that the system quasi-potential function $U(q)$ is the sum $U(q) = U_\uparrow(q) + U_\downarrow(q)$, where $U_\uparrow$ and $U_\downarrow$ represent the quantity of PABS secreted and utilized by the regulating mechanisms respectively:

$$U_\uparrow(q) = \frac{\alpha}{q^m} \quad (m > 0) \quad , \quad U_\downarrow(q) = \begin{cases} \beta \cdot q^n & (n > 0) \quad \text{for } q \le q_C \quad , \\ U_C = \text{const} & \text{for } q > q_C \quad , \end{cases} \tag{E1.1}$$

where α and β are some positive constants (see Fig. 1).

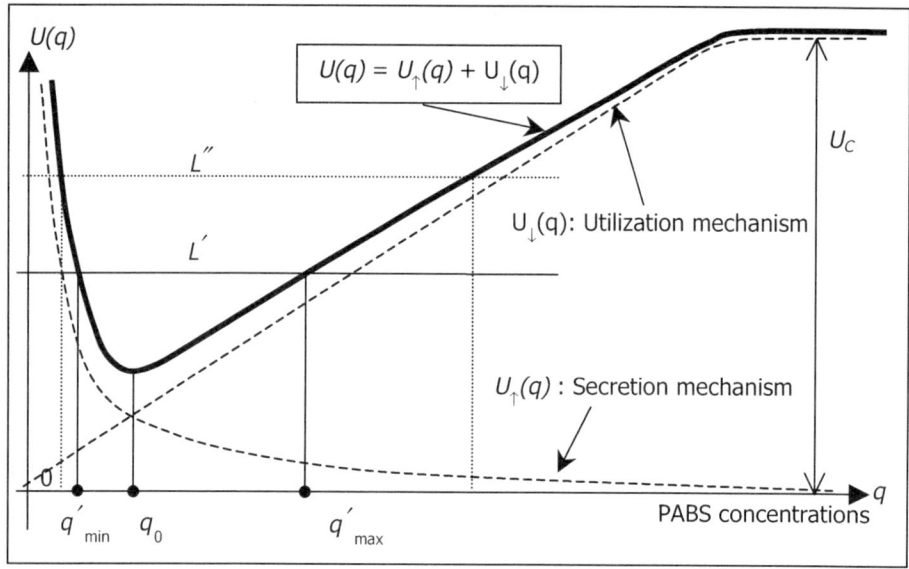

Fig. 1. The quasi-potential U(q) of the system regulating PABS concentrations.

Considering the normal state of the system as a state that corresponds to the lowest level L_0 and substituting (E1.1) into (3.6)

$$\frac{\partial^2 \Psi_0}{\partial q^2} - \frac{1}{a^2 b^2}\left[\frac{\alpha}{q^m} + U_\downarrow(q) - L_0\right]\Psi_0(q) = 0 \quad , \tag{E1.2}$$

we get the far asymptotics of the eigenfunction $\Psi_0(q)$:

$$\Psi_0(q) \xrightarrow[q \to \infty]{} \exp(-kq) \quad , \tag{E1.3}$$

where the real factor k is

$$k = +\sqrt{\frac{U_C - L_0}{a^2 b^2}} \quad . \tag{E1.4}$$

Let us suppose that when $q \to 0$ an asymptotic behavior of $\Psi_0(q)$ is

$$\Psi_0(q) \xrightarrow[q \to 0]{} q^s \quad (s \geq 0) \quad . \tag{E1.5}$$

Then, by substituting (E1.5) into (E1.2) we receive

$$s(s-1) = \frac{\alpha}{a^2 b^2} \cdot q^{2-m} \quad (q \to 0) \quad . \tag{E1.6}$$

Therefore, with $0 < m < 2$ we will have $s=1$, and the eigenfunction $\Psi_0(q)$ will take the form

$$\Psi_0(q) = q \cdot R(q) \cdot e^{-kq} \quad , \tag{E1.7}$$

where $R(q)$ satisfies the following conditions:

$$R(q) \xrightarrow[q \to 0]{} const \quad ,$$

$$R(q) \xrightarrow[q \to \infty]{} q^w \ (0 \le w < \infty) \quad .$$

(E1.8)

From the oscillation theorem follows that $\Psi_0(q)$ must have the same sign with all q, hence $\Psi_0(q)$ gets the maximum (or the minimum) when q equals some "equilibrium" concentration q_0. This produces the equality

$$k = q_0^{-1} \quad ,$$

(E1.9)

if we put $R(q) = A = const.$ Therefore, we obtain that the membership function $\mu_0(z)$ takes the form

$$\mu_0(z) = |\Psi_0(z)| = A \cdot q_0 \cdot z \cdot e^{-z} \quad ,$$

(E1.10)

where z are dimensionless concentrations

$$z = \frac{q}{q_0} \quad .$$

(E1.11)

We can find constant A from the condition

$$\mu_{max} = \mu_0(z)\big|_{z=1} = 1 \quad ,$$

(E1.12)

which finally gives us the form of the membership function for the set of the normal PABS concentrations, stated as follows:

$$\mu_0(z) = z \cdot \exp(1 - z)$$

(E1.13)

(see Fig. 2).

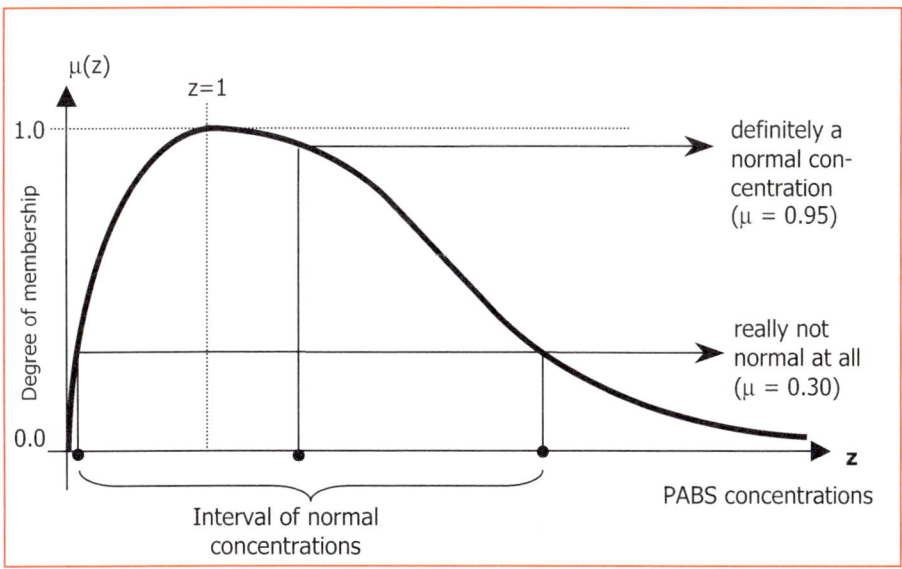

Fig. 2. The membership function for the normal PABS concentrations.

The curve described by expression (E1.13) is in quite good agreement with the experimental results published in the papers devoted to measurements of PABS concentrations (for example, see [1-2]).

Example 2. The Set of Old Persons

Perhaps, one of the most commonly used examples of a fuzzy set is the set of old persons, and so we should try the operator method of fuzzification on it. We will begin by looking into how people answer a question, which regards a subject they do not know for sure. Apparently, in this case people are guided by some value of doubt that arises when they look over possible answers. Namely, the answer seems to be right when the doubt gets minimal. Suppose, all the possible answers are the points of the continuous variable q. Then we can represent the value of doubt as a function of q. This function $U(q)$ takes the minimum in the point q_0, which is the apparently right answer. It is clear, that the function of doubt $U(q)$ cannot have a peaked configuration in the point q_0 if knowledge of the subject questioned is inexact. Therefore, the more uncertain knowledge, the wider the minimum of the function of doubt $U(q)$.

Let us assume now that people are being asked a question what person can be called young. In order to build the fuzzy model of this decision making process, we select the simplest function of doubt $U(q)$ that takes the form of parabola:

$$U(q) = \alpha^2 q^2 \quad , \tag{E2.1}$$

where q is the person's age, α is some positive constant. Substituting (E2.1) into (3.6) we will get:

$$\frac{\partial^2 \Psi(z)}{\partial z^2} + \left(\lambda - z^2\right)\Psi(z) = 0 \quad , \tag{E2.2}$$

where the dimensionless variables z and λ are

$$z = \sqrt{\frac{\alpha}{ab}}\, q \quad , \quad \lambda = \frac{L}{\alpha \cdot ab} \quad . \tag{E2.3}$$

Solving the equation (E2.3) and taking the eigenfunction $\Psi_0(z)$ corresponding to the minimal level of doubt $\lambda_0 = 1$. We finally obtain the set of old persons, which is described by the formula:

$$\mu(z) = 1 - \exp\left(-\frac{z^2}{2}\right) \quad . \tag{E2.4}$$

By its shape, this membership function (E2.4) is resembles those ones usually pictured in papers on fuzzy logic (see, for example [3-6]), and, when adjusted, it gives fairly realistic numbers. For instance, if we state that a person younger than 25 years old is really not very old at all ($\mu \leq 0.3$), we will get that all people older than 70 years old are definitely old ones ($\mu > 0.95$).

Conclusion

As one can notice, the core of the operator method of fuzzification, proposed in this paper, is the construction of the quasi-potential function $\mathbf{U}$. Hence both the advantage and disadvantage of the method follow. The advantage of the method is in an ability to base the membership function on the information concerning a given system. Therefore, by this method, fuzzification appears as an objective fact in our real world. However, the disadvantage is that the proposed method of fuzzification will not operate when the quasi-potential **U** cannot be composed (in virtue of the lack of knowledge, for instance).

References

1. D.D. Bikle (Editor), Assay of the Calcium Regulating PABSs, Springer Verlag, 1983.

2. T. Chard, An Introduction to Radioimmunoassay and Related Techniques (Laboratory Techniques in Biochemistry and Molecular Biology (Cloth), Vol. 6, Pt. 2), Elsevier Science Ltd., 1995.

3. Bezdek, C. James, Fuzzy Models – What Are They, and What?, IEE Transaction on Fuzzy Systems, 1:1, pp. 1-6, 1993.

4. R. Jang, N. Gulley, Fuzzy Logic Toolbox for use with MathLab®, The Mathworks Inc., 1995.

5. G. J. Klir, U.S. Clair, B. Yuan, Fuzzy Set Theory: Foundations and Applications, Prentice Hall, 1997.

6. H.T. Nguyen, E.A. Walker, A First Course in Fuzzy Logic, CRC Press, 1999.

A System for Monitoring Nosocomial Infections

E. Lamma[1], M. Manservigi[2], P. Mello[1], S. Storari[1], F. Riguzzi[3]

[1] D.E.I.S., Università di Bologna,
Viale Risorgimento 2, 40136 Bologna, Italy
{elamma,pmello}@deis.unibo.it, sstorari@iol.it
[2] DIANOEMA S.p.A. Via Carracci 93, 40100 Bologna, Italy
mmanservig@dianoema.it
[3] Dipartimento di Ingegneria, Università di Ferrara,
Via Saragat 1, 44100 Ferrara, Italy
friguzzi@ing.unife.it

Abstract. In this work, we describe a project, jointly started by DEIS University of Bologna and Dianoema S.p.A., in order to build a system which is able to monitor nosocomial infections. To this purpose, the system computes various statistics that are based on the count of patient infections over a period of time. The precise count of patient infections needs a precise definition of bacterial strains that is found by applying clustering to data on past infections. Moreover, the system is able to identify critical situations for a single patient (e.g., unexpected antibiotic resistance of a bacterium) or for hospital units (e.g., contagion events) and alarm the microbiologist.

1 Introduction

A very important problem that arises in hospitals is the monitoring and detection of nosocomial infections. A hospital-acquired or nosocomial infection is a disease that develops after the admission to the hospital, and is the consequence of a treatment, not necessarily a surgical one, or work by the hospital staff. A community infection, instead, is an infection acquired by the patient before the admission to the hospital. Usually, a disease is considered a nosocomial infection if its symptoms appear more than 48 hours after the admission to the hospital.

Nosocomial infections are much more dangerous than community infections because they are caused by bacteria that are much more resistant to antibiotics. Usually nosocomial infections are resistant to more than one antibiotic, while community infections are resistant to a single or very few antibiotics. As a consequence, the cure of a community infection normally does not pose problems while it may prove difficult to cure nosocomial ones. In Italy, this problem is very serious: actually almost 15% of the patients admitted to hospitals develop a nosocomial infection. In order to monitor nosocomial infections, the results of microbiological analyses must be carefully collected and analysed.

In Italy, a great number of hospitals manages analysis results by means of a software system named Italab C/S, developed by Dianoema S.p.A. Italab C/S is a Laboratory Information System based on a Client/Server architecture, which manages

R.W. Brause and E. Hanisch (Eds.): ISMDA 2000, LNCS 1933, pp. 282–292, 2000.

all the activities of the various analysis laboratories of the hospital. Analysis results are collected from automatic analyzers connected to the system or from manual input. The results are then checked for validity and stored in a relational database. In the past, we have designed and implemented an expert system for the validation of clinical analysis [4].

In this work, we describe a project, jointly started by DEIS University of Bologna and Dianoema S.p.A., in order to build a system which is able to monitor nosocomial infections. In particular, on the basis of the microbiological analysis results stored in the Italab C/S relational database, the system must:

1. provide statistics about the number of nosocomial infections in the various areas of the hospital;
2. identify critical situations for a single patient (e.g., unexpected antibiotic resistance of a bacterium) or for hospital units (e.g., contagion events) and alarm the microbiologist.

Statistics about infection frequencies are useful from two points of view: on one hand they can be used in order to monitor the diffusion of nosocomial infections over time in the hospital, on the other hand they are a valid help for clinicians to perform a first diagnosis. In this task it is very important to correctly count of the number of infections in each area of the hospital over a period of time. In order to avoid counting a mutation of a bacterium as a new infection, data mining techniques (and clustering, in particular) have been applied in order to find group of similar bacteria (strains). In sections 2, 3 and 4, we briefly report about the first results we have obtained by applying clustering on the microbiological data collected along two years in an Italian hospital.

In order to address the latter task, instead, we will adopt a knowledge-base approach and build a surveillance expert that is able to identify critical situations and correspondingly generate alarms (see section 5).

2   Microbiological Data Analysis

Italab C/S stores all the information concerning patients, the analysis requests, and the analysis results. In particular, data for bacterial infections includes:

- information about the patient: sex, age, hospital unit where the patient has been admitted;
- the kind of material (specimen) to be analysed (e.g., blood, urine, saliva, pus, etc.) and its origin (the body part where the specimen was collected);
- the date when the specimen was collected (often substituted with the analysis request date);
- for every different bacterium identified, its species and its antibiogram.

For each isolated bacterium, the antibiogram represents its resistance to a series of antibiotics. The set of antibiotics used to test bacterial resistance can be defined by the user, and the antibiogram is a vector of couples (antibiotic, resistance), where four types of resistance are possibly recorded: R when resistant, I when intermediate, S when sensitive, and null when unknown.

The antibiogram is not uniquely identified given the bacterium species but it can vary significantly for bacteria of the same species. This is due to the fact that bacteria of the same species may have evolved differently and have developed different resistances to antibiotics. Bacteria with similar antibiograms are grouped into "strains".

From these data, infections are now monitored by means of a Italab C/S module called "Epidemiological Observatory" that periodically generates reports on the most frequent infections detected in the hospital. In particular, for each area of the hospital, the system must show the n (where n is configurable by the user, usually 10) bacterium species most frequently infecting the area. For each species, the system must show:

- the name of the species,
- the percentage of isolated bacteria belonging to that species over the total number of isolated bacteria,
- the resistance of the bacteria to antibiotics, i.e., for each antibiotic, the percentage of found bacteria that are resistant, intermediate and sensitive.

This information is useful because it allows to monitor the behavior of nosocomial infections over time. Moreover, it allows the clinician to give the patient an "empirical therapy": whenever a patient shows the symptoms of an infections, the clinician is able to give him immediately an antibiotic cure by considering the symptoms and the frequency of the candidate infections in the area of the hospital, without waiting for microbiological analysis results that usually take two to three days to come back from the laboratory. Then, when the analysis results become available, he will be able to provide the patient a more accurate cure in case the empirical therapy had not the desired effect.

In order to count the number of bacteria for each species, the "Epidemiological Observatory" analyses the data regarding the positive culture results of a particular time period (3 or 6 months). Every identified bacterium is compared with the other bacteria found on the same patient in the previous N days (usually N is 10). The bacterium is counted provided that its strain is different from that of bacteria of the same species found on the patient in the previous N days. This is because, in case the strain is the same, the new bacterium is considered as a mutation of the previous one rather than a new infection.

In order to detect when two bacteria belong to the same strain, Italab C/S uses a very simple similarity function that computes the percentage of antibiotics in the antibiogram having different values for the two bacteria. If this percentage is below a user defined threshold (usually 30%), then they belong to the same strain.

However, this approach for detecting when two bacteria belong to the same strain is quite rough: it is not universally accepted by microbiologist and does not seem to work in all possible situations (different hospitals, different units within a hospital).

In order to improve the accuracy of the system in recognising strain membership, we defined, helped by microbiologists, a new strain membership criteria.

The first step consists in identifying all existing strains in a target hospital. In some cases, strain descriptions can be provided by the microbiologist, in other cases this is not possible and clustering is applied to all the antibiograms found in the past for every bacterium species. Each cluster found is considered as a strain and its description is stored by the system.

A new bacterium is considered as a new infection provided that no bacterium of the same species and strain is found in the same patient in the previous N days. The new bacteria is classified as belonging to a strain by using a membership function that depends on the strain description used.

In order to find bacterial strain, the clustering algorithm is executed on data regarding the positive cultures (only bacterial specie and relative antibiogram) of a large period of time (ex. 12 months) that have been found at the hospital where the system will be installed.

Applying clustering to find bacterial strain is useful also because it can give the microbiologist new insights about the hospital population of bacteria and their resistance to antibiotics.

In order to test this approach for strain identification, we have performed a number of prototypical clustering experiments on data from various bacterial species. In this experimental phase we have used Intelligent Miner by IBM [3] for its free availability to academic institutions and its powerful graphical interface. However, clustering in final system will be performed by special purpose code.

3   The Demographic Clustering Algorithm

The demographic clustering algorithm that is enclosed in Intelligent Miner [2] builds the clusters by comparing each record with all clusters previously created and by assigning the record to the cluster that maximizes a similarity score. New clusters can be created throughout this process.

The similarity score of two records is based on a voting principle, called Condorset [2]. The distance is computed by comparing the values of each field, assigning it a vote and then summing up the votes over all the fields. For categorical attributes, the votes are computed in this way: if the two records have the same value for the attribute, it gets a vote of +1, otherwise it gets a vote of −1. For numerical attributes, a tolerance interval is established and the vote is now continuous and varies from -1 to 1: -1 indicates values far apart, 1 indicates identical values and 0 indicates that the values are separated exactly by the tolerance interval. The overall score is computed as the sum of the score for each attribute.

In order to assign a record to a cluster, its similarity score with all the clusters is computed. To this purpose, the distribution of values of each field for the records in the cluster is calculated and recorded. The similarity between a record and a cluster is then computed by comparing the field values of the record with the value distribution of the cluster. In this way, it is not necessary to compare the record with each record in the cluster.

The algorithm assigns the record to the cluster with the highest similarity score. In case the score is negative for all clusters, then the record is a candidate for forming a new cluster. In this way, the number of clusters does not have to be known in advance but can be found during the computation.

This process is repeated a fixed number of times ("phases") and clusters are updated until either the maximum number of phases is reached or the maximum number of clusters is achieved or the clusters centres do not change significantly as measured by a user-determined margin.

4 Results

We have considered all the bacteria belonging to the species Staphilococcus Epidermidis. The dataset contains 1961 records having the attributes described in section 1. They have been collected from the 5th of March 1997 to the 20th of November 1999 at Le Molinette Hospital in Turin, Italy.

Table 1. Resistance to antibiotics of Staphilococcus Epidermidis on all the dataset

Antibiotics	S	R	I	null
AMIKACINA	35,1%	61,4%	0,9%	2,6%
AMOXI/A.CLAVULANICO	20,2%	74,2%	-	5,6%
AMOXICILLINA	0,9%	98,9%	-	0,2%
CEFAZOLINA	20,7%	79,0%	0,1%	0,2%
CEFOTAXIME	16,5%	60,1%	0,3%	23,1%
CEFUROXIME PARENTERALE	20,7%	79%	-	0,3%
CIPROFLOXACINA	29,6%	66,2%	3,9%	0,2%
CLINDAMICINA	49,7%	48,8%	1%	0,5%
COTRIMOXAZOLO	48,4%	50,9%	0,5%	0,2%
DOXICICLINA	85,7%	13,8%	0,4%	0,1%
ERITROMICINA	29,1%	69,1%	1,5%	0,2%
GENTAMICINA	32,1%	65%	2,8%	0,1%
GENTAMICINA_HL	-	-	-	100%
IMIPENEM	20,8%	78,8%	0,2%	0,2%
MEZLOCILLINA	0,7%	22,1%	-	77,2%
NETILMICINA	34,1%	61,7%	1,7%	2,5%
NITROFURANTOINA	-	0,1%	-	99,9%
NORFLOXACINA	-	-	-	100%
OFLOXACINA	33%	65,6%	1,1%	0,3%
OXACILLINA	21,1%	78,8%	-	0,1%
PEFLOXACINA	28,6%	69,3%	1,9%	0,2%
PENICILLINA_G	1%	98,8%	-	0,2%
PIPERACILLINA	0,1%	-	-	99,9%
RIFAMPICINA	54,6%	21,9%	0,5%	22,9%
STREPTOMICINA_HL	0,1%	-	-	99,9%
TEICOPLANINA	99,3%	0,2%	0,4%	0,1%
TIAMFENICOLO	86,7%	30,2%	0,9%	0,2%
VANCOMICINA	99,8%	-	-	0,2

We first report the distribution of attribute values relative to the complete dataset. In table 1 the percentage of R, S, I and null values are reported for each of the 23 antibiotics that have been tested.

As in the PTAH system [1], an additional feature was computed for each record: the level of resistance, that represents the percentage of antibiotics for which the bacterium was resistant over the total number of antibiotics whose resistance was known (R, S, I). Figure 1 shows the distribution of the resistance level in the dataset: the X axis reports the level of resistance while the Y axis reports the percentage of records in the dataset having that resistance level.

An experiment was performed where the number of phases was set to 3. In this case, 9 clusters were found with a global Condorset value of 0.843. The clustering has been performed by considering only the record fields relative to antibiotics resistance.

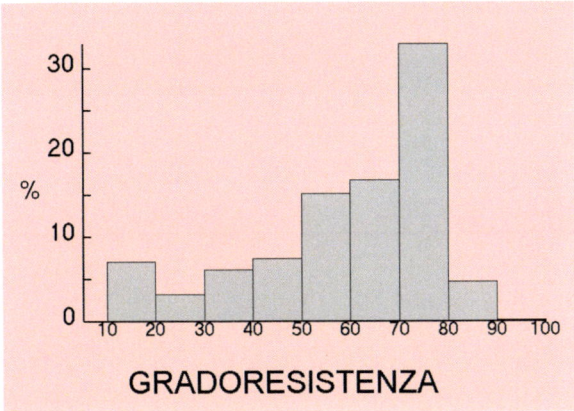

Fig. 1. Distribution of bacteria resistance level (GRADORESISTENZA in Italian)

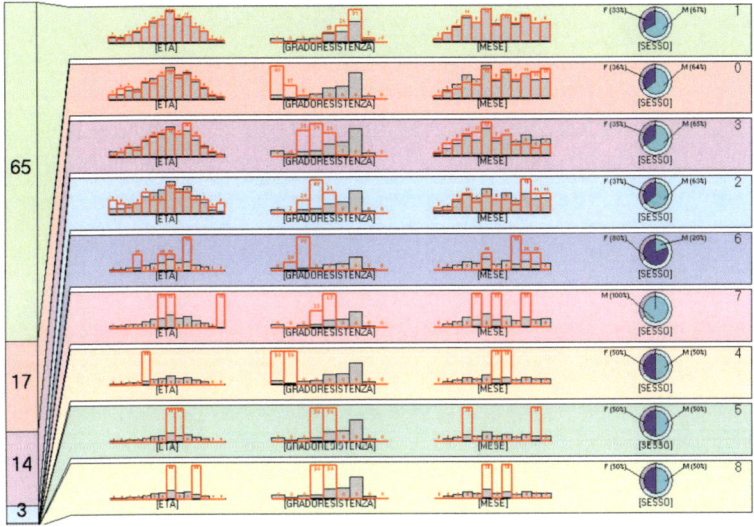

Fig. 2. Value distribution in the clusters

Figure 2 shows a graphic representation of all the clusters, where the number on the left represents the percentage of records in each cluster and the number on the right is the cluster identifier. Within each cluster, the distribution of values for a variable is depicted by a sub-chart, either a histogram for numeric variables or a pie-chart in the case of categorical variables. The sub-charts have an overlay structure that enables them to depict the distribution of the associated variable within both the individual cluster and the overall population for comparison purposes. As regards the histograms, the filled histogram is the distribution of values over all the data, while the empty histogram is the distribution of values in the cluster. As regards the pie-charts, the internal pie is referred to the cluster, while the external ring is referred to the overall dataset.

The variables whose distribution is depicted in Figure 2 are: ETÀ (age), GRADORESISTENZA (resistance level), MESE (month) and SESSO (sex).

Table 2 shows the modal values of antibiotic reactions in the 9 clusters.   The second row shows the number of elements of each cluster and the last the average resistance level of the cluster.

Cluster 1 is the biggest and is the one with the highest level of resistance (average of 69.4 %).

Figure 3 shows the resistance level to antibiotics in cluster 1. From this figure we can observe that in cluster 1 the percentage of resistant bacteria is higher for all antibiotics with respect to the complete dataset except for Doxiciclina for which the percentage of sensitive bacteria is higher. Cluster 0 has the same behaviour with R substituted for S: Doxiciclina is the only antibiotics for which the percentage of resistant bacteria is higher.

Clusters 3 and 2 are characterised by values of the resistance level that are intermediate between those of cluster 1 and 0. Clusters 4, 5, 6, 7 and 8 contain few elements and this means that some antibiograms are significantly different from all the others.

Table 2. Modal values of the resistance for each cluster.

Cluster →	0	1	2	3	4	5	6	7	8
Dimension →	339	1266	65	276	2	2	5	3	2
AMIKACINA	S	R	R	S	S	R	S	S	R
AMOXI_A_ CLAVULANIC	S	R	S	R	S	R	S	R	R
AMOXICILLINA	R	R	R	R	R	R	R	R	R
CEFAZOLINA	S	R	S	R	S	R	S	R	S
CEFOTAXIME	S	R	S	R	S	R	S	R	R
CEFUROXIME_ PARENTE	S	R	S	R	S	R	S	R	S
CIPROFLOXACINA	S	R	R	S	R	R	R	S	I
CLINDAMICINA	S	R	R	S	S	S	R	S	S
COTRIMOXAZOLO	S	R	R	S	R	S	S	R	R
DOXICICLINA	S	S	S	S	S	S	S	R	S
ERITROMICINA	S	R	R	S	R	R	R	S	R
GENTAMICINA	S	R	R	S	I	R	S	I	R
IMIPENEM	S	R	S	R	S	R	S	R	S
MEZLOCILLINA	R	R	R	R	-	R	S	-	-
NETILMICINA	S	R	R	S	S	R	S	S	R
OFLOXACINA	S	R	R	S	R	R	R	S	R
OXACILLINA	S	R	S	R	S	S	S	R	S
PEFLOXACINA	S	R	R	S	R	R	R	S	R
PENICILLINA_G	R	R	R	R	R	R	R	R	R
RIFAMPICINA	S	S	S	S	R	R	R	S	S
TEICOPLANINA	S	S	S	S	S	S	S	S	S
TIAMFENICOLO	S	S	S	S	S	S	S	R	S
VANCOMICINA	S	S	S	S	S	S	S	S	S
Resistance level	14,7	69,4	44,8	44,2	20,8	50,9	32,7	51,4	47,9

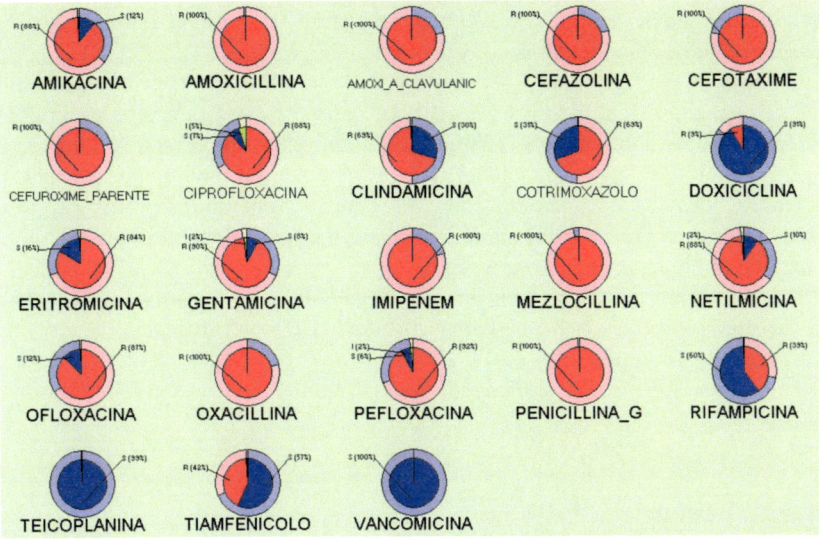

Fig. 3. Resistance to antibiotics in cluster 1

On the basis of these results, some comments can be made. We expected that the majority of bacteria from the same species had similar behaviour and that, more rarely, we could find "abnormal" bacteria that had become more resistant. On the contrary, by clustering the Staphylococcus Epidermidis bacteria, we have found that the majority of bacteria is highly resistant and that rarer cases are characterised by a higher sensitivity to antibiotics. This is probably due to the nature of this bacterium. In fact, another clustering experiment performed over *Escherichia Coli* bacteria has shown that bigger clusters have a lower resistance level and smaller cluster have a higher resistance.

5   Surveillance Expert System

Given a newly isolated bacterium, the system must provide the following alarms:
1. unexpected resistance to an antibiotic,
2. contagion by a multi-resistant bacterium,
3. ineffective therapy.

The first alarm is given if the new isolated bacterium is resistant to an antibiotic to which it is normally sensitive. This is important in order to timely alert the microbiologist about the appearance of an unexpected resistance. To this purpose, the system should store, for each species, the list of antibiotics to be monitored.

The second alarm is given if a bacterium belonging to the same strain was previously found on another patient in the same hospital area within a given period X (usually 30 days). This case indicates that there has been a contagion among the two patients and therefore it must be signaled so that future contagia are avoided. The alarm must be given only if the isolated bacterium is resistant to more than two antibiotics because otherwise it is considered not dangerous.

In the case of the third alarm, the system looks if another bacterium was isolated for the same patient in a previous period Y (usually 30 days, more for some chronic infections). In case a previous bacterium was found, its antibiogram is compared with the one of the current bacterium and an alarm is generated if the number of resistances is increased. The system should show the species and antibiograms of the two bacteria. Moreover, the system should compare the species of the two bacteria and produce one of the following two alarms:

1. if the species are different, then the system should alert the user that the therapy was ineffective because the patient was infected by two different bacteria but it was cured for only one,
2. if the species are the same, then the system should indicate that the therapy has failed.

6   Related Works

PTAH [1] is a decision support system that was designed for helping medical doctors in the prescription of antibiotics for the cure of nosocomial infections. It has been evaluated in the General Hospital Jesenice in Slovenia on data collected since 1994. PTAH can perform four type of analyses:

- resistance level over time,
- hierarchical clustering of antibiograms,
- similarity of antibiograms,
- effectiveness of antibiotics over time

Each analysis is performed over data regarding a single bacterium species at a time.

The resistance level for a bacterium is plotted over time in order to identify occasional and partly periodic appearances of highly resistant bacteria. This allow medical doctors to identify possible inefficiencies in the antibiotic therapy that have caused the appearance of highly resistant bacteria.

Besides identifying time trends of resistance level, PTAH performs clustering of antibiograms. The clusters are hierarchically organized: low level clusters are grouped into higher level cluster and so on up to the root cluster that contains all the data. The hierarchy enables the user to study the clusters at different level of granularity. In this way it is possible to discover the different types of resistance vectors and to evaluate their frequency.

The third type of analysis is aimed at showing the similarities of antibiograms in order to identify possible infection diffusion in the hospital. To this purpose, a two dimensional graph is plot where each horizontal line corresponds to a resistance vector and the X axis is associated to time: each point in the graph represents an antibiogram at a given moment in time. Antibiograms are ordered on the Y axis in a de-crescent way according to their resistance level. Two points are connected by a line if the antibiograms differ for at most one element and have a time difference smaller than a given threshold. In this way, it is possible to identify moments in time where the same bacterium was found with similar characteristics at several patients thus leading to the identification of a possible epidemic: groups of point vertically aligned indicate the presence of a set of similar bacteria at the same time and the higher they are in the graph the more dangerous they are.

The antibiotic effectiveness is analyzed by plotting over time the cumulative or moving average percentage of antibiograms that are resistant to a given antibiotic. In this way it is possible to identify when the effectiveness of an antibiotic becomes too low so that it can be dismissed for medical and financial reasons.

We owe to PTAH a number of inspiring ideas, first of all the introduction of the resistance level variable for a bacterium that is very useful for providing an indication of the dangerousness of bacteria, and also the clustering of bacteria. Differently from PTAH, we do not cluster only resistance vectors but also data regarding the patient: this data turned out to be important since the most significant variables for the clustering are age, resistance level, month and sex. Moreover, we do not use hierarchical clustering as PTAH does: this is due to the fact that the results here presented are obtained from a first study, in the future we plan to adopt as well a hierarchical clustering algorithm because we think that the results will probably be easier to be interpreted by a medical doctor.

7 Conclusions

This paper describes a project, jointly started by DEIS University of Bologna and Dianoema S.p.A., in order to build a system for monitoring nosocomial infections. This function is really important because of the high risks and costs associated to nosocomial infections.

Computing the frequency of infections in the various areas of the hospital is really important for monitoring nosocomial infections. The behavior over time of this frequency may highlight possible hygienic problems. Moreover, it can be used for an early diagnosis and therapy.

In order to correctly compute infection frequencies, it is important not to count twice bacteria belonging to the same strain. To this purpose, we have adopted clustering for performing the identification of the bacterial strains. We report on a first experiment in using clustering on data regarding the Staphilococcus Epidermidis bacteria.

Another important aspect of infection monitoring consists in generating alarms regarding newly identified bacteria. Alarms are raised in case a unexpectedly resistant bacterium is found, in case a contagion among patients of a unit is detected or in case the therapy is found to be ineffective.

Acknowledgements

We are grateful to Dr. Serra (Le Molinette Hospital, Turin), Dr. Furlini (S.Orsola Malpighi Hospital, Bologna) and Dr. Andollina (Officine Ortopediche Rizzoli, Bologna) for helpful discussions. This work has been partially supported by DIANOEMA S.p.A., Bologna, Italy and by the MURST project "Intelligent Agents: Interaction and Knowledge Acquisition".

References

1. M. Bohanec, M. Rems, S. Slavec, B. Urh, "PTAH: A system for supporting nosocomial infection therapy", in N. Lavrac, E. Keravnou, B. Zupan (eds) "Intelligent Data Analysis in Medicine and Pharmacology", Kluwer Academic Publishers, 1997
2. Cabena, Hadjinian, Stadler, Verhees, Zanasi, "Discovering Data Mining – from concept to implementation", Prentice Hall – IBM
3. Intelligent Miner, http://www.software.ibm.com/ data/iminer/fordata
4. Evelina Lamma, Paola Mello, Sara Monesi, Sergio Storari: "An expert system approach for clinical analysis result validation", Proceedings of International conference on Artificial Intelligence, IC-AI'2000, 26-29 giugno 2000

A Data Mining Alternative to Model Hospital Operations: Filtering, Adaption and Behaviour Prediction

David Ria~ ñoand Susana Prado[2]

[1] Universitat Rovira i Virgili, 43006 Tarragona, Spain,
drianyo@etse.urv.es,
WWW home page: http://www.etse.urv.es/~drianyo
[2] Inform´atica El Corte Inglés, Bolivia 234, 08020 Barcelona, Spain
susana_prado@ieci.es

Abstract. The historical evolution of all the patients admitted to a hospital is a source of information that can be studied with intelligent data analysis methods. The transitions of the patients between the hospital services can be represented by a graph structure that is modified to reflect only the interesting information and also to represent the possible behaviour of a concrete patient. The hospital intelligent system HISYS1 incorporates a filtering and an adaptation stages to achieve these activities.

1 Introduction

In a hospital there are two communities that can benefit of the intelligent data analysis: the administration community and the clinical community. Although these communities are concerned with different aspects of the hospital daily work, there are some activities in which they are very related. So, while the administration community deals with the hospital aspects of costs, organisation, reserves, or scheduling, the clinical community deals with diagnoses, prescriptions, patient evolution, or test analysis. In spite of that, practically all the clinical actions have a direct effect on the cost of the patient treatments, and they can affect the scheduling of the administration community which can decide to experiment new lines of treatment or to suggest some physicians to change their procedures, etc.

The historical data of all the patients that have been accepted to a hospital, and the treatments they have received are usually kept in the hospital databases in order to make the annual balance of the hospital and also because of legal reasons. These data represent a clear reflection of the hospital operation, and the intelligent analysis of those data can give rise to clinical behaviour models that, on the one hand, the administration community can use to know if the hospital is working efficiently and, on the other hand, the clinical community can use to predict the behaviour of the new admitted patients and advance the cheapest of the best treatments.

R.W. Brause and E. Hanisch (Eds.): ISMDA 2000, LNCS 1933, pp. 293–299, 2000.

Moreover, these models of behaviour can be used to study the real expenses of the hospital. Many hospitals in Europe, the USA, and Australia use the *Diagnostic-Related Group* model (DRG) to compute their costs. This model [6] is based on a classification of patient groups that are homogeneous with respect to the hospital resource consumption. DRG depend on the patient's age, sex, primary diagnosis, secondary diagnoses, procedures, and discharge reasons. Each DRG is given a fixed cost. The hospital stores the number of cases attended for each DRG and supplies the list to the *National Health-Care Financing Administration* of the country of the hospital. This organisation pays all the DRG cases back to the hospital, using the tables of DRG costs.

Some of the benefits of using DRG to calculate hospital costs are: DRG are based on millions of cases that come from hundreds of hospitals; periodic revisions can be automated; the number of cases is limited to a manageable number which is easy to remember by doctors; patients in a class have similar expected consumption; DRG are medically coherent, that is to say, they are able to define a common language between the administration and the clinical communities; DRG reduce the variance of cases below the variance of the rest of classifications that are not based in iso-consumptions [1], and they are very friendly to calculate hospital costs.

On the contrary, DRG has received several criticisms from the administration and clinical communities since the estimated costs are sometimes away from the real costs which depend on the patient treatments and procedures.

In [10] we propose the hospital intelligent system HISYS1 that does not only calculate the real costs in the hospital, but also it can supply information about the internal operation of the hospital. Here, we extend this work with the incorporation of both a filtering and an adaptation stages to the system that are very useful to transform general models of the hospital behaviour to particular aspects of the hospital and to particular patient cases.

For the sake of comprehension section 2 explains the HISYS1 system briefly. It also describes the new stages in detail. Section 3 describes how these stage are used to filter, adapt and predict the behaviour of the patients of the *Hospital Joan XXIII* in the city of Tarragona, Spain. Finally, section 4 shows the conclusions of this work and some ideas to extend the system.

2   Technical explanation

When a patient is admitted to a hospital, he or she receives an admission number and a *primary diagnosis*, which are the same until he or she leaves the hospital. Moreover, while the patient is in the hospital he or she uses to pass through several departments or hospital services where he or she can receive several *secondary diagnoses* which are related to the complications of the patient in the hospital and also to the patient's own pathologies as diabetes, asthma, HIV, etc. Simultaneously, all the medications, tests, and treatments are also registered under the generic name of *procedure*. If the main reason of a patient admission is to have a medical treatment, this is called the *primary procedure*. The rest of treatments, which can be needed because of the patient evolution though the hospital services, are called *secondary procedur es* The list of transitions of a patient for a given admission is called an *episo de* Each episode has attached a service and sev eral secondary diagnoses and procedures that are stored in the hospital database.

This information can be analysed with intelligen t methods in order to learn the behaviour of a hospital. Traditionally, these methods are classified into those which generate knowledge in the form of a decision tree [7, 8], a set of production rules [4, 9], a Bay esian classifier [2, 3] or an artificial neural netw ork.

The next subsections show the structure that HISYS1 uses to model the hospital operation, and how this structure is transformed to focus the attention in particular aspects of the hospital and to adapt the hospital behaviour to the new patients.

2.1   The HISYS1 system

In [10] the episodes in the database are used to represent the transitions of the patients as a path in a graph structure in which nodes represent admissions, hospital services and disc harge reasons, and arcs represent patient transitions within the hospital. For example, figure 1 shows the graph of the patients which are admitted to the *Hospital Joan XXIII* in 1999 with primary diagnosis *Chronic Obstructive Bronchitis*.

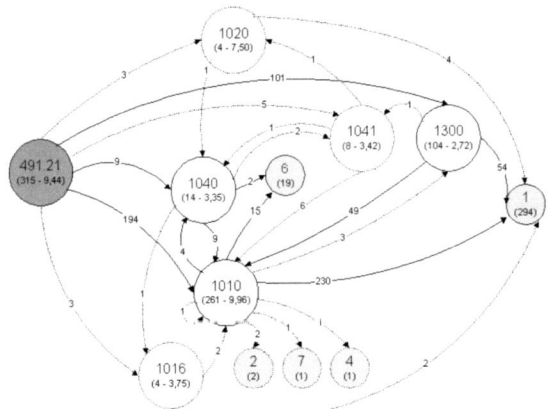

Fig. 1. The *Chr onic Obstructive Bonchitis* (Code 491.21) graph showing some of the hospital services: In ternal Medicine (1010), Cardiology (1016), Pnephrology (1020), In tensiv e Care (1040), Intermediate Care (1041), Emergency (300); and discharge reasons: home (1), transfer to acute hospital (2), transfer to social hospital (4), *exitus* (6), and escape (7).

Each node in the graph stores information about the n umber of patients visiting the node, the accumulate number of days and cost of the stay, and the sets of secondary diagnoses, procedures and physicians involved. As far as the arcs are concerned, they store the detailed information of the patients that have passed through them: admission number, sex, age, ZIP code, cost, physician in charge, number of days, and the sets of secondary diagnoses and procedures. This reinforces the elements that are more visited in the graph and permit the administration and clinical communities to have a criterion to recognise which are the important elements and behaviours.

Once the graph is generated, the CN2 [4] inductive learning algorithm is applied to distinguish between the outgoing arcs of each node. This way, we obtain a set of rules that define the behaviour of the patients when they are accepted to the hospital and when they leave a hospital service. This knowledge is organised in the hierarchical structure that is shown in figure 2.

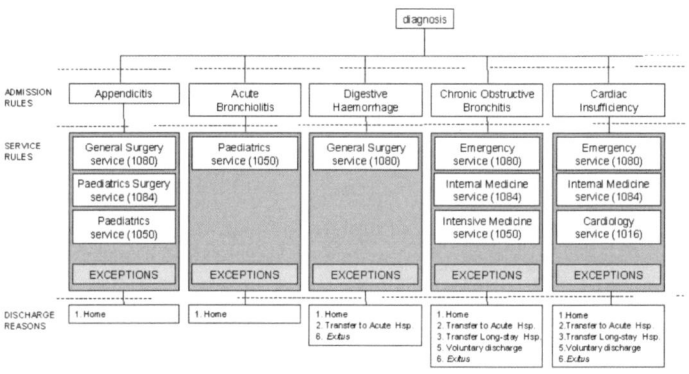

Fig. 2. The HISYS1 rule-set architecture

The four horizontal lanes contain the rule sets. The first lane (diagnosis) separates the patients depending on the primary diagnosis. The second lane (admission rules) decides which is the hospital service that the patient is assigned to. The third lane (service rules) describes the transitions of the patients within the hospital services. And the forth lane (discharge reasons) indicates which is the discharge reason of the patients.

The rule-set architecture of figure 2 is a dynamic representation of the graphs that HISYS1 supplies in order to predict the local behaviour of the new patients. So, if a patient is admitted with primary diagnosis *Chronic Obstructive Bronchitis*, the admission rules suggest which is the input service of the patient. Once the patient is in a service, the rule-set related to that service is used to predict the next service that will attend the patient, or the discharge reason.

Although the hospital managers and physicians show ed their interest in the predictive capacity of HISYS1, they soon proposed the adaptation of the system to their particular needs. While hospital managers are interested in the marginal study of some aspects of the global graph structure, the physicians are concerned about the patients as individuals and they proposed the adaptation of the global graph structures to a concrete graph structure that represents the feasible beha viours of a concrete patient. The next subsections describe ho w the HISYS1 system achiev es these goals with the filtering and the adaptation stages.

2.2 The filtering stage

The graph structures that HISYS1 generates contain all the historical information about the behaviour of all the cases with a particular primary diagnosis: patient's admission number, sex, age, ZIP code, cost, ph ysician in charge, number of da ys, secondary diagnoses, primary procedure, and secondary procedures. F or administration reasons, it is suitable to ha vea mechanism to separate some aspects of the graph information that are not relev an tfrom those which are relev an t for the managemen analysis which is being carried out at that moment.

During the filtering stage, the irrelev an tinformation is remov ed from the graph. The nodes and arcs that lose all the information are remov ed from the graph. Finally, only those elements that are relevan t remain in the filtered graph. In section 3 we describe some tests of the filtering stage.

2.3 The adaptationge

When a new patient arriv es to the hospital the HISYS1 rule-set architecture of figure 2 can predidte patien   t transitions betw een the hospital services. This process has an alternative which is mre in teresting to the clinical communit y and which consistsin the   adaptation of the general graph representing all the patients to a new graph that represents only the behaviour alternatives of the new patient. This w ayeac h new patient is able to ha vehis or her particular graph

The adaptation stage that HISYS1 implements is based on a distance function and a threshold value. The distance function tak es in to consideration the patient's sex, age, and set of secondary diagnoses, as equation 1 shows. Alternative distance functions have been tested with worse results.

$$dist(i,j) = \frac{1}{6}\left(diff(sex_i, sex_j) + 2\frac{|age_i - age_j|}{100} + 3\left(1 - \frac{|sd_i \cap sd_j|}{|sd_i \cup sd_j|}\right)\right) \quad (1)$$

$$diff(a,b) = \begin{cases} 0 \; a = b \\ 1 \; a \neq b \end{cases}$$

F or all the arcs in the general graph, the distance betw een the new patien t and the patients stored in the arcs is calculated. Only those arcs which have a patient which is closer to the new patient than the threshold value are maintained. Disconnected nodes are also removed. The final graph is a description of the behaviour of all the patients that are similar to the new patient. Under the *gener alityprinciple* of the nearest neighbour algorithms [5], patients which are similar can have similar behaviors.

3   Application

The filtering and adaptation stages of the HISYS1 ha ve been applied to the study of the patients with a *Chronic Obstructive Bronchitis* (COB) in the *Hospital Joan XXIII* in Tarragona, Spain, in 1999.

The filtering stage has been applied to study the behavior of the patients according to their sex, age, and the physicians which attend them. The graphs obtained sho w ed thatthere are less COB cases for women (59 cases) than for men (256 cases), the women graph is simpler than the men graph, and women follo w a normal cycle while men sho w abnormal cycles with complications. A similar situation w asobserved for people belo w60 (28 cases) which sho w eda simple graph with normal cycles. On the contrary , people abo ve 60 (287 cases) sho w ed complicated cases. Finallythe filter of physicians was useful to discov er that the patients of one of the doctors had a mean stay 10 days higher than the stays of other patients. This w asbecausethese patients w ereadmitted before some tests were done when the normal behavior is to admit them after the tests are done.

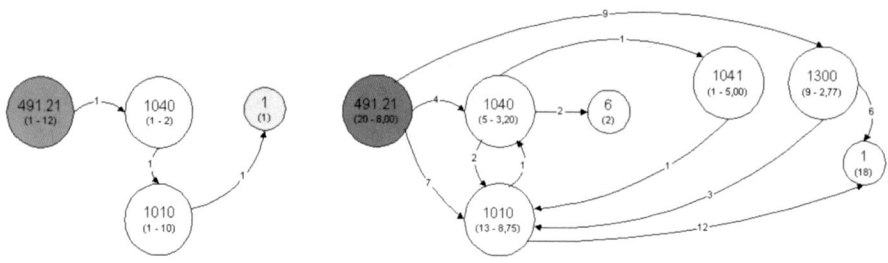

Fig. 3. Adapted *Chr onic Obstructive Bronchitis* graphs with thresholds 2.0 and 4.0

The adaptation stage has been applied to the general graph obtained for 300 historical COB cases. See figure 1. This graph has been adapted to 15 different cases using the thresholds 0.2, 0.3, 0.4, 0.5, and 0.6. One of the cases is shown in figure 3 for a test patient which has passed though the hospital services 1040, 1041, and 1010. Figure 3 shows that a threshold 0.2 is too restrictive, and 0.4 con tains the real behavior of the patient.

4 Conclusions and future work

The system HISYS1 has been enriched with filtering   stage that is able to focus the information of the general graph on the aspects that the administration or clinical communities are interested. An adaptation stage has been also implemented. This stage transforms the general graph into a particular graph showing the possible behaviors of a concrete patient. A distance function has been defined that, together with a threshold value, define the input to the adaptation stage.

There are some aspects that should be changed in the system: the distance function must be improved and the weights of the features involved in the function calculated by some optimisation algorithm. More tests of the filter and adaptation stages should be done on other primary diagnoses as appendicitis, acute bronchiolitis, digestive haemorrhage, cardiac insufficiency, etc. and the results analysed by the clinical community.

This work has received the support of the Spanish CICyT project SMASH (cod. TIC96-1038-04), the A CŒS project of the Unviersitat Rovira i Virgili, and the technical support of IECISA and the *Hospital Joan XXIII*.

References

1. Casas, M.: Los grupos relacionados con el diagn´osticoexperiencia y perspectivas de utilisaci´ on. Ed. Masson S.A. (1991) ISBN: 84-311-0578-X
2. Cheeseman, P., Kelly , J., Self M., Stutz, J., Tylor, W., and Freemann, D.: Autoclass: a Bayesian Classification System. Fifth Int. Conference on Machine Learning, Morgan Kaufmann Publishers, (1988), 54-64
3. Cheeseman, P., and Stutz, J.: Bayessian classification (Autoclass): Theory and results. AAAI Press, The MIT Press, (1996), chapter 6.
4. Clark, P., Nibblet, T.: The CN2 induction algorithm. Int. Journal of Machine Learning $3(4)$, (1989) 261–283
5. Dasarathy, B. V.: Nearest neighbour norms: NN pattern classification techniques. Los Alamitos, Ca: IEEE Computer Society Press (1991)
6. Fetter, R. B., Youngsoo, S., Freeman, J. L., Averall, R. F., Thomson, J. D.: Case mix definition by diagnosis-related groups. Med Care. **18** (1980) 1 53
7. Quinlan J. R.: Induction of decision trees. Int. Journal of Machine Learning **1** (1986), 81–106
8. Quinlan J. R.: C4.5: Programs for machine learning. Morgan Kaufmann, San Mateo, California, 1993.
9. Ria˜ no, D.: On the process of making description rules. Lecture Notes in Artificial Intelligence **1624**, *In* Collaboration between Human and Artificial Societies, Julian A. Padget (Ed.) (1999), 182–197
10. Ria˜ no, D., Prado, S.: A data-mining alternative to model hospital operations: clinical costs and predictions. Int. Conference in Data Mining, Cambridge, UK (2000) 63–72

Selection of Informative Genes in Gene Expression Based Diagnosis: A Nonparametric Approach

Martin Beibel

Universität Freiburg, Institut f¨ur Mathematische Stochastik, Eckerstr. 1, D-79104
Freiburg, Germany, beibel@stochastik.uni-freiburg.de

Abstract. We study a nonparametric approach to cancer classification
using data from DNA microarrays. We compare our approach to the
approach of [4].

1 Introduction

DNA microarrays allow the monitoring of the expression levels of thousands of genes simultaneously. Golub et al developed in [4] a systematic approach to the classification of cancer subtypes on the basis of such data. They distinguished two major issues: the discovery of previously unknown subtypes (class discovery) and the assignment of tumor samples to already known subtypes (class prediction). Here we focus on *class prediction* in the case of a *binary* classification. To build and construct a prediction scheme a set of samples is needed for which the classification into the two subtypes is precisely known. Typically this dataset is divided into two subsets: a *training set* and a *test set*. First the training set is used to construct a prediction rule. The performance of the obtained rule is then judged by its performance on the test set. The construction of a prediction rule in our context usually proceeds in two steps. Given the large number of genes and the relatively small number of samples one first singles out a small set of (say 50) most informative genes. The expression levels of the selected genes are then used as a basis for the construction of a prediction rule.

We compare two approaches: the one introduced in [4] and an alternative approach we propose. [6] motivates the approach in [4] with a model assuming normality of the (transformed and normalized) gene expression levels. The motivation behind our proposal is to use a distribution free approach. In fact, our method is invariant under monotone transformations of the gene expression levels. We use two datasets to asses the performance of both rules: the data of [4] (available at http://www.genome.wi.mit.edu/MPR) and the data of [1] (available at

R.W. Brause and E. Hanisch (Eds.): ISMDA 2000, LNCS 1933, pp. 300–307, 2000.
© Springer-Verlag Berlin Heidelberg 2000

`http://llmpp.nih.gov/lymphoma`). In both cases we use the data as they are supplied. For the data of [4] this means that we do not employ any filtering or normalization. Note that these data are raw expression levels.

2   The prediction rules

Suppose we have n samples at hand for the training set. For each gene g we then have expression levels $X_1(g), \ldots, X_n(g)$, where $X_i(g)$ is the expression of gene g in sample i. Moreover we know for each sample whether it belongs to the first subtype (`class 0`) or the second subtype (`class 1`). Let c_i denote the class number of sample i.

2.1   The Golub et al approach

Let $n_0 = \#\{i|c_i = 0\}$ and $n_1 = \#\{i|c_i = 1\}$ be the number of samples from `class 0` and `class 1` in the training set. Let

$$\mu_0(g) = \frac{1}{n_0} \sum_{i|c_i=0} X_i(g), \ \mu_1(g) = \frac{1}{n_1} \sum_{i|c_i=1} X_i(g),$$

$$\sigma_0^2 = \frac{1}{n_0-1} \sum_{i|c_i=0} (X_i(g) - \mu_0(g))^2, \ \sigma_1^2 = \frac{1}{n_1-1} \sum_{i|c_i=1} (X_i(g) - \mu_1(g))^2$$

denote the mean and variances of the expression levels of gene g over the training set samples coming from `class 0` and `class 1`. In [4] the following measure $P(g,c)$ of association between the expression levels and the class distinction is considered: $P(g,c) = [\mu_0(g)-\mu_1(g)]/[\sigma_1(g)+\sigma_2(g)]$. $m/2$ genes with the highest values of $P(g,c)$ and $m/2$ genes with the lowest values of $P(g,c)$ are then selected for a suitable number m. Suppose we select genes $g_1, \ldots, g_m$. A new sample with expression levels $\tilde{X}(g_j)$ $(1 \leq j \leq m)$ is then classified as follows. Let $m(g_j) = 0.5*(\mu_0(g_j)+\mu_1(g_j))$ and $V_j = V(g_j, \tilde{X}(g_j)) = P(g_j,c)(\tilde{X}(g_j) - m(g_j)$. V_j can be considered as the 'vote' of gene g_j. Let $V = \sum_j V_j$ denote the sum of all votes. If $V < 0$, then the new sample is classified as `class 0` otherwise as `class 1`. The strength of a prediction is measured by the relative margin of victory given by $PS = |V/\sum_j |V(g_j)||$.

2.2   The cutpoint approach

Let h be a real number and suppose we divide the training set in to two groups according to whether (for a fixed gene g) $X_i(g) \leq h$ or $X_i(g) > h$.

We call h a cutpoint. The basic idea behind our approach is to classify the samples according to whether $X_i(g) \leq h$ or $X_i(g) > h$ for a suitable cutpoint h. A measure for ho ww ellthis distinction agrees with the distinction of the samples into class 0 and class 1 is giv en ly the deviance $D(g, c, h)$

$$D(g, c, h) = n_{<0} \log \frac{n_{<0}}{n_<} + n_{<1} \log \frac{n_{<1}}{n_<} + n_{>0} \log \frac{n_{>0}}{n_>} + n_{>1} \log \frac{n_{>1}}{n_>},$$

where

$$n_< = \#\{i | X_i(g) \leq h\}, \quad n_> = \#\{i | X_i(g) > h\},$$

$$n_{<0} = \#\{i | X_i(g) \leq h, c_i = 0\}, \quad n_{<1} = \#\{i | X_i(g) \leq h, c_i = 1\},$$

$$n_{>0} = \#\{i | X_i(g) > h, c_i = 0\}, \text{ and } n_{>1} = \#\{i | X_i(g) > h, c_i = 1\}.$$

See [2] for the use of such a measure for the construction of classification trees. Note that $D(g, c, h) \leq 0$. $D(g, c, h) = 0$ holds if the cutpoint h completely separates the tw o classesclass 0 and class 1.

We take the maximum $D(g, c)$ of $D(g, c, h)$ ov er all possible cutpoirts h as a measure of how well the tw o classesclass 0 and class 1 can be distinguished on the basis of the expression levels of gene g. See [3] and [5] for such a maximization approach. It is clearly sufficient to consider the (at most) $n - 1$ midpoints of the ordered observations for the computation of this maximum. Let $h^*(g)$ be a cutpoint for which the maximum is attained. Let $s^*(g)$ be -1 if $n_{<0}/n_{<1} < n_{>0}/n_{>1}$ and $+1$ otherwise. This means that $s^*(g) = -1$ if the relative proportion of samples from class 0 among the samples i with $X_i(g) \leq h^*(g)$ is smaller than the relative proportion of samples from class 0 among the samples i with $X_i(g) > h^*(g)$. In this case it is natural to classify a new sample as class 0 if its expression level for gene g is higher than $h^*(g)$ and as class 1 otherwise. If $n_{<0}/n_{<1} \geq n_{>0}/n_{>1}$ and so $s^*(g) = +1$, it is natural to classify a new sample as class 0 if its expression lev el for gene g is low erthan $h^*(g)$ and as class 1 otherwise.

In order to combine the information from different genes, m Genes with the highest v alues of $D(g, c)$ are selected for a suitable n umber m. Suppose we select genes $g_1, \ldots, g_m$. A new sample with expression levels $\tilde{X}(g_j)$ ($1 \leq j \leq m$) is then classified as follows. Let $V_j = V(g_j, \tilde{X}(g_j)) = s^*(g_j)(\tilde{X}(g_j) - h^*(g_j))$. If $V_j < 0$, then gene g_j 'v otes' for class 0 and otherwise for class 1. Note that $V_j < 0$ if either $s^*(g_j) = -1$ and $\tilde{X}(g_j) > h^*(g_j)$ or $s^*(g_j) = +1$ and $\tilde{X}(g_j) < h^*(g_j)$. Now eac h of the genes $g_1, \ldots, g_m$ casts its vote and we combine these votes as follows: we decide for the class which gets the majority of the votes. The strength of a prediction is measured by the percentage of votes for the winning class.

3   Numerical Results

T o compare the tw o approaches we repeated the following bootstrap procedure a 100 times for eac h data set and predictor. In eac   h run w e
randomly divided the available data in to a training set and a learning
set. Each sample had a chance of 2/3 to be assigned to the training set
and a chance of 1/3 to be assigned to the test set. Samples were allocated
independently of each other. A predictor was then constructed using the
training set and test set error rates were obtained. We considered the

1. rate of correct classifications
2. rate of correct and 'trusted' classifications
3. rate of incorrect but 'trusted' classifications .

F or the Golub et al approach predictions with a prediction strength
$PS \geq 0.3$ were considered as 'trusted'. Accordingly, for the cutpoint approach, predictions with a percentage of v otes for the winning class of
at least 0.65 w ereconsidered as 'trusted'. We considered four different
v alues for the n umber m of selected informative genes; namely $m = 10$,
$m = 20$, $m = 50$ and $m = 100$. We report below he empirical means of
the rate of correct classifications and the rate of correct and 'trusted' classifications o v erthe 100 simulations. The results on the rate of incorrect
but 'trusted' classifications are summarized in boxplots. All computations
w ere performed using S-PLUS version 3.4.

3.1   The Golub et al Data

The dataset in [4] consists of gene expression data from bone marrow and
blood samples from patients with acute leukemia. The patients were distinguished in to cases of acute lymphoblastic leukemia (ALL) and acute
my eloid leukemia (AML). In [4] 38 samples w ereused as a training set
and 34 samples as a test set. We combined the tw osets and assigned
samples randomly to a training set and a test set as described abov e. The
results are given in Tables 1 and 2 and Figure 1 below.

T able 1. Mean of rate of correct classifications – Golub et al data

	m = 100	m = 50	m = 20	m = 10
Golub et al. approach	0.97	0.96	0.95	0.94
cutpoint approach	0.96	0.96	0.97	0.96

T able 2. Mean of rate of correct 'trusted' classifications – Golub et al data

	m = 100	m = 50	m = 20	m = 10
Golub et al. approach	0.89	0.88	0.88	0.87
cutpoint approach	0.81	0.84	0.91	0.91

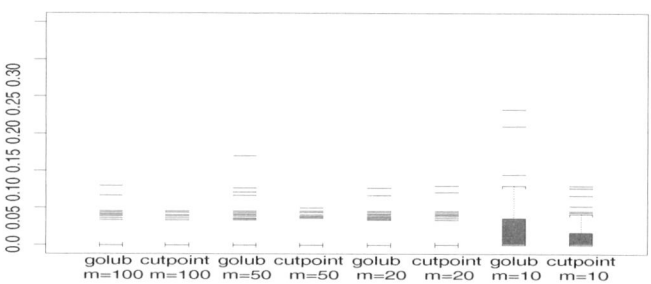

Fig. 1. Rate of incorrect but 'trusted' classifications – Golub et al data

3.2   The Alizadeh et al Data

Alizadeh et al studied in [1] gene expression data from adults with diffuse large B-cell lymphoma (DLBCL). They identified tw omolecularly distinct forms of DLBCL which they termed 'Germinal center B-like DLBCL' and 'activated B-like DLBCL'. We used the data related to Figure 3b in [1] which give the expression levels for 2984 genes in 42 samples. We randomly assigned these samples to a training set and a test set as described above. This dataset has missing values. We did not exclude genes with expression lev els missing for some samples. In calculating $P(g, c)$ and $D(g, c)$ on the training set for a particular gene g w e only considered those samples for which an expression lev el of that gene w asa v ailable. F or the classification of a test set sample, w e only used v otes of those selected genes g_j for which an expression level was a v ailable for that particular sample. The results are given in Tables 3 and 4 and Figure 2 below.

T able 3. Mean of rate of correct classifications – Alizadeh et al data

	m = 100	m = 50	m = 20	m = 10
Golub et al. approach	0.97	0.97	0.93	0.91
cutpoint approach	0.92	0.93	0.89	0.88

T able 4. Mean of rate of correct 'trusted' classifications – Alizadeh et al data

	m = 100	m = 50	m = 20	m = 10
Golub et al. approach	0.81	0.85	0.85	0.84
cutpoint approach	0.48	0.59	0.71	0.73

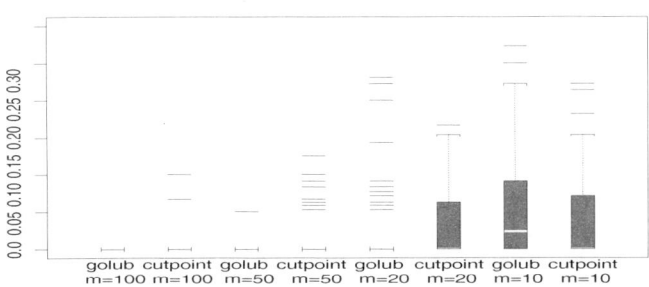

Fig. 2. Rate of incorrect but 'trusted' classifications – Alizadeh et al data

4   Discussion

Our results indicate a certain robustness of the approach of Golub et al. In fact, the nonparametric competitor which w e propose does not perform better than the method of Golub et al for the ra w data of [4]. F or the transformed and normalized data of [1] the method of Golub et al. is considerably superior. In particular the rate of correct 'trusted' classifications is significantly lo w er.This is probably due to the loss of information in our approach caused by largely neglecting the actual value of the gene expressions.

The numerical results on the performance of both classification rules in Subsection 3.1 and Subsection 3.2 are not en tirely comparable. The combined data from [4] consist of 72 samples whereas the data from [1] consist of 42 samples. The training sets in Subsection 3.1 therefore are on av erage considerable larger than the training sets in Subsection 3.2.To account for this difference we repeated the bootstrap approach of Section 3 for the data from [4] with a smaller probability p for each sample to be assigned to the training set. Now eac hsample had a chance of $p = 1/3$ to be chosen for the training set. T able5 below giv esthe av erage value of the rate of correct classifications for each prediction rule over 100 runs with $p = 1/3$. The results indicate that the inferior performance of our cutpoint approach for the data from [1] is not due to the smaller number of samples. Probably our approach has more difficulties to cope with the relatively large number of missing values in this data set.

Table 5. Mean of rate of correct classifications (for $p = 1/3$) – Golub et al data

	m = 100	m = 50	m = 20	m = 10
Golub et al. approach	0.94	0.94	0.92	0.91
cutpoint approach	0.91	0.93	0.92	0.92

Increasing the number m of selected informative genes does not greatly improve the overall performance of both predictors. More precisely, increasing m does increase the rate of correct classifications somewhat. Moreover the rate of incorrect but 'trusted' classifications decreases considerably. The rate of correct 'trusted' classifications, however does not increase with growing m. In particular, for the cutpoint approach this rate even decreases significantly when m increases. This behaviour might be due to the fact that in both approaches the combination of the votes of different genes does not take into account the possible correlation between these votes. Finding appropriate ways to incorporate this correlation into a prediction rule will be a topic of future research.

One might think of using classification trees rather than our related cutpoint approach. However our experience indicates that classification trees do not perform as well as our proposal for the type of problem at discussion. Growing classification trees on our training sets typically leads to trees with a small number of splits (often only one or two). Therefore a single classification trees is not able to effectively combine the additional information provided by the expression levels of several genes and there is a tendency to overfitting on the training set.

We applied 50 runs of the bootstrap procedure of Section 3 to select training sets using the combined data of [4] and constructed classification trees on the basis of the training sets and determined the rate of correct classifications on the corresponding test sets. In order to speed up the computations we preselected a set of 3360 genes on the basis of a variation filter. This resulted in an average rate of correct classifications of 0.86. 12 out of the 50 trees had exactly one split, 35 had exactly two splits and the remaining 3 had exactly three splits. Figure 3 below shows

a typical tree with tw osplits. The corresponding training set consists of
47 samplost of   which 30 are ALL (=class 0) and 17 AML (=class
1).The ratios given below the nodes are the misclassification rates on the
samples of the training set at that particular node. The first split already
separates 29 ALL samples from the 17 AML samples. The second split is
only needed to distinguish the last ALL sample from the 17 AML samples. This particular tree correctly classifies 21 out of the 25 samples of
the corresponding test set.

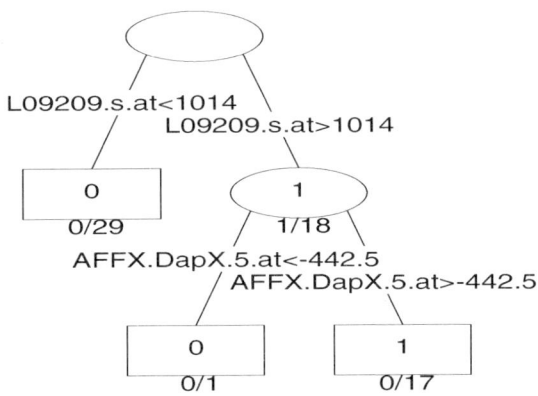

Fig. 3. Example of a classification tree – Golub et al data

References

1. Alizadeh, A. A. et al: Distinct types of diffuse large B-cell lymphoma identified b y
   gene expression profiling. Nature **403** (2000) 503–511
2. Ciampi, A. et al: Recursive partioning: a versatile method for exploratory data
   analysis in Biostatistics. in *Biostatistics* (eds. I. B. MacNeill and G. J. Umphrey).
   (1987) D. Reidel Publishing, New York
3. Gail, M. H. and Green, S. B.: A generalization of the one-sided tw o-sample
   Kolmogorov-Smirnov statistic for ev aluating diagnostic tests. Biometrics**32** (1976)
   561–570
4. Golub, T. R. et al: Molecular classification of cancer: class disco very and class
   prediction by gene expression monitoring. Science **286** (1999) 531–536
5. Miller, R. and Siegmund, D.: Maximally selected chi-square statistics. Biometrics
   38 (1982) 1011–1016
6. Slonim, D. K. et al: Class prediction and disco very using gene expression data.
   Manuscript a vailablæt http://www.gen ome.wi.mit.edu/MP R

Principal Component Analysis for Descriptive Epidemiology

A. Giuliani and R. Benigni

Istituto Superiore di Sanita', Comparative Toxicology and Ecotoxicology Lab.
Viale Regina Elena 299, 00161 Roma, Italy
alessandro.giuliani@iss.it

Abstract. The Principal Component Analysis (PCA) of the tumor frequency distribution across Europe highlighted the existence of a strong and reliable deterministic structure organizing the spatial variability of the relative frequency of the different tumors. The analysis highlighted 5 principal "macrocauses" organizing the spatial variability of tumor incidences for both sexes. These "macrocauses" were demonstrated to be relatively time invariant and pointed to still undiscovered cancer determinants. From a general data analysis point of view, this work proves the ability of PCA of detecting very small signals out of noise and indicates the utility of the technique in epidemiological studies.

1 Introduction

The epidemiological studies are the main tools used by medical science to control at the population scale for the relevance of hypotheses and models generated in the laboratories. The basic scheme of epidemiological studies derives from classical inferential statistics in which the hypothesis of interest is proven through the demonstration that the variance of a given observable (e.g. the incidence of a particular pathology) "explained" by the parameter of interest (e.g. the exposure to a chemical agent or the presence of a given genotype) is much greater than the variance due to all the other causes not explicitly taken into account and thus considered as noise [8].

This general scheme is implemented through the definition of experimental groups characterized by different levels of the parameter of interest (e.g. exposed and not exposed to a chemical agent or drug and placebo administered patients) and controlling for the existence of a statistically significant excess of the between-groups variance over the within-group variance for the observable of interest [8].

This scheme is very efficient when in presence of a single causative agent far exceeding all the others as for explanation power : this is the case of infective diseases in which the microorganism responsible for the disease exceeds all the other concomitant causes.

In the case of multifactorial non infective diseases like cancer , the situation is much more entangled and this is the reason for only a comparatively minor

R.W. Brause and E. Hanisch (Eds.): ISMDA 2000, LNCS 1933, pp. 308–313, 2000.

portion of carcinogenic agents (like cigarette smoke or asbestos) were detected. In the case of multifactorial processes, the classical epidemiological approach is based on a covariance-like scheme in which the effect of each putative agent is "depurated" by the "confounding effect" of concomitant factors that could mask a real action or, on the contrary, could render significant a spurious correlation. The disentanglement of an underlying cause from the spurious concomitant events is efficient only when in presence of additive effects, while in the case of complex and nonlinear interactions between concomitant causes the process provokes a drastic lowering of the power of the test, thus making the proof of any medical hypothesis practically unfeasible [10].

This is the reason for sentences like "epidemiology faced its limits" [10].

From an engineering point of view, the need for an increased power of epidemiological studies can be considered, in metaphorical terms, as an SNR (signal-to-noise-ratio) maximization problem. Based on this analogy, we looked for analysis tools able to maximize the SNR of epidemiological studies.

We selected Principal Component Analysis (PCA) for its intrinsic nature of filter for correlated (and thence signal-like) information [2], [7]. Moreover we had previously demonstrated the ability of the technique to detect signals with very low SNR (less than 0.001) [3].

What we needed for the technique to be properly applied was a variability space in which to express the relevant epidemiological information. The chosen space was constituted by the tumor registries collected by IARC (International Agency for Research on Cancer) on different tumors incidence data relative to 71 European locations [4],[5]. These registries report the relative incidence in the population of 87 (42 male and 45 female) tumor types. The quality of the data is strictly controlled by IARC and each register is based on a basin of around 1 million people so giving reliable estimates even for very rare tumors [4], [5]. The data refer to the occurence of primary tumors (each individual is scored for only one tumor); this implies that the between-tumors correlations highlighted by PCA are external to the individuals and point to distinct (given the mutual orthogonality of components) macro-causes unifying the different tumor types [1]. The presence of two distinct data collections (old: 1981-1985 and new: 1986-1991 periods) allowed us to check for the temporal invariance (and thus for the deterministic character) of the extracted components.

Our results pointed to the existence of 10 components (5 for male tumors and 5 for female tumors) of tumor profile that remained markedly invariant during the time. Only one of the extracted components was already recognized by medical science, while the others pointed to still undiscovered cancer determinants. The male and female solutions were in turn demonstrated to be the image of the same underlying structure, consistently with the hypothesis that the components measure environmental determinants experienced by both sexes even if with different modalities.

These observations allow for a research program to be initiated to give a name (and thus prefiguring a positive preventive action) to the extracted components.

2   Materials and Methods

2.1   Data

Out of the European regions, 71 had cancer registries approved by IARC for the 1986-1991 period: 48 out of 71 were in common with the 1981-1985 collection and were used for the temporal correlations. The data are normalized as for the age structure of the different populations, to eliminate the possible bias due to the marked age dependance of cancer.

The data were expressed in terms of the relative percentage of each tumor type, the total number of tumors per area scaled to 100, to eliminate the burden of the variance due to the general differences in average tumor incidence between areas.

2.2   Statistical Methodology

The unit/variable matrices having as rows (statistical units) the different locations and as columns the different tumors were analyzed by two independent PCA for both sexes. The number of components to be extracted was decided by means of the scree test [7]. This test is based on the observation that random noise has a flat eigenvalue spectrum [2], this allows to stop the components extraction when the component number vs. eigenvalue curve reach a plateau (noise floor).

The procedure was applied to both 1981-1985 and 1986-1991 compilations (48 registries in common) and the extracted components ($PROM\#/PROF\#$ for 1981-1985 male/female data and $NEOM\#/NEOF\#$ for 1986-1991 male/female data) were correlated through time by means of Pearson correlation coefficients and Canonical Correlation [7]. The recognition of temporal invariance of the extracted components was taken as a proof of the deterministic character of the component themselves in addiction to scree test. This implies that the real dimensionality of the system is underdetermined but we preferred to base our considerations on a statistically robust ground than giving an exact estimate of the number of tumor macro-causes.

The first five principal components relative to the entire 1986-1991 data set (71 locations) were globally consistent with the reduced set ones and were denominated $EUROM\#$ and $EUROF\#$ for male and female respectively. These components were the input variables of a "second order" PCA to check for the commonality of the environmental factors experienced by the two sexes. Given the orthogonality of principal components, the minimal dimension of this data set is five (equal to each set dimensionality), thus, the demonstration of an effective dimensionality of five with actual data corresponds to a proof of the unitary character of male and female tumors.

3   Results and Discussion

The scree test suggested a minimalist five component (around 45% of the total variance explained) and a maximalist ten component (around 67% of the total variance explained) solution for all the four data sets.

The temporal canonical correlation for the five component space for both the male and female data sets was very high and statistically significant, with the two main canonical variates showing a correlation of 0.97 and 0.96 for males and 0.96 and 0.87 for females ($p < 0.0001$). This result points to a general invariance of the tumor macro-causes while the relative importance of the single components in explaining the spatial variability of the tumor profiles changed along the years: the first component (in order of explained variance) of the male old data set ($PROM1$) was correlated (Pearson $r = 0.87, p < 0.0001$) with the second component of the male new data set ($NEOM2$), while $PROM2$ was correlated at $r = 0.92$ with $NEOM1$ and $NEOM3$ was correlated at $r = 0.74$ with $PROM4$. In the female data set two main principal components maintained their relative importance invariant across the years ($r(NEOF1, PROF1) = 0.92, r(NEOF2, PROF2) = 0.75$).

The inspection of the component loadings allowed us to identify $NEOM1$ (and consequently $PROM2$) with the already recognized association linking the so called "head and neck" cancers [6] unified by the common major causative agent of the combined alcohol and tobacco use [9]. The other associations are still unrecognized and ask for further studies to identify the respective causative agents.

Having proven the marked temporal invariance of the picture, we concentrated on the 71 locations relative to the 1986-1991 data set in order to get a proof of the soundness of our interpretation of principal components as macro-causes organizing the spatial variability of tumor profiles. In a previous work [1] we demonstrated that the areas expressed in the component space had a marked cluster structure (k-means clustering of locations on the 5 component space) almost exactly following the "cultural" boundaries of Europe. The clustering pointed to a "Mediterranean" cluster unifying Italian and Spanish locations, a Northern Europe cluster (British Isles + Denmark), a Scandinavian cluster, a Eastern Europe cluster and a pure French cluster . The male and female component spaces generated almost equivalent classifications pointing to a general commonality of the hidden structure represented by the components [1]. This result is consistent with the general hypothesis of "components = environmental macro-causes of cancer", because both males and females experience the same external environment (or life-style from the point of view of the subjects) even if at different "degrees", i.e. with the same determinants influencing at different proportions the male and female populations.

If this is the case, we expect the 10-dimensional space spanned by the 5 male components ($EUROM1 - EUROM5$) plus the 5 female components ($EUROF1 - EUROF5$) to have an effective dimensionality of five, i.e. the minimal possible dimensionality given the mutual internal orthogonality of the male and female component space. The "second order" PCA applied on that space confirmed the sketched hypothesis: Figure 1 reports the percentage of variability explained by extracted components as a function of the component number and it is evident the abrupt change of explained variance after component five, reminescent of the passage from "signal" to "noise floor" [2].

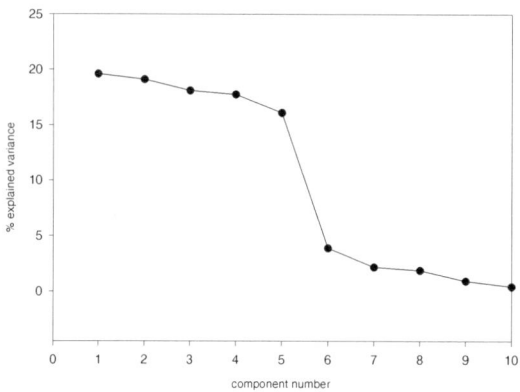

Fig. 1. Percentage of the explained variability as a function of component number

4   Conclusion

The proposed approach increases the sensitivity of epidemiological investigations through two basic , somewhat related, mechanisms: a) filtering out noise keeping only the correlated portion of information , b) eliminating all the "intrinsic" determinants of carcinogenesis like differential genetic susceptivity by concentrating on spatial-based tumor associations.

This allows to concentrate on pure environmental determinants of cancer filtering out all the other confounding factors. We could try and give a rough quantitative idea of the signal enhancement exerted by PCA. As first, we must consider that the transpose of the matrix we used for the analysis (i.e. the matrix having as variables the locations and as rows the tumor types) has a first component explaining the 90% of total variability , so pointing to a general invariance of the tumor profile in humans. This means that, given we concentrated on the spatial variability of tumor profile, our starting material corresponds to the 10% of the total variability carried by the studied compilations . Then we select only the 45% of this residual variability , correspondent to the five extracted components, thus each component retains only, on average, a vanishingly small 1% of total information.

It is remarkable that such low-power signals, completely undetectable by means of classical methods, were neverthless demonstrated to be very reliable across years and sexes.

However this huge increase in power has a drawback: the difficulty of "giving a name" to the extracted components and then to identify the correspondent causative agents and to plan corrective actions. We are now doing some ecological studies [1] to correlate the extracted components with socio-economic determinants, but notwithstanding the observation of relatively strong correlations between pathology and socio-economical components, the picture offered by the socio-economic indices is still too coarse-grain for a reliable biological (and more important operative) hypothesis to be sketched.

The path in front of us is probably long and difficult, but surely worth of being undertaken.

References

1. Benigni, R., Giaimo, R., Matranga, D., Giuliani, A. : The cultural heritage shapes the pattern of tumour profiles in Europe: a correlation study. J. Epidemiol. Community Health **54** (2000) 262-268.
2. Broomhead DS., King, GP. : Extracting qualitative dynamics from experimental data. Physica D **20** (1986) 217-236
3. Giuliani, A., Colosimo, A., Benigni, R., Zbilut JP.: On the constructive role of noise in spatial systems. Physics Lett. A **247** (1998): 47-52
4. IARC : Cancer Incidence in Five Continents Vol. VI, Lyon (1992)
5. IARC : Cancer Incidence in Five Continents Vol. VII, Lyon (1997)
6. Negri E., La Vecchia, C., Levi, F., Franceschi, S., Boyle, P.: Comparative descriptive epidemiology of oral and oesophageal cancers in Europe. Eur. J. Canc. Prev. **5** (1996): 267-279
7. Preisendorfer, RW.: Principal Component Analysis in Meteorology and Oceanography. Development in Atmospheric Science 17, Elsevier, Amsterdam (1988)
8. Remington, RD., Schork MA.: Statistics with applications to the biological and health sciences, Prentice Hall, Englewood Cliffs, NJ (1970)
9. Schlecht, NS., Franco, EL., Pintos, J., Negassa, A., Kowalski, LP., Benedito, VO.: Interaction between tobacco and alcohol consumption and the risk of cancer in the upper-digestive tract in Brazil. Am. J. Epidemiol. **150** (1999): 1129-1137.
10. Taubes, G. : Epidemiology faces its limits. Science **269** (1995): 164-169.

Author Index